D1526088

About the editors

COLIN A. ROSS, MD, is the Director of the Dissociative Disorders Unit of the Charter Health System of Dallas, Texas, and Associate Clinical Professor of Psychiatry at the Southwestern Medical Center in Dallas. He is the 1994 President of the International Society for the Study of Multiple Personality and Dissociation. Among his published works is *Multiple Personality Disorder: Diagnosis, Clinical Features, and Treatment* (Wiley).

ALVIN PAM, PhD, is Assistant Professor in the Department of Psychiatry, Albert Einstein College of Medicine, Bronx, New York, and Acting Director of Psychology at the Bronx Psychiatric Center in New York City.

10/2/95

PSEUDOSCIENCE IN
BIOLOGICAL PSYCHIATRY

PSEUDOSCIENCE IN BIOLOGICAL PSYCHIATRY

BLAMING THE BODY

Colin A. Ross and Alvin Pam

John Wiley & Sons, Inc.

New York • Chichester • Brisbane • Toronto • Singapore

RC
344
.R67
1995

This text is printed on acid-free paper.

Copyright © 1995 by John Wiley & Sons, Inc.

All rights reserved. Published simultaneously in Canada.

Reproduction or translation of any part of this work beyond
that permitted by Section 107 or 108 of the 1976 United
States Copyright Act without the permission of the copyright
owner is unlawful. Requests for permission or further
information should be addressed to the Permissions Department,
John Wiley & Sons, Inc., 605 Third Avenue, New York, NY
10158-0012.

This publication is designed to provide accurate and
authoritative information in regard to the subject
matter covered. It is sold with the understanding that
the publisher is not engaged in rendering legal, accounting,
or other professional services. If legal advice or other
expert assistance is required, the services of a competent
professional person should be sought.

Library of Congress Cataloging in Publication Data:

Ross, Colin A.
    Pseudoscience in biological psychiatry : blaming the body / Colin
A. Ross and Alvin Pam.
        p.   cm.
    Includes index.
    ISBN 0-471-00776-5 (cloth)
    1. Biological psychiatry—Philosophy.   2. Biological psychiatry—
Social aspects.   3. Psychiatric errors.   4. Mental illness—
Etiology.   I. Pam, Alvin.   II. Title.
    [DNLM: 1. Biological Psychiatry.   2. Models, Psychological.   WM
100 R823p 1995]
RC344.R67   1995
616.89—dc20
DNLM/DLC
for Library of Congress   94-27307

Printed in the United States of America

10 9 8 7 6 5 4 3 2 1

THE AUTHORS

COLIN ROSS, M.D., is director of the Dissociative Disorders Unit at Charter Hospital of Dallas, and Clinical Associate Professor of Psychiatry at Southwest Medical Center in Dallas, Texas.

ALVIN PAM, PH.D., is Director of Internship Training at the Bronx Psychiatric Center, and Assistant Professor of Psychiatry (Psychology) at Albert Einstein College of Medicine, Bronx, New York.

ADDITIONAL CONTRIBUTIONS BY

ELLEN BORGES, PH.D., Sociology, is a member of the Associate Faculty at Goddard College in Plainfield, Vermont.

SUSAN E. DEVINE, R.N., M.S.N., Director of the New Haven Court Clinic of the Connecticut Mental Health Center and Yale University, New Haven, Connecticut.

SUSAN KEMKER, M.D., Staff Psychiatrist, North Central Bronx Hospital, Bronx, New York.

ALI KHADIVI, PH.D., Associate Clinical Psychologist at Bronx Lebanon Hospital, and Adjunct Assistant Professor of Clinical Psychology, New School for Social Research, New York City.

DAVID K. SAKHEIM, PH.D., in Private Practice in South Windsor, Connecticut, and Consultant to the Trauma Resolution Program at Elmcrest Hospital, Portland, Connecticut.

HARRY WEINER, M.D., Director of Professional Information for a major pharmaceutical company in New York City.

CONTENTS

ACKNOWLEDGMENTS

Dr. Ross would like to thank Aleen Davis, the Administrator at Charter Behavioral Health System of Dallas, for providing him with a nine-week sabbatical, during which he completed his two chapters. Dr. Pam would like to thank Dr. Herman van Praag for his support and encouragement.

INTRODUCTION

Alvin Pam

IN WHAT SENSE IS BIOLOGICAL PSYCHIATRY A "PSEUDOSCIENCE"?

Biological psychiatry is devoted to the investigation of constitutional determinants of psychological disorders, with a goal of devising corresponding preventive or remedial measures for whatever may be amiss in the human organism. This task is carried out using scientific method, which involves empirical research, statistical analysis, and formal inferential logic. In many respects, biological psychiatry has adhered to scientific standards—for example, the field of psychopharmacology has been rigorous in its testing of new drugs. Although it is true that even this applied field has its detractors—most recently, Breggin (1991)—such charges as misuse of medications and "toxic psychiatry" do not constitute an attack on the scientific foundation of psychopharmacology. Rather, debate about efficacy, side effects, and the role of drugs in psychiatric treatment is consonant with the spirit of scientific research, ultimately fostering the development of more effective new compounds with reduced toxicity profiles.

So where is the "pseudoscience"? The purpose of this book is to show that biological psychiatry—presently the dominant force within the discipline of psychiatry—is dominated by a reductionist ideology

1

that distorts and misrepresents much of its research. This ideology goes far beyond a mere conceptual frame for the treatment of patients; it defines *somatic variables* as the prepotent factor in the etiology of "abnormal" behavior. According to its tenets, the individual with behavior problems must suffer in some way from defective protoplasm, a constitutional predisposition to mental illness. The psychiatric symptoms of patients thus warrant research into etiology and treatment along the same lines as the physical symptoms of patients in general medicine. Given this stilted, unidimensional, and mechanistic worldview, research in psychiatry has been geared toward discovering which aberrant genetic or neurophysiological factors underlie and cause social deviance. In such investigations, the ideology implicitly structures the experimental methodology and the inferences drawn from the data. The resultant body of work forms a professional "literature," which then becomes the basis not only for the training of apprentices in psychiatry, but also for the education of the public on psychiatric matters. It becomes part of the culture. At the same time, biological psychiatry is a product of its culture. Unless challenged, contemporary culture will progressively regard *homo sapiens* as *homo biologicus*—something on the order of a highly evolved, intricately wired, and socially verbose fruit fly.

The "model of man" propounded by biological psychiatry is a parochial medical approach to psychopathology, but it has vast implications for other disciplines, most notably the social sciences. In addition, it has significant public health, legal, and political ramifications. In the course of pursuing its goals, biological psychiatry claims for itself a scientific status based on empirical research, so that its findings are beyond criticism from any other discipline. Accordingly, these findings can only be criticized, according to biological psychiatry, from inside biological psychiatry—that is, through new information provided by fresh research, innovations in methodology, and reviews or reevaluation of old data. The nature of knowledge in the field has disturbing elements of ontological solipsism.

It follows from the above that a critique of biological psychiatry must start with an assessment of its scientific status. Is the methodology sound? Are the inferences valid? Is the "model of man" compelling? The present book begins with a chapter by Pam, who evaluates the field's methodology and inferential logic. Pam concludes that this body of work has all the accoutrements of science but is grossly lacking in the most elementary aspects of experimental design and interpretation of data. He offers evidence that biological psychiatry does little to criticize its own premises and thus recapitulates the same errors over time.

Moreover, it wields a strong public-relations arm, which manipulates the press into heralding its "breakthroughs," although very little of scientific merit is actually occurring. In its march toward scientific "progress," biological psychiatry tends to endorse fads—if one may speak of research efforts in this way—that momentarily "explain" in sophisticated terms the physiological etiology and mechanics of various syndromes and diagnoses. Later, such results are not replicated, and specific hypotheses quietly fade away while the general theoretical approach remains.

Pam cannot focus on the current state of each area of biological research because his chapter would soon be outmoded by the flood of new papers. Instead, he points out unchecked errors in procedure and logic that can be found across many studies in different areas and represent pervasive "blind spots" in a prolific literature. The chapter is an expansion and updating of a monograph originally published in *Acta Psychiatrica Scandinavica* (1990) and is intended for an audience interested in psychiatry but not necessarily wanting a technical exposition of research design and findings. However, the chapter does serve as a rough primer in how to evaluate research.

BLAMING THE BODY

Biological psychiatry has always had to perform social functions that are supportive of established authority, especially in times of marked social inequality or retrenchment. In its search for such biological defects as genetic anomalies, abnormal brain morphology, and neurotransmitter dysregulation as primary etiological factors, biological psychiatry tends to "blame the body" for disturbed behavior, rather than the family or society. This perspective lets the social surround escape unscathed from any blame or responsibility, no matter how much psychological disorder is in its midst. The inherent bias in a reductionistic biological psychiatry is that no one—not even the afflicted individual—is accountable for his or her behavior, because abnormal behavior is presumed to have some impelling pathophysiological cause. Human choice and values are negated, and the sociocultural status quo remains intact. Thus, an overly biologized psychiatry becomes an instrument with which to repress alternative psychosocial models of psychopathology.

Since Freud, symptoms have been understood as a nonverbal protest: a symptom conveys the bitter message that developmental needs have not been met, resulting in unmistakable signs of suffering, as well as metaphorical acting-out. However, biological psychiatry does not accept the Freudian perspective that symptoms are a desperate, counterproductive, indirect communication. Rather, in response to a patient's symptoms, a biological psychiatrist typically offers a medication that will "correct" a putative biochemical imbalance. Given such a narrow base for clinical intervention, the prescribing of a psychotropic medication (which may be pragmatically quite helpful) may produce a destructive end result. This is because dispensing a pill can reinforce a pseudoscientific biological determinism that covers over or distorts the patient's actual social situation. In such cases, even good psychopharmacology can be bad medicine!

Biological factors enter into all behavior, including symptoms, but only rarely are the cause and significance of a patient's behavior primarily biologically driven. It is more accurate to view the body as *mediating* the expression of affect and purpose for the whole organism. Thus, contrary to the model of humans upheld by biological psychiatry, in which such agencies as genes, lesions, or neurotransmitters direct behavior, this book supports an alternative "trauma model" in which psychopathology is usually caused by external events precipitating a psychological crisis. The body activates and adjusts itself as it deals with the crisis, and it adapts itself quasi-permanently—as a result of the crisis—to a different experience of the environment. Treatment should inclusively address three factors in each case: (a) the noxious aspects of the environment, (b) the tendency to psychologically construe the environment as "noxious," and (c) the restoration of normal as opposed to stress-related somatic functioning. Only the latter requires medication, and medication may not be necessary if the first two aspects are ameliorated.

In short, we argue for the biopsychosocial paradigm that is, ostensibly, universally accepted by mental health professionals. However, this book would not be necessary if adherence to the paradigm were truly universal. We believe that biological psychiatry has made a travesty of the biopsychosocial paradigm, either by largely omitting psychosocial factors in its clinical formulations or by downgrading them to mere incidental "triggers."

THE PLAN OF THE BOOK

The organizational schema of this book needs to be outlined at this point. As stated above, the point of inception is the critique by Pam, a clinical psychologist, of the methodology and inferences of current research in biological psychiatry. The purpose of his chapter is to raise serious concerns in the reader's mind about the validity of relatively unchallenged data and conclusions, and the bias implicit in much of biological psychiatry's research.

Chapters 2 and 3 are by Ross, a psychiatrist specializing in the treatment of dissociative disorders. Chapter 2 reviews cognitive errors that are part-and-parcel of the training of psychiatric residents; they are imbibed without much discussion of the validity of these "scientific" assertions. Ross analyzes current biological psychiatric lore about the etiology of mental illness and the workings of "human nature"—both reduced by biological psychiatry to simplistic biomedical paradigms. Chapter 3 reviews articles published from 1990 to 1993 in the prestigious *American Journal of Psychiatry*, illustrating the extent to which psychiatry is now under the sway of biological determinism. Ross analyzes many of the articles to show that the methodology, statistics, and inferences are substandard, or the findings trivial or inconclusive, although the papers reinforce the image of psychiatry as a biomedical science.

Chapter 4 has ironic dimensions. Wiener, a physician employed at a major pharmaceutical company, has an interest in psychiatric genetics. He takes up the challenge proffered by Cloninger (1993), who stated that several key variables in a biopsychosocial model of depression "have been shown to be heritable, including those usually interpreted as nongenetic environmental factors, such as stressful life events and social supports" (p. 1138). Cloninger asserted that so-called "environmental" variables may actually be genetic in nature, because familial influences on a growing child could be produced by a genetic predisposition to depression. This is an extreme version of biological determinism. Cloninger's claim would provoke many a social scientist to scream, but Wiener has an unorthodox theory of genetic transmission of personality traits that accords with Cloninger's approach—although it is doubtful that Cloninger would accept it! The reader is invited to see what flaws, if any, can be found in Wiener's exposition. Ross and Pam think it is as plausible as that offered by Cloninger and other bioreductionist researchers studying psychiatric genetics.

Chapter 5, by Borges, a sociologist, is a review of biological psychiatry in the light of class, racial, and sexist tensions within society. Borges argues that biological psychiatry largely ignores these issues, as if its scientific contribution is "objective" and so does not occur within a cultural matrix. Borges contends that unstated social values and vested interests are endemic in the research of biological psychiatry.

In Chapter 6, Kemker and Khadivi—a psychiatrist and a psychologist respectively, involved in the training of psychiatric residents—apply

Ross's perspective to the clinic, showing how residents are inducted into the culture of uncritical biologism, and how hospitals are affected when biological psychiatrists take over residency programs and treatment services. Kemker and Khadivi's sense is that psychiatrists who came into the field primarily to work hands-on with patients are often unhappy with the biological reductionism rampant today.

Sackheim, a psychologist in private practice, and Devine, a nurse, have contributed Chapter 7, which argues that the trauma model alone does justice to the traumatic experiences of mental patients, whereas the biomedical model ignores the social conditions that give rise to psychopathology, or tries to remedy the situation with medication, no matter what the social conditions. Like Ross, Sackheim and Devine are very much engaged in the dissociative disorders field, in which the emphasis on childhood trauma has generated the main source of opposition to the medical model within the mental health field.

In the final chapter, Ross outlines a trauma model of psychopathology that offers an alternative to biological reductionism.

The purpose of this book, then, is twofold: (a) to provide a critique of biological psychiatry in its current form, and (b) to suggest an alternative trauma model that is truly biopsychosocial in nature.

The authors would like to thank Herb Reich, Senior Editor at John Wiley & Sons, for his editorial support and his willingness to take on this project.

REFERENCES

Breggin, P. (1991). *Toxic psychiatry.* New York: St. Martin's Press.

Cloninger, C. R. (1993). Editorial: Unraveling the casual pathway to major depression. *American Journal of Psychiatry, 150,* 1137–1138.

Pam, A. (1990). A critique of the scientific status of biological psychiatry. *Acta Psychiatricia Scandinavica, 82* (Suppl. 362), 1–35.

1

BIOLOGICAL PSYCHIATRY: SCIENCE OR PSEUDOSCIENCE?

Alvin Pam

In a century of outstanding scientific progress, different branches of medicine have developed diagnostic and therapeutic techniques that have made previously dreaded diseases far more treatable, and in some cases even eradicable. As of this moment, similarly impressive progress is being reported in many areas of investigation by biological psychiatry; for example, preliminary findings on genetic markers for depression and schizophrenia have been published, both panic and obsessive-compulsive reactions have been induced in the laboratory by chemical means, and neurotransmitter abnormalities are under scrutiny in alcoholism, suicide, and other psychiatric disorders. Indeed, one takes for granted that progress will go on until constitutional mechanisms have been specified for every syndrome so that, in the near future, remedial pharmacological or other interventions can be applied. An indispensable formulary is already available for the treatment of most conditions, and the new drug treatments have resulted in much less reliance on institutional management and qualitatively better lives for mental patients. It is understandable that biological psychiatry takes much pride in this recent record of accomplishment.

However, all may not be as roseate as might appear at first blush. I do not refer to the lack of exact knowledge as to just what genetic or biochemical defect is involved in psychiatric disorders because causes are complex and it will take considerable time to work out intricate psychophysiological sequences. What I mean is much more fundamental: biological psychiatry cannot fulfill its mission properly because in its current state it has more the accoutrement of a scientific discipline than the substance. To be sure, this statement will raise skeptical eyebrows. It will be the burden of this chapter to spell out the grounds for such a broad iconoclastic assertion. To wit, I will be charged to show: (a) that the methodology of biological psychiatry is sufficiently flawed as to call into doubt the preponderance of its accepted findings, and (b) that an approach to psychopathology largely based on biological determinism introduces an ideological slant that selectively shapes the research that is done. Both of these criticisms already inhere in Gerard's avuncular dictum to the field of psychiatry—"no twisted thought without a twisted molecule" (Abood, 1960)—or van Praag's variant: "strange people, strange substances" (1977). When an approach to psychopathology is based on reductionist thinking, it projects a worldview that proclaims, in effect, *biology is destiny*. Because research activity inevitably will be influenced by such an implicit bias, my contention is that a biology-based orientation to what is called "mental illness" has generated an experimental methodology expressly crafted to emphasize the crucial role of somatic variables, with resultant data circularly used to validate a reductionist theory.

To demonstrate this thesis, the present chapter must chiefly be concerned with a critique of the methodology. For purposes of organization, I have adopted Akiskal and Webb's (1978) fourfold classification of methods of research into the "psychobiological interface": (a) pedigree studies, (b) pharmacological response studies, (c) neuropsychological–neurophysiological findings, and (d) biochemical correlates of emotion. Despite unavoidable overlap, their division of the scope of the field is as serviceable as any. I will review, in turn, historically significant investigations in each of the four topical areas so as to detail distinct limitations of the research, some inherent in the methods themselves and others arising from faulty application that may have gone unscrutinized. The methods in themselves are valid if there are biological variables to measure, but use of the methods (producing a copious literature) hardly constitutes ipso facto proof that the sought-after biological variables exist! With this warning in mind, it will quickly become apparent, as one reads along, that past and present research in all four areas has frequently led to dubious conclusions asserting the existence of requisite, usually prepotent biological factors.

My review will not attempt to be comprehensive in its treatment of any particular syndrome, nor will there be a sustained effort to keep up with the current status of research into the various psychopathologies (such an ambitious undertaking on my part would soon be out of date anyway). Instead, my focus is on analysis of technical fallacies endemic across research studies, as well as spurious inductions drawn as a product of investigator bias, overgeneralization, and markedly lower research standards than Lewontin, Rose, and Kamin (1984) believe would be tolerated anywhere else in science.

As analysis of representative work within the four areas will show, failure to meet standards of scientific quality can be mainly attributed to the misconceptions, prejudices, and tunnel vision that biological psychiatrists have brought into their research in the form of unexamined and sometimes untenable *ideological* premises (Ingleby, 1980, 1981). Because virtually every psychiatric disorder is largely imputed to constitutional dysfunction, the problem is presumed to be "inside" the body of the patient rather than the product of an "outside" interaction. In this medical-model view, the immediate surround becomes in essence no more than a fortuitous "trigger" for a decompensation that was always latent within the patient's physical being. Such an approach can be characterized as a "blame-the-victim's-body" philosophy. Personal problems become tantamount to biological problems; indeed, the appropriateness and morality of action are soon converted via "the medicalization of social deviance" (Conrad, 1980) into a matter of laboratory values within normal limits. The question is never asked as to whether the body can indeed **cause** rather than merely *mediate* a psychiatric symptom—as if the body, which actualizes what we do, also tells us how to live (Lipowski, 1989). Ross (1986) has chided many of his colleagues for intrinsic reductionism: the *idée fixe* within the psychiatric field that a physical abnormality causes at least a predisposition in nearly all forms of psychic disorder, culminating in a search for the defining biological marker:

> [D]ealing with symptoms or syndromes as if they were specific diseases reflects a trend in psychiatry to regard mental illnesses as . . . biological entities, definable by laboratory tests, treatable in accordance with these tests, and monitored in the course of treatment primarily by calibration of test results. But in this surrealistic world of pseudo-entities, the psychiatrist abdicates reality to embrace biological reductionism. (p. 431)

The chapter concludes by summarizing both methodological and ideological errors typically encountered in research which, taken collectively, grievously compromise the scientific standing of biological psychiatry. Recommendations are then made; they are intended to improve the contribution of biological psychiatry to the mental health field by dint of establishing more stringent criteria for research design, interpretation of data, and theory construction.

PEDIGREE STUDIES

The aim of pedigree studies is to determine whether the onset of a given diagnostic condition is associated with some form of genetic diathesis. Examples of fruitful investigation have been the discoveries of the exact mode of chromosomal transmission of Huntington's chorea, phenylketonuria, and other rare and well-defined neurological diseases. Biological psychiatry has always striven to find similar genetic transmission for the so-called "functional" disorders, and almost every psychiatric category has been the target of pedigree studies, with positive findings reported and generally accepted by the field for most of the major diagnostic groupings. Pedigree studies can be classified into three classic subtypes: (a) consanguinity research, (b) co-twin control cases, and (c) adoption comparisons. Each will be discussed in order, and then the latest addition to the subtype methodology—the genetic marker design—will be addressed. For ready reference, this section on pedigree studies will be schematically presented as outlined in Table 1.1.

Consanguinity Research

Family inheritance is investigated in two ways: by tracing the psychiatric genealogy of an indexed subject, the "propositus," who has the disorder (design A), and by noting the correspondence of a given diagnosis with degree of kinship (design B). The earliest investigations of this type were carried out by American adherents of the eugenics movement started in Great Britain by Sir Francis Galton. Influenced by social Darwinism, these pioneer researchers declared they aimed to "purify the race" by identifying those individuals who were biologically unfit to be parents, with the purpose of weeding them out of the nation's reproductive pool. But first they had to show that specific forms of human "degeneracy" (as they called most of the mental disorders) were indeed inherited conditions. The maiden study, *The Jukes* (1887), was by a prison superintendent, Richard Dugdale. His data showed extremely high rates of criminality and social parasitism through many generations traced in the Jukes' genealogy, and he concluded that inherited and therefore

Table 1.1. Paradigms and Respective Power of Pedigree Methodology

Method	Design	Power
Consanguinity, research	A. Psychiatric genealogy	Inconclusive
	B. Concordance rates	Inconclusive
Co-twin control studies	C. Monozygotic (MZ) vs. same-sex dizygotic (DZ) twins	Inconclusive
	D. Concordance rates for MZ twins reared apart	Powerful but impractical
Adoption comparisons	E. Collaterals: comparison of rates for biological vs. adoptive relatives, especially parents	Suggestive
	F. Descendants: comparison of rates for children of index parents vs. children of controls	Suggestive
	G. Cross-fostering: rates of children of index parents and control adoptive parents vs. children of control biological parents and index adoptive parents	Powerful
Genetic marker studies	H. Identification: correlating a genetic marker with presence of the diagnosis	Powerful
	I. Prospective–longitudinal: predicting which members of a family unit will develop the disorder in adulthood	Conclusive

untreatable antisocial tendencies made such families severe social liabilities. The Jukes study was generally accepted by the academic community for about 50 years, but was ultimately considered embarrassing and unworthy of scientific attention because it did not control for the effects of poverty and parental modeling. The mere fact that some form of psychopathology "runs in families" does not necessarily support a genetic etiology, because the psychopathology could be explained on the basis of environment alone. What remains pertinent about the Jukes study even today is that a genealogical methodology does not—either explicitly or implicitly—demonstrate there has been genetic transmission, in particular when family, cultural, and economic factors conduce to the psychopathology.

The next major report by a eugenics-oriented researcher was by Henry Goddard, a psychologist at Vineland State School in New Jersey, published as *The Kallikak Family* (1912). The propositus, Deborah Kallikak, was brought for admission at age 8 because her mother's new husband would not accept an illegitimate child. Deborah was diagnosed "mentally deficient" and was taken off her mother's hands for what proved to be a lifelong stay at Vineland. Goddard attributed the patient's condition to inherited tendencies going back to the American Revolution when a young soldier-ancestor had an affair with a "feeble-minded" barmaid, resulting in a line of mental retardates originating from the child of this brief union ("Old Horror," as he was later called); after a respectable marriage, another line descended from the same soldier resulted in an eminent New Jersey family. The two branches did not know they had a common progenitor. Goddard concluded from this pedigree study that mentally retarded persons should not be allowed to reproduce—and this reading of his data meant in practice that the staff at Vineland was instructed to do their utmost to prevent the rather beautiful Deborah Kallikak from having any opportunity for a sexual experience, marriage, or discharge from the institution (Smith, 1985). In 1927, the U.S. Supreme Court went further and approved new laws for sterilization because science had now shown that mental deficiency was inherited! The eugenics movement applauded Justice Holmes's brief in *Buck v. Bell*, which declared: "Three generations of idiots is enough"; selective sterilization was seen as a necessary first step toward civilized control of reproduction (Kevles, 1985). As might be expected, forced sterilization in the United States over the three decades it was legal was very disproportionately directed at single-parent African American women on welfare in the South (Chase, 1977).

Extremely admired and influential for many years following its publication, the Kallikak book is nowadays rarely cited, for it has become a prototype of how *not* to trace psychiatric inheritance. Goddard's tracking of ancestry involved reaching a diagnosis on scanty information, mostly hearsay gossip from aged relatives or neighbors, with classification reached by an untrained investigator told only to look for any signs of "mental deficiency." This procedure violated the research canon of "blind" diagnosis. Worse yet, Goddard misled critics by falsely alleging that he knew the name and biography of the barmaid (Smith, 1985) and by retouching the photographs of the "bad" Kallikak branch to make them look sinister (Gould, 1981)! Beyond methodology, his genetics are remarkably confused, as described by Scheinfeld (1939):

> Granted "Old Horror" was a degenerate because of bad heredity (and there is yet no evidence that "degeneracy" is inherited), by what gene mechanism did he become that way? No single dominant gene could produce any such complex condition, nor is there any known gene that can singly produce even feeble-mindedness. Recessive genes would have had to be involved. Which means that as such genes must come from both parents for the effect to assert itself [within one generation], no matter how chock-full of "black" genes the feeble-minded mother was, the worthy [father] had to be carrying such genes if the condition of his presumptive son, "Old Horror," was due to heredity. And that would mean, in turn, that the "good" Kallikaks also received some of those "black" genes! (pp. 361–363)

Yet, no subsequent descendant of the "good" Kallikaks ever displayed "feeble-mindedness," although they numbered in the hundreds by the time Goddard did his survey. Moreover, many members of the "bad" Kallikaks were found to be unlikely cases of retardation (indicating investigator bias) by Smith when he retraced and added to the family history 73 years after the appearance of Goddard's book. The final irony is that Deborah herself was not retarded: she could read well, write creatively, read music and play the cornet, embroider dresses, do excellent carpentry and wood carving, sew well enough to make shirts, and wait tables (Chase, 1977)! She had a mental-age score of 9 years when tested by Goddard in 1911, but Chase has noted, "As with so many other second-rank psychologists then and since, Goddard was never to learn how to differentiate between a living person and that person's IQ test score" (p. 146).

Currently, only certain forms of mental retardation are regarded as due to chromosomal abnormalities. Whereas serious retardation is now attributed to either inborn or incurred neurological deficit, mild cases—the vast majority—are seen as usually stemming from psychosocial deprivation or a mixture of deprivation and minimal brain damage (Scott & Carran, 1987). However, in the earlier years of the century, a eugenic conception of "intelligence" had a profound impact on American thinking about mental retardation, with far-reaching social and political consequences (Gould, 1981). Congress even apportioned its 1924 immigration quotas on Goddard's "inherited mental deficiency" research, which was based on giving IQ tests to mostly non-English-speaking arrivals from various nations. Goddard had found Italians, Jews, Poles, and Greeks much less endowed with "innate potential" than longer-established immigrants from the British Isles, Germany, or Scandinavia. Prospective citizens from Asia, Africa, and Latin America were considered to dilute the quality of the national stock to a degree inimical to civilized standards. Educational and cultural parameters were not considered in obtaining these results. However, Goddard did state that low-IQ citizens could serve a useful purpose in doing the menial labor! Ultimately, his research was discounted as hopelessly classist and racist. At best, Goddard had shown that mental retardation, like criminality, tends to "run in families," but once again a genetic interpretation of the data did not hold up to critical scientific scrutiny.

This brings us to the beginnings of the modern era in psychiatric pedigree research, that is, to work that followed the lead of Dugdale and Goddard but was on a more sophisticated plane in terms of experimental technique and statistics so as to still be cited in contemporary textbooks and review articles. In the area of schizophrenia research, Franz Kallmann (1938, 1946) took up the eugenics cause, contending from the family genealogies he investigated that schizophrenia was inbred and thus constituted a reproductive threat to society. He too did hearsay diagnosis of distant or dead relatives, while relying on hospital psychiatrists to diagnose the close relatives of patients they were treating (hardly a "blind" procedure). He did several concordance studies, arriving at figures higher than any subsequent researcher—for instance, his 68% concordance rate for the child of two schizophrenic parents compares with a risk of 34–44% in four other studies, according to Lewontin et al. (1984). Kallmann's studies contain, at most, perfunctory reports on methods, and only seldom does he provide the case histories that might permit readers to form their own ideas about social context, clinical course, or diagnosis. He does not deal with the genetically impossible fact of a schizophrenic who has no family history through many generations on either side (unless schizophrenia is a mutation), occurring in 36% of his own sample of 589 twins where sufficient information was available and later estimated to occur in up to 60% of cases of schizophrenia (Smythies, Coppen, & Kreitman, 1968). No explanation is offered as to why schizophrenia does not weed itself out of the human population by virtue of having no evolutionary value for survival, while reproduction rates are known to be low (Rosenthal, 1971). Like his predecessors who upheld eugenics, Kallmann never considered early environmental factors in accounting for how psychopathology is passed from one generation to the next.

In contrast to the homage Kallmann continues to receive as the first biological psychiatrist to research schizophrenia in many extensive, systematic, and technically advanced pedigree studies, his contribution has been called "bloodcurdling pseudoscience" by Lewontin et al. (1984). Kallmann's mentor, Ernst Rudin, developed psychiatric genetics as a new form of science at the University of Munich and later served the Nazis when they came to power—indeed, Rudin helped draw up the 1933 German sterilization law for mental patients, as a member of a committee chaired by Heinrich Himmler.

Kallmann imbibed the hereditary "taint" hypothesis propounded by Rudin to explain all types of mental disorder, but his own career in Germany was blocked because he was Jewish. He was forced to interrupt his investigation of schizophrenia as an inherited disease until after emigration to the United States in 1936. According to his widow, Kallmann somewhat modified his research conclusions for humanitarian reasons: he attributed schizophrenia to a "recessive" gene to evade mass sterilization. But Lewontin et al. (1984) showed that Kallmann never compromised the rigors of science for any humanitarian aim. In an early paper, he argued for sterilization of schizophrenics *and* their apparently healthy siblings—just because schizophrenia was "recessive." Two Nazi geneticists had to oppose him to protect the large proportion of the German people involved! Perhaps in reaction to the Nazis, who escalated from the forced sterilization of 225,000 mental patients to "euthanasia," killing 400,000 mental patients in 1939–1940, Kallmann gave up his advocacy of sterilization and wanted the State to regulate the marriages of schizophrenics and their children and to use institutionalization in the last resort to enforce birth control (as Goddard had mandated for Deborah Kallikak). His attitude toward schizophrenics, and his notion of their "treatment," was quite frankly proclaimed (Kallmann, 1938):

> Since there is thus far no accurate means at our disposal for preventing the incidence of the schizophrenic psychosis in a tainted individual, it seems to be even more expedient and more urgent to carry out restrictive measures against the inheritance of the taint. In this way psychiatry would accomplish its part in making the biological quality of future generations an important matter for medical . . . activity, by decreasing not only the number of schizophrenic patients, but also the number of heterozygotic taint-carriers, such as schizoid eccentrics, criminal adventurers, or other members of the lunatic fringe. (p. 3)

Note the ascription of political or social deviance to the schizophrenic "taint." Kallmann simplistically blamed "bad" genes for much of what he thought degenerate in an otherwise estimable society (overlooking any input that society itself may have had in bringing on "degeneracy"). Contemporary genetic research into psychiatric disorder has considerably cleaned up its act since the days of Kallmann, in an effort to redeem itself from the stigma of past associations. Modern eugenicists, such as Gottesman and Erlenmeyer-Kimling (1971), lament that hardly anyone these days continues to mind the quality of the human gene pool because the old eugenics ideology attracted bigots and zealots eager to save future generations from a flood of so-called hereditary defects or taints, leading to "such humanity-shattering excesses (in the name of eugenics) as genocide in Nazi Germany, compulsory sterilization laws, and an immigration quota system [in the United States] based on national origin" (p. S1). Given the mortification of the scientific community after World War II as to this historical ramifications of psychiatric genetics, Kallmann's connections to the eugenics movement in general and to Rudin in particular have had to be studiously ignored if his work is still to be respectfully quoted in nearly every review on the inheritance of schizophrenia. And so it is! In other words, Kallmann's family concordance rates are removed from their eugenics context and then treated as bona fide, though outdated scientific data. For example, Liston and Jarvik (1976) are typical of the many authors who laud Kallmann's contribution to psychiatric genetics; moreover, in the course of their appreciation of Kallmann as a scientist, they also go the atypical route of openly granting similar recognition to Rudin:

> Rudin and Kallmann were pioneers on the frontiers of medical genetics. The trails they blazed were necessarily crude, and their early hypotheses and conclusions may seem rough-hewn today. While these two scientists, their contemporaries, and their successors may not have proved "conclusively" and to everyone's satisfaction that schizophrenia is an inherited disease, they have come close; and the paths they cleared are now leading to new and continuing research challenges in the genetics of schizophrenia. (p. 92)

I take strong exception to this sort of tribute to Kallmann *qua* scientist, for there have been reasons all along to discredit Kallmann's work, apart from his eugenics ideology. On grounds of lack of a methodology section alone, his results are automatically suspect—his reports should not have been accepted for publication, and no reputable researcher should cite his statistics without caveat. Indeed, the problem of statistics without accompanying procedures and data was recently brought home to the scientific community by the Cyril Burt scandal (Burt supplied data on the inheritance of intelligence in bogus twin studies) so that the finding that intelligence is mainly inherited has had to be reviewed (Kamin, 1974). Getting back to Kallmann, his studies were not "blind" and he seemed to have had diagnostic suspicions about the relatives of schizophrenics that constituted a stereotype on the same order as Goddard's. Moreover, the figures Kallmann presented are routinely inflated: he used an abridged Weinberg method for age correction, setting the age group at risk for schizophrenia as being 15 to 44, so that nonschizophrenic relatives still in that age group could be tabulated into the totals as half-schizophrenics, because they had not yet had adequate time to demonstrate that some 50% of them were indeed whole schizophrenics (Neale & Oltmanns, 1880)! When the usual Weinberg formula is applied based on a risk period of ages 15 to 40, the reported rates fall drastically (for example, the famous .86 concordance for MZ twins drops to .69). Further, it should be realized that the usual Weinberg calculation is already an overcorrection because the risk period for onset of schizophrenia is by and large between ages 15 and 25.

Kallmann's interpretation of data is as problematic as his methodology. He maintained he had demonstrated that concordance rates for relatives of schizophrenics were significantly higher than the almost 1% rate (.0085) expected in the general population, increasing to its highest level in first-degree relatives. In other words, genetic theory correctly predicted that siblings, parents, and children (first-degree relatives) would have higher rates than grandparents, uncles, aunts, nieces, nephews, and half-siblings (second-degree relatives) whose rate, in turn, would be higher than the 1% general rate. However, shortcomings in this approach can be seen in Slater's (1968) summary of many studies, including Kallmann's (see Table 1.2).

Many inconsistencies in genetic predictions are contained in Table 1.2. Rates for children of schizophrenics are strikingly higher than for

Table 1.2. Expectations of Schizophrenia for Relatives of Schizophrenics

Relationships	N	Schizophrenic	Expectation (%)
Parents	6,331	243	3.8
Siblings	7,571	659	8.7
Children	1,149	138	12.0
Uncles, aunts	3,376	68	2.0
Half-siblings	311	10	3.2
Nephews, nieces	2,315	52	2.2
Grandchildren	713	20	2.8
Cousins	2,438	71	2.9

Data from E. Slater, "A Review of Earlier Evidence on Genetic Factors in Schizophrenia," in *The Transmission of Schizophrenia,* edited by D. Rosenthal and S. Kety, 1968, Oxford, England: Pergamon Press.

siblings, who in turn have markedly higher rates than parents. All of these collaterals are first-degree relatives. Further, parents' rates, between 3 and 4%, are barely higher than the 2 to 3% expectation for second-degree relatives, and the rates for the latter are themselves only slightly above the baseline 1% in the general population. Only with a very large N based on combined samples can statistical significance be reached that contradicts quite small differences among baseline, second-degree relatives, and parents. Further, the magnitude of Mendelian ratios is not at all approximated. Given a dominant model of heredity, expectancy rates are about 50% for first-degree relatives and about 25% for second-degree relatives. Given a recessive model, expectancy rates for first-degree relatives are about 25%; siblings are somewhat more vulnerable to the disorder than either parents or children, and the latter two groups should be about equally vulnerable. However, children's rates are more than three times higher than parents' rates, which means that growing up with a schizophrenic parent puts one at far greater risk for schizophrenia than being the parent of a schizophrenic child—a fact that argues for nurture rather than nature because parents control the home environment. If there is assortative mating (meaning a schizophrenic has an above-average chance of marrying another schizophrenic), as is almost certainly the case, distribution of a recessive gene in the mate can no longer be presumed random and expectancy rates will correspondingly rise; thus, when both parents are known to be schizophrenics, the expected rate reaches 100%. None of the figures in Slater's above-cited list are anywhere near the magnitudes predicted by Mendelian theory. For example, Slater's data showed only a 36% incidence for the offspring of two schizophrenics.

Explanations within biological psychiatry for the shortfall in expected magnitudes are of two kinds: (a) that environment plays some part in the pathogenesis—but this glibly slips in the presumption that genetic factors already account for the rest; and (b) that "incomplete penetrance" complicates the genetic effect, without any basis for this assertion other than conjecture and the plotting of graphs for hypothetical distributions. Even a convinced hereditarian like Rosenthal had to admit that explanation (b) was problematic: "Although the concept of [reduced penetrance] could and perhaps should be useful . . . , many geneticists feel that it is too often used to make ignorance respectable, and that in human genetics, it has been abused to the extent that it is in danger of falling into disrepute" (1970, p. 29). Dumont (1984) added that incomplete penetrance is an "apologetic compromise" to hold onto a genetic approach that is unsupported either by data or by the science of genetics (". . . to assume the structure [of a gene] can 'cause' the structure [of behavior] is an error of such magnitude as to be some-thing like a thought disorder itself" (p. 332)).

The most serious breach in inductive logic committed by Kallmann was his use of kinship concordance rates to demonstrate genetic transmission of psychopathology. We have already noted that no fam-ily inheritance study can control for environment in human research; such data, therefore, are nowhere near "suggestive"—they are at best inconclusive and at worst misleading (as in the Jukes and Kallikak studies). This inferential limitation holds with respect to any consan-guinity finding, even if the design and technique employed in the in-vestigation were scientifically impeccable. Because environmental theories also predict that specific disorders will "run in families," ge-netic researchers can mention family genealogy and concordance rates to show that transmission by heredity is not excluded as a possi-ble cause, but they must still bring to bear evidence from more power-ful methodologies in order to prove a psychiatric condition is inbred. As will be seen, this is far from the case with consanguinity research even today.

Co-Twin Control Studies

The next line of evidence in pedigree studies is comparative rates for a psychiatric disorder in MZ twins vs. same-sex DZ twins (design C), but especially comparing diagnoses of MZ twins reared apart (design D). Kallmann (1946) did an extensive and much quoted study in the area of schizophrenia, giving the aforementioned concordance rate of 86% for MZ twins whether raised together or apart. Nevertheless, closer in-spection throws serious doubt on the validity of this figure, not count-ing the Weinberg inflation. Kallmann defined "identical twins reared apart" by the criterion of at least five years' separation prior to the on-set of schizophrenia in one of them! Because his sample averaged 22 years of age at onset, with 12 years' average separation, it can be sur-mised that "reared apart" meant separation at an average of 10. In fact, even separation as late as this made a difference in Kallmann's concor-dance rates: 92% for MZ twins still living together but 78% for "reared apart" MZ twins. In any event, Kallmann's statistics are now regarded as "preposterous" in the opinion of Lewontin et al. (1984), who showed that the four most recent studies average out of 26% for MZ twins reared together.

Moreover, it is a misinterpretation of the higher concordance of MZ twins as compared to same-sex DZ twins to infer that hereditary fac-tors are responsible. When cases are examined, it often appears that the schizophrenia is a *folie à deux,* or some variation of a shared paranoia where each twin plays a central part in the other's delusional system (Jackson, 1960). Two recent books on twin symbiosis, by Wallace (1986) on elective mutism and Sacks (1985) on idiot-savants, describe ineffable communicative bonds between MZ twins for which there is no analogue between DZ twins. In short, because twins—especially MZ twins—share their childhood environment, it is not legitimate to construe differential rates of concordance as proof of genetic etiology. Such interpretation of data becomes another version of the "runs in the family" fallacy.

Proponents of the hereditarian point of view are mindful of this restriction in pedigree methodology but have made strenuous efforts to nullify it. An entire line of research has been devoted to what is called the "equal environments assumption" (Plomin, DeFries, & McClearn, 1980, p. 295)—namely that shared family environment is comparable for MZ and same-sex DZ twins. Kendler, Neale, Kessler, Heath, & Eaves (1993) listed four lines of empirical evidence for the "equal environments assumption." Each is described here briefly.

1. It is acknowledged that psychological similarity in twins is influenced by the similarity of their treatment by the social surround, but this situation is seen as an epiphenomenon brought about by their degree of physical resemblance. For example, Zerbin-Rudin (1972)—the daughter of Ernst Rudin—attempted to refute any environmental explanation of greater concordance rates in MZ than in DZ twins for schizophrenia by the following reasoning:

> The large difference between the concordance figures for MZ and DZ twins cannot be explained exclusively by the more similar environment of MZ twins. If MZ twins create a similar environment through their greater similarity, they do so because of the greater inherited similarity in their appearance and response modes. Thus, in a roundabout way, we still come back to the importance of heredity. (p. 48)

Kendler (1987), in a reprise of Zerbin-Rudin, again contended that the environmental similarity of MZ twins is the result and not the cause of their similarity. To support his position, Kendler cited one study in which physical resemblance of MZ pairs did not correlate with concordance for schizophrenia. But it is unclear just what this is supposed to prove: bonds between MZ twins are partly a product of physical resemblance inducing others to treat them as a unit, but they are also a product of intimate contact and common experience—even if the twins can be told apart on sight.

2. The second method used to support the "equal environments assumption" involves direct observation of twins in the family setting. The method readily acknowledges that the social surround tends to treat twins, especially look-alikes, as a "unit," but a crucial distinction is drawn between events where the family arranges such similarity for twins (the "imposed environment") and events where the family is responding to behavior initiated by the twins (the "elicited environment"). In this vein, Morris-Yates, Andrews, Howie, and Henderson (1990) studied 343 same-sex twin pairs, checking the similarity of their early environment against their scores in adulthood on neuroticism, anxiety, and depression scales. As these researchers expected, MZ twins were treated much more similarly than DZ twins—a finding that, if taken at face value, would invalidate the "equal environments assumption." But, in their view, such a reading of the data would be false: their sample showed no correlation between imposed similarity and subsequent intrapair psychopathology and only a few barely significant correlations between elicited similarity and later psychopathology. In short, the measures they used seemed to indicate that a similar early environment did little to presage concordance in psychopathology in adulthood. However, this result still did not quite rescue the "equal environments assumption" from their own contrary data. The researchers then further inferred that because similarity imposed by the environment had no effect on concordance rates but similar treatment elicited by the twins' behavior from the environment did have some effect, the latter was arguably "a consequence of their genetic identity" (p. 325). Thus, they concluded that the "equal environments assumption" is valid—the twins make the environment similar! This twist put on the data is based on the premise that one can easily discern which behavior is "imposed" or "elicited"—although any family therapist will insist that encounters between parents and children are interactional. Moreover, twin co-behavior that "elicits" similar treatment from significant others is not a self-evident product of common genetic factors as soon as the twins are two people with a shared history and many conjoint interests.

3. The third method involves the correlation of similarity of environment with later indexes of personality, intelligence, and psychopathology. Because MZ twins have been repeatedly found to have a more similar environment both in childhood and adulthood than DZ twins,

this research has to be done separately for each group. According to Kendler (1987), the combined results of various studies are unclear: some found no correspondence while others did.

4. The fourth method involves a comparison of trait similarity as a function both of "real" zygosity, as assessed by investigators, and "perceived" zygosity, as reported by twins or their parents.

When families, the community, and the twins themselves expect MZ twins to be more similar than DZ twins, and if this expectation influences trait similarity, then falsely classified MZ and DZ twins become crucial tests of nature versus nurture. Plomin et al. (1980) reviewed research on "mislabeled zygosity," occurring in 40% of pairs in the major study they cited (Scarr & Carter-Saltzman, 1979), and noted that those who falsely thought they were MZ or DZ twins resembled their biological groups on intelligence and personality tests more than their supposed groups—a finding that runs counter to what environmental theory would have predicted. "We can conclude from this [that the environmental variable of] labeling twins as identical or fraternal has little effect on their behavioral similarity" (Plomin et al., p. 296). However, although the MZ twins who thought they were DZ were less alike than correctly classified MZ twins, they were also more alike than correctly classified DZ twins—an equivocal result. In contrast, the DZ twins who thought they were MZ were more dissimilar on personality tests than either correctly classified MZ or DZ twins—a perplexing result that throws into doubt any simple interpretation of these data. The conclusion by Plomin et al.—that labeling has little effect on similarity—seems to be an overgeneralization based on one more or less favorable study.

In a more recent study using this same approach, Kendler, Neale et al. (1993) found mislabeled zygosity in 15% of female twin pairs and found no evidence for a significant influence of perceived zygosity on major depression, generalized anxiety disorder, phobia, bulimia, and alcoholism. Limitations of the study were: the small number of cases in each of the five diagnostic categories (only 15% of this sample were considered mislabeled zygosity as compared to 40% in the Scarr and Carter-Saltzman research); possible errors in investigator-assigned zygosity because blood specimens were not always taken; and the inclusion of twins who did not know their zygosity in the same statistical category as twins who disagreed about their zygosity.

Whatever the merits of current "perceived zygosity" research, social labels of MZ or DZ twinship are only one source of twin homogeneity—as noted above, due weight must also be given to the extent of intimate contact and common experience as formative factors. In this vein, Carson and Sanislow (1993) showed that concordance rates for schizophrenia are consistently higher for DZ twins than for siblings in general, pointing to the relevance of proximity to each other and shared life events in determining vulnerability to schizophrenia (and presumably other psychiatric disorders).

To date, I know of no paper that has reviewed research on the "equal environments assumption" as a body. Instead, various reports cite various favorable studies, but unless the research as a whole is examined, the contradictions between even the favorable studies go unexamined. For example, Livesley, Jang, Jackson, and Vernon (1993) used the co-twin control method to ascertain the genetic contribution to personality disorders, claiming a heritability range from 0 to 64% for different subtypes. They mentioned the equal environments assumption as critical to their methodology (p. 1827) and were able to state that they found no significant differences between their samples' MZ and DZ twins in terms of similarity of early environments! Although it is not said, this is the opposite of nearly all other studies. Ford (1993) argued that the physical resemblance of MZ twins calls forth similar treatment, but regarded this phenomenon as an environmental variable; Zerbin-Rudin (1972) considered it a genetic variable. Different studies using different measures, usually self-report scales, report different results for concordance rates for psychopathology. This entire research area is a muddle, but one only sees in the literature that the equal environments assumption is being supported in study after study. I contend that most of these studies are not solid and that there is sophistry in the way inferences are drawn from data. In short, if the equal environments assumption does not hold, as I believe it does not, it becomes impossible to disentangle joint environment from joint heredity, so that co-twin control studies are finally just as inconclusive as other subtypes of consanguinity research.

Nevertheless, if MZ twins are truly reared apart from birth, then it does become theoretically possible to do conclusive genetic investigation. Kallmann's dishonest definition of "reared apart" can be somewhat forgiven because necessity breeds a contrived solution—the research is invaluable and there simply are not enough cases to be found. In one U.S. nationwide survey (Newman, Freeman, & Holzinger, 1937), a mere 19 cases of MZ twins separated in very early life were identified, and none was schizophrenic. When Jackson (1960) raised questions about the genetic etiology of schizophrenia, he was able to locate only two concordant cases of MZ twins reared apart in the entire world literature! Given the crucial theoretical importance of these two cases, Jackson provided clinical vignettes, and these can be checked against the original published reports.

One of them, written by Kallmann (1938) based on his work in Germany, concerned 22-year-old Kaete and Lisa, born to a psychotic unmarried mother who could not take care of them. The twins were soon sent away, one to each of the mother's brothers, both of whom were described by Kallmann as "eccentric borderline cases." Kaete developed catatonic symptoms after the birth of an illegitimate child at age 15 and showed a deteriorative course in hospital except for a brief remission at age 16. Lisa showed "increasing helplessness and emotional indifference" and was placed at age 17 in the same Berlin hospital as her sister, also with a diagnosis of schizophrenia. This case is concordant for schizophrenia but has several drawbacks as a "genetic" study: the twins were separated from a disturbed mother at an unspecified point in childhood, may have been reared in problematic foster homes, and had contact during their upbringing—scarcely conditions for a test of nature vs. nurture, especially when the subjects are in the care of their mother's siblings as the "environmental" aspect of the study!

The second case, reported by Craike and Slater (1945), actually called the concordant twin psychoses *"folie à deux."* Edith and Florence were separated at 9 months of age when their mother died, and did not meet again until age 24. Edith remained with her father and a new stepmother; at age 8, she was placed in a children's home for "anxious behavior" and stayed till 19! Her first paranoid symptoms occurred at age 20 while she was living with her father (who was described in the case study as a "brutal" man, without further details). She soon had to leave, eventually making her way as a domestic in London. When she encountered her twin sister there by chance, Edith accused Florence of "spying" on her and she held onto this idea ever after, but Edith was never hospitalized despite many peculiarities. Florence, however, was hospitalized at age 51, which is how the case came to the attention of Craike and Slater. Florence was sent to an aunt in London after her mother's death. She remained there, also working as a domestic, until her aunt's death in 1944, whereupon she promptly developed paranoid symptoms about her twin sister. This was the first time she had been symptomatic in her life, and the delusions quickly cleared in psychiatric treatment. Craike and Slater concluded that Edith was more disturbed than Florence and that both shared a schizophrenic disease. It can be objected that the history supports no such diagnosis for either twin, and they may have been contamination of independent diagnosis because the sisters were known to be MZ twins. Moreover, both twins were raised by relatives, and one had to deal with an apparently abusive father and spent 11 years of childhood in an institution.

Juel-Nielsen (1965) again searched the world literature on MZ-twins-reared-apart and found 2 more concordant and 3 discordant cases, for a box score of 4/7 concordant at that time. The third concordant pair came from Kallmann and Roth (1956): one twin developed schizophrenia in childhood and the other at age 18. Because no additional information was provided by these authors, we are without any case history material. The fourth pair, reported by Slater (1961), was greatly elaborated on and progressively brought up to date by Shields (1962) and Gottesman and Shields (1972, 1982). This case concerned Nicholas and Herbert, the illegitimate and soon-placed offspring of a Chinese–English adolescent about whom nothing seems to be known concerning psychiatric history. Nicholas was in three foster homes until age 4; Herbert was in two Roman Catholic nurseries until the same age. They met for the first time when they were evacuated from London during the Blitz. Upon their return to the city, their grandmother took custody, from ages 6 to 7. Nicholas was then sent to a stable foster home; Herbert remained with his grandmother, who was then remarried. At age 22, Herbert was hospitalized with an unusual clinical picture: Slater mentioned catatonic symptoms, delusional thinking, then "hysterical pseudodementia," which led to speculations about a "Ganser state or buffoonery syndrome." In the end, Slater reluctantly came to a diagnosis of schizophrenia. Upon learning that an MZ-twin-reared-apart existed, Slater immediately arranged for a psychiatric interview of this collateral and was no doubt amazed to hear that the twin had just been hospitalized himself with a diagnosis of schizophrenia! The background to these two first psychiatric admissions was as follows: on December 22, the two brothers had seen each other for the first time since age 7, and Nicholas learned that their mother had just visited England (she now resided in the United States) and spent time with Herbert. On January 5, Nicholas was admitted to hospital; on January 8, Herbert was admitted. Neither brother recovered and 20 years later they were still institutionalized. This case illustrates a more or less simultaneous schizophrenic break in identical twins who had very little contact up to age 22, and represents the best evidence from a co-twin control case for the genetic point of view. But their very unstable early history might account for the psychopathology of the brothers. There is also the common denominator of the grandmother (psychiatric history also unknown), who played a role in the upbringing of both boys. As for a precipitant, one can only wonder what the impact of their mother's surprise visit was on the child she saw, who then quickly communicated what had occurred to the child she had not seen.

In 1972, Gottesman and Shields reported more new cases and gave 7/11 as the concordance tally at that time; in 1982, these authors again surveyed the world literature and adjusted the count to 7/12 concordant cases. Their new material came from Inouye and Mitsuda in Japan, who discovered more MZ-twins-reared-apart in their country than the rest of the world combined! However, it was not a matter of Japanese willingness to separate MZ twins as was initially speculated; the large number of cases were mainly the result of overzealous reporting and shoddy selection. Of 15 pairs, only 1 had been separated at birth and only 4 before age 5; most were reunited after 2 years apart, and little or no history was offered to assess their environment or how they were diagnosed.

In summary of the co-twin control studies, it is doubtful whether one can argue that reared-together MZ vs. DZ twin comparisons can be imputed to a genetic differential: environment of MZ twins appears to be much more similar than that of DZ twins, even leading in some instances to an uncanny psychological symbiosis. Further, investigation of MZ-twins-reared-apart research has yielded far too few cases to draw conclusions: of only 12 known cases in the world in 1982, 5 were discordant; of the remaining 7, just the above-described 3 were presented in sufficient depth to be scientifically useful. Moreover, in these 3 cases, we have seen that the children were raised over many years by uncle, aunt, father, or grandmother—a gross violation of the essential design of any nature–nurture experiment. Independent diagnosis has also been a concern in 2 cases reported in the literature.

The MZ-twins-reared-apart research is theoretically powerful, but in practice the method amounts to naturalistic observation. Because the rare cases "just happen," they cannot be screened to assure an environment good enough to be conducive to the future mental health of each of the twins. Indeed, the cases are *by defintion* confined to twins whose mothers could not or would not take care of them, with the twins separated from each other (but not necessarily at birth) and often ending up in precarious foster situations or institutions. It therefore follows that no reputable scientific paper should uncritically cite concordance rates for MZ-twins-reared-apart whenever essential case history data are lacking, or when such data are ignored in reaching a genetic interpretation.

Adoption Comparisons

As with MZ-twins-reared-apart research, adoption comparisons are theoretically capable of settling the nature–nurture debate; moreover, the problem of getting sufficient cases is readily solved by using a population pool of *all* children adopted at an early age (not just MZ twins), which allows latitude in sampling and the establishment of control groups. Hence, adoption comparisons today rightfully comprise the principal evidence for a genetic cause or for predisposition to a psychiatric disorder.

With regard to schizophrenia, the series of Danish papers by the American research team of Kety, Rosenthal, and Wender in conjunction with several Danish colleagues are of surpassing importance. However, some earlier studies are also reputable, most notably that of Heston (1966), where we shall start. Heston traced the history of 58 children born to schizophrenic mothers in Oregon state hospitals between 1915 and 1945. These children had been placed in foster care no more than 2 weeks after birth. Their 58 matched controls in the study were children who had been placed for adoption by the same agencies very soon after their birth, but whose mothers lived in the community and, as far as was known, were not schizophrenic. The results for the index and control samples were reported in Table 1.3.

Heston concluded that the finding of statistic significance for schizophrenia supported a genetic etiology. However, such significance may be an artifact of a flaw in research design: in Heston's study, there is abundant evidence of *selective adoption*—the bane of all adoption studies. Prospective foster parents knew the background of each child, and the children of state-hospital mothers were much harder to place. Half the index cases and none of the control cases spent 2 years or more in institutions because of placement problems (Heston, Denney, & Pauly, 1966). In addition, Heston did not take into account that pregnant schizophrenics may not have received adequate prenatal care

Table 1.3. Adopted Children to Schizophrenic and Nonschizophrenic Mothers

	Index Adoptees (N = 58)	Control Adoptees (N = 58)
Death in childhood	9	5
Lost to follow-up	2	3
	Index Group (N = 47)	Control Group (N = 50)
Schizophrenia	5	0*
Mental retardation	4	0
Sociopathic	9	2*
Neurosis	13	7

* Statistical significance at .05 level.

Modified from "Psychiatric Disorders in Foster Home Reared Children of Schizophrenic Mothers" by L. Heston, 1966, *British Journal of Psychiatry, 112*, pp. 820, 822.

(Rosenthal, 1971), nor that schizophrenic mothers are prone to extraordinary rates of birth complications that can lead to neurologically impaired neonates (Mednick, 1970). In connection with possible prenatal or perinatal damage, it can be pointed out that the childhood death rates were inordinately elevated in both groups, but were almost twice as high in the index subjects (9/58 = 16%). Finally, the data do not support a purely schizophrenic interpretation but rather indicate, from a genetic point of view, that there is a nonspecific polypathological diathesis for those children who survived until adulthood (31/47 were schizophrenic, retarded, sociopathic, or neurotic, compared to 9/50 control cases). In short, Heston showed that schizophrenic women were likely to produce children exceptionally vulnerable either to early death or subsequent emotional disturbance. Further, it was not demonstrated that this latter outcome was a product of genetic influence: comparatively poor adult adjustment could have been explained by a combination of neurological deficit and the difficulties of placing "bad seed" children.

This brings us to the studies conducted in Denmark, where the national health register permits researchers to check the diagnosis of virtually any adult in the population who came to psychiatric attention. Published largely between 1968 and 1974, the series can be conceptualized as consisting of three interlocking investigations:

1. Kety, Rosenthal, Wender, and Schulsinger (1968)—a study of *collaterals* (design E in Table 1.1); identified a sample of diagnosed schizophrenics who had been adopted in very early life, then proceeded to a comparison of rates of schizophrenia in their biological vs. adoptive relatives;

2. Rosenthal, Wender, Kety, Welner, and Schulsinger (1971)—a study of *descendants* (design F); identified a sample of adopted-away children of diagnosed schizophrenics, then proceeded to compare rates of schizophrenia in this cohort vs. those of adopted-away controls born of nonschizophrenic parents;

3. Wender, Rosenthal, Kety, Schulsinger, and Welner (1974)—a *cross-fostering* study (design G); compared rates of schizophrenia when adoptive but not biological parents had been diagnosed schizophrenic vs. rates when biological but not adoptive parents were so diagnosed.

It should be mentioned that a "schizophrenic" parent in any of the Danish series need not have been so at the time of the child's birth, adoption, or even childhood—on average, the diagnosis was given 11 years after a child's birth. No history was provided for any case. Let us now consider the results of the Danish series.

The Kety et al. (1968) study located 33 adoptees who were diagnosed schizophrenic as adults, and matched a control group of 33 other adoptees never so diagnosed. The average age of separation from the natural mother was 3.5 months for the former and 4.1 months for the latter, with age at transfer to an adoptive home 18.3 and 16.0 months respectively. The researchers traced 150 biological relatives (parents, siblings, and half-siblings) of the index cases and 156 control relatives. They found only 2 diagnoses of schizophrenia among all relatives, one in each group; in both groups, they found less than the 1% expected rate of schizophrenia in the general population! They then pooled together a larger nosological category—"schizophrenic spectrum disorder"—which included chronic and acute schizophrenia, borderline states, schizoid and inadequate personality, and uncertain schizophrenic or borderline conditions. With a bigger net, they caught more fish: 13 of the biological relatives of the index group (9%) were within the new "spectrum," as compared to only 3 (2%) of the biological relatives of the control cases. This difference was statistically significant.

The Rosenthal et al. (1971) study located adoptees given up by a parent who was at some time diagnosed schizophrenic, and matched a control group of other adoptees who had no known schizophrenic parent—a design quite similar to that of Heston's investigation. However, whereas Heston's subjects were separated from their natural mothers days after birth, the median age of separation was 5.9 and 5.8 months respectively for the two Danish groups. In their preliminary report (Rosenthal et al., 1968) the researchers found only 1 case of a schizophrenic adoptee from a schizophrenic parent; nevertheless, invoking the "spectrum," they had a Danish colleague do "blind" interviews with the now grown-up children and had suggestive but not statistically significant results (13/39 index cases vs. 7/47 control cases). Shortly afterward, data from more cases were available and a final report was issued (Rosenthal et al., 1971); with an increased N, significance was now claimed (34/76 index cases vs. 12/67 control cases).

The Wender et al. (1974) study compared 69 children born to "schizophrenic spectrum" biological parents but raised by nonschizophrenic adoptive parents (the index group) with 28 children born to nonschizophrenic biological parents but raised by schizophrenic spectrum adoptive parents (the cross-fostered group); there were also 79 children from nonschizophrenic biological and adoptive parents (the control group). The median age of separation from the natural mother was 5.9

months for the index group, 4.5 months for the cross-fostered group, and 5.8 months for the control group (with a range for the latter from 5 days to a striking 7 years). Based on a new and apparently unvalidated "global psychopathology" interview-based scale (which for unstated reasons supplanted the previous history-based diagnosis of a schizophrenic spectrum disorder), no difference was found between the scores of the cross-fostered and control groups, just as would be predicted by genetic theory. More importantly, the mean score of the index group was significantly higher than that of the other two groups, *but only if* the latter groups were combined to make a large enough N. The combining of scores was done, and thus the reported results support the genetic hypothesis of the study. However, the price paid to obtain this outcome was costly: significance was achieved by sacrificing the cross-fostering design in the final statistical analysis, thereby rendering the findings equivocal.

Whatever their shortcomings, the Danish reports are without question the most comprehensive pedigree studies yet done. Snyder (1976) declared that they stand as a landmark contribution. Konner (1982) held the Danish adoption series to be "the best study so far in the whole field of human behavior genetics, and as close as human studies are likely to come to experimental rigor" (p. 97). Crowe (1982) hailed their collective findings as resolving the nature–nurture controversy so far as schizophrenia is concerned. Wender (1976) stated on behalf of the research team: "We failed to discover any environmental component" (p. 23). Wender and Klein (1981) extrapolated from the Danish adoption data that 8% of the general population are genetically predisposed to develop a personality disorder within the schizophrenic spectrum; only medication could correct the underlying biochemical problems. Rosenthal (1971) attributed 73% of the etiological variance for schizophrenia to genetic factors. Neale and Oltmanns (1980) stated: "If any doubt remained concerning the importance of genetic factors in schizophrenia, it was abolished by the [Danish] adoption studies" (p. 215). Strong claims from many quarters!

However, granted the deserved accolades for a prodigious investigation, the Danish adoption research is hardly beyond very serious reproach and does not singlehandedly settle the nature–nurture controversy. It cannot be contended that the series shows the heritability of schizophrenia; at best, two of the studies show the heritability of "schizophrenic spectrum disorder"—a vague and possibly non-homogenous condition. Even scholars as meticulous as Neale and Oltmanns elide this distinction, as can be noted in the statement quoted above. Moreover, biological psychiatrists often uphold and glorify the

Danish studies by virtually disregarding the major criticisms that have found their way into the professional literature. Already, four devastating critiques have been published that should not be overlooked, especially in that the last three even impugn the scientific integrity of the Danish research team.

The first critique, by Benjamin (1976), noticed that none of the biological parents of schizophrenic children in the Kety et al. (1968) study was schizophrenic, and that statistical significance came from 9/13 schizophrenic spectrum biological relatives who were half-siblings by the father (see Table 1.4). In short, second-degree relatives had higher rates than first-degree relatives, and this result, Benjamin points out, is a violation of the principle that genetic effects increase with greater consanguinity. The study's conclusion is therefore invalid on its face.

In a second important critique of the Danish series, Lidz, Blatt, and Cook (1981) complained that in the Rosenthal et al. studies (1968, 1971) the researchers allowed cases of manic-depression to get mixed into the schizophrenic spectrum, and that these cases made the difference in achieving significant results because manic-depressive parents were just as fecund as schizophrenic parents in breeding offspring in the schizophrenic spectrum (see Table 1.5)! Because manic-depressive and schizophrenic genetic processes are held to be distinct, this study too can be considered invalid on its face. In addition, Lidz et al. called on the Danish team to publish the results of psychological testing they administered to all subjects so as to provide an independent means to reach blind diagnosis. The insinuation here was that the researchers were suppressing information presumably unfavorable to their genetic hypothesis.

In a third critique, Cassou, Schiff, and Stewart (1980), a team of experts from the French National Institute of Medical Research, concluded that the Danish studies were inadequate and misleading; they even questioned the probity of the researchers for making claims to blind diagnosis that were belied, in their opinion, by the way cases were reassigned and statistics juggled. Cassou et al. also held that adoption studies are automatically invalid if case histories are not presented as to the circumstances in which a child is separated from its mother, as well as how the child subsequently fares in placement, so readers can judge whether that youngster was neglected, abused, or otherwise damaged before or after adoption, as well as whether the adoption was traumatic in itself. They refer to the probandi as *"enfants abandonnés,"* subtly indicating by this choice of terminology the irony of using throwaway kids as proof that schizophrenia is genetically transmitted! Another issue surrounds *when* children are placed: few

Table 1.4. Diagnosed Mental Illness in the Biological Families of Index and Control Cases

Proband Diagnosis	Schizophrenic Spectrum Disorders in the Biological Family					
	Probands			Controls		
	Parents	Sibs	1/2-sibs	Parents	Sibs	1/2-sibs
B1						
B2						
B3	B3		D1			
B3			B3			
B1		C				
B1	D3					
B1						
B1						
B1				B1	B3	
B2						
B3	C					
B1						
B3						
B2						
B1						
B1						
B2						
B1			B3,B3,B3			
B2						
B3						
B3						
B1			B1			
B3						
B2						
B1			D3			
B3*						
B3*						
B2				D3		
B3						
B1						
B1						
B1						
B1						
B3			B3,D3			
Totals	3+	1+	9 = 13	2+	1+	0 = 3
	Proband biological relatives = 150			Control biological relatives = 156		

Legend:
B1 = chronic schizophrenia
B2 = acute schizophrenic reaction
B3 = borderline schizophrenic or schizoid
C = inadequate personality
D1 = uncertain chronic schizophrenia
D2 = uncertain acute schizophrenic reaction
D3 = uncertain borderline schizophrenic or schizoid

* Only one of a pair of MZ twins was counted as a proband.

Data from "The Types and Prevalence of Mental Illness in the Biological and Adoptive Families of Schizophrenics" by S. Kety, D. Rosenthal, P. Wender, and F. Schulsinger, in *The Transmission of Schizophrenia* (pp. 354–355), edited by D. Rosenthal and S. Kety, 1968, Oxford, England: Pergamon Press.

Table 1.5. A. Consensus Diagnosis of Sick Parents

Diagnosis	N
B1	36
B2	7
B3	3
B1/B3	2
B1/B2	6
B2/B3	2
D	1
B1/D	1
B/M	1
D/M	1
M?	1
M	8
Total	69*

Table 1.5. B. The Percent of Schizophrenia Spectrum Diagnoses in the Offspring, According to the Subcategory Diagnosis of the Parent

Parental Diagnosis	Number of Cases Examined	Number in the Spectrum	Percent in the Spectrum
B1	24	7	29%
B2	5	1	20
B3	2	1	50
B/	3	2	67
M or M?	5	2	40
Controls	47	7	15
Total/Average %	86	20	23%

Legend: B1 = chronic schizophrenia
B2 = acute schizophrenic reaction
B3 = borderline schizophrenic
D = doubtful schizophrenia
M = manic-depressive psychosis

* [Note by A.P.:] Of the 69 parents, 8–11 were manic-depressive, or between 11 and 16% of the total.

Data from "Schizophrenics' Offspring Reared in Adoptive Homes," by D. Rosenthal, P. Wender, S. Kety, F. Schulsinger, J. Welner, and L. Ostegaard, in *The Transmission of Schizophrenia* (pp. 382, 388), edited by D. Rosenthal and S. Kety, 1968, Oxford, England: Pergamon Press.

were taken at birth and thus many spent their first 6 months with their natural mothers—the "bonding phase" during which a disturbed woman might well have the most harmful impact on her progeny's development (Magid & McKelvey, 1987). There were even some children who spent well beyond 6 months with their natural mothers before being placed for adoption; in general, index cases were placed later and adopted earlier than control cases throughout the Danish series. One must wonder what the research criterion was for "early" separation, especially when we see that at least one child was included who was given up for adoption at nearly age 7.

The fourth critique was by Lewontin et al. (1984), who went so far as to insist that the data can be used to demonstrate that environment is decisive for schizophrenia, not genetics! They argue from the findings of the Danish studies themselves: virtually no schizophrenic parents produced schizophrenic children and virtually no schizophrenic children came from schizophrenic parents. Despite the negative impact adoption can have—Henig (1988) reported that 1 to 2% of Americans growing up in adoptive homes represent 10% of psychiatric inpatients—Kety's review of the Danish data (1983) makes it clear that the adopted-away offspring of schizophrenics fare much better in adulthood compared to their home-raised brethren! The adopted-away offspring had lower rates in adulthood than the baseline expectancy for schizophrenia in the general population (Lidz & Blatt, 1983)! Thus, the most important finding of the Danish studies may be an environmental effect: not being raised by one's schizophrenic parent turned out to be salutary in terms of ultimate mental health. Lewontin et al. also believed that the Danish researchers twisted their data to reach congenial conclusions—for example, by reporting pseudointerviews with dead or absent relatives based on suppositions as to what they would have said (p. 224). In addition, Lewontin et al. offered evidence of glossing over the key issue of selective adoption: they show that 24% of adoptive homes for index cases had a foster parent who had been in a mental hospital vs. 0% for control cases (p. 223). The issue of selective adoption is further exacerbated by the fact that, in Denmark, foster care agencies deliberately place children in accord with social characteristics of their biological parents (Hutchings & Mednick, 1975), a factor that was unaddressed by the researchers.

But the Danish studies cannot so easily be paradoxically used to support environmental causality. Proponents of the genetic point of view maintain that the schizophrenic spectrum is not very different from Meehl's "schizotypy" or Heston's "schizoidia" and that the heritability of the schizophrenic spectrum is borne out in several smaller replications of the Danish design (Heston, 1970) and the more recent Roscommon family study (Kendler et al., 1993a, 1993b). At this moment in time, we can only wonder whether the glass is half-full or half-empty. Despite the vehemence of such as Paul Meehl (1972), who asserted it was not interesting to talk to anyone who disputed the contention that schizophrenia was inherited, the genetic etiology of the disorder is still nothing more than a hypothesis. Just as Jackson said in 1960, one can merely repeat in 1994 that a hereditary predisposition to schizophrenia is not a proven scientific fact.

Genetic Marker Studies

A new methodology in family pedigree studies is represented by the search for anomalies on particular chromosomes that can be traced across generations (design H in Table 1.1). With modern technology, a molecular design can now be utilized, specifying the mechanism within the DNA by which hereditary transmission of psychiatric disorders takes place. Such an approach forms the basis of a paper by Egeland et al. (1987), linking manic-depressive disorder to a single gene on the short arm of chromosome 11; this work was done on subjects from the Amish community in Pennsylvania.

After making allowance for the natural enthusiasm greeting a promising new avenue for research, some of the same old problems in pedigree studies are already evident in the professional response to Egeland: her results were initially accepted as if genetic transmission were an *a priori* truth just waiting to be shown, with scientific criticism suspended just as has generally been the case with the Danish adoption series. Egeland's findings should have been seen as merely speculative—the "marker" she observed may or may not have to do with genetic transmission of depressive traits. Definitive confirmation depends on replication of the data across many investigations, as well as on *predictions* based on the putative genetic marker as to which family members would be vulnerable in the future (design I), to be ascertained by longitudinal research. Pending such data, scientific acceptance of her results must be held in abeyance. In contrast, from the very date of publication, there was already reason for skepticism: in the same issue of *Nature* in which Egeland reported her findings, a similar study done in Iceland (Hodgkinson et al., 1987) found no linkage to chromosome 11 but concluded that ". . . mutations at different loci are responsible for the manic-depressive phenotype in the Amish and in Iceland" (p. 805). Both papers brim with high-tech molecular biology, but taken together they stand in contradiction. Although Egeland pointed to family history as proof that depression is inherited, the idea of a "mutation" can make any family history superfluous. The proposition that different ethnic groups have their own distinct genetic channels to manic-depression utterly denies the biological unity of the human species and runs counter to the basic premise of anthropology, which accounts for differences between ethnic groups on cultural rather than constitutional grounds. It boggles the mind to see "mutation" given as a reason for different results across populations when common sense would simply take this to be a failure of one study to replicate another, throwing doubt on the findings of one or the other. Moreover, the technology that is supposed to finally identify the predisposing gene for manic-depression did not consistently implicate chromosome 11, nor did Egeland's research confirm the presence of anomalies on chromosomes that had been specified in other research. The "News and Views" editor of *Nature,* Robertson (1987), synthesized the findings, citing two more marker studies not supportive of Egeland's chromosome 11 but concluding that therefore several genes must be causally involved in manic-depression—in other words, everybody could be right! No one considered in this issue of *Nature* that perhaps the data indicated that medical genetics are not germane to the study of depressive disturbance, and may even be neo-Lamarckian by viewing symptoms possibly acquired in the course of noxious family circumstances as genetically transmissible.

Following Egeland's model, linkage studies for schizophrenia have now also appeared in print. Bassett, McGillivray, Jones, and Pantzar (1988) encountered an odd-looking first admission while on psychiatric duty in a Canadian hospital and learned the patient had an uncle similarly odd-looking and emotionally disturbed: both men had a flat head, widely spaced eyes, protuberant ears, short stature, obese body, fusion of fingers, shortened toe, left kidney abnormality, small phallus, and—intriguingly—onset of schizophrenia at age 20. The rest of their immediate family was free of physical or mental deviance. On cytogenetic study, anomalies were noted in the 5q segment of chromosome 5 in the two men, but not in the rest of the family, except for their mother–sister who was a "balanced translocation carrier." Based on her "one-in-a-million" chance discovery, Bassett suspected that she had stumbled across the genetic mechanism predisposing to schizophrenia! However, she did not provide any case histories of the two probandi, nor did she conjecture whether their physical peculiarities in some neurological or psychological way contributed to the onset of schizophrenia. Even the question as to how they could possibly be prototypes for the schizophrenic condition did not arise—after all, very few schizophrenics look this way! She simply took for granted that a partial trisomy chromosome 5 resulted in deformity *and* schizophrenia.

This cause–effect logic can be criticized as nothing but the circumstantial evidence of a correlation in a single family pedigree.

Bassett's encounter with her unusual patient soon led to a funding grant for the next research step: an investigation of 7 families in Iceland and Britain, with 2 families showing evidence of chromosome 5 abnormality in their schizophrenic members (Sherrington et al., 1988). However, another study coreported in the same issue of *Nature* (Kennedy et al., 1988) did not find evidence for chromosome 5 abnormality in schizophrenic Swedish families, but once more speculated that mutations could account for differences between ethnic groups. The "News and Views" editor, this time Lander (1988), again posited that different genes could independently cause schizophrenia, so that all the marker studies might be valid despite the obvious problem of nonreplication. The incongruent findings were presented as if important progress had been made in the genetics of schizophrenia. Noting these scientific developments, on November 10, 1988, the front page of *The New York Times* announced that the chromosomal aberrations leading to schizophrenia may have been discovered!

The next year, these early genetic marker studies had to be retracted for both manic-depression and schizophrenia (Schmeck, 1989). The indisputable failure to replicate was the main problem. In addition, prospective–longitudinal data showed that 2 subjects from Egeland's Amish pedigree *without* the chromosomal abnormality developed manic-depressive disorder. From a research point of view, Egeland had properly applied scientific standards and accordingly withdrew her hypothesis. However, because of this failure, eminent biological psychiatrists are now convinced that multiple sites must be involved in manic-depression and that ". . . scientists will tease out the genes that go afoul in mental disease, if only they are meticulous in their hunt" (Angier, 1993). Based on consanguinity studies like those reviewed in this chapter, such psychiatrists are convinced that there must be a genetic cause, so that when no specific gene can be implicated, there must be several genes. It appears that the old abuse of the concept of reduced penetrance to explain away data inconsistent with genetic theory has now been replaced by reliance on a faith in "polygenetic transmission" to deal with contradictory or inconclusive results (Bader, 1990).

A still more recent genetic marker study (which also made the front page of *The New York Times*) will be discussed later in the chapter, along with alcoholism, in the section on neuropsychological-neurophysiological findings. In addition, some pedigree studies of psychiatric syndromes not yet addressed will be evaluated, within the context of discussing these particular syndromes.

PHARMACOLOGICAL RESPONSE

One line of inquiry into the etiology of a psychiatric disorder is *pharmacological challenge:* determining whether any drug can incite the condition, taken to imply that some chemically similar internal hyperfunction is the biological cause of the condition. Another related line is *psychopharmacology:* determining whether there is a therapeutic effect from administration of a drug, taken to imply that the drug must be compensating for an internal deficiency (or countering a hyperfunction) that is the cause of the condition. These approaches taken together comprise the research methodology of *pharmacological response;* they both share the assumption that psychiatric dysfunction has a biochemical basis (probably involving neurotransmitters), with the corollary that drug treatments can be developed to correct homeostatic dysregulation and thus restore mental health. The most obvious problem in this conceptualization is biological reductionism—the attribution of psychological symptoms not to past or present environmental events but to some putative bodily abnormality. The rather simplistic designation of "biochemical imbalance" as the cause of mental disorder has become an unfortunate characteristic of contemporary theorizing in biological psychiatry, usually with the main supportive evidence being response of some patients to a medication. For the general public, the concept of biochemical imbalance dispenses even with that evidence (see Mankoff's cartoon below). Lipowski (1989) found the concept to be counterproductive, both in

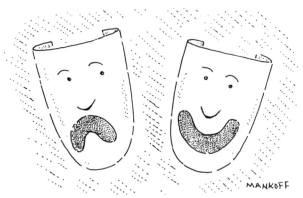

*"Oh, yeah? Well, I think you're the one with
the biochemical imbalance."*

Source: Drawing by Mankoff; © 1992, *The New Yorker Magazine, Inc.*

terms of its effect on treatment and its narrowing of the scope of scientific thinking:

> Another current fad is to tell patients that they suffer from a chemical imbalance in the brain. The explanatory power of this statement is of about the same order as if you said to the patient: "You're alive." It confuses the distinction between etiology and correlation, and cause and mechanism, a common confusion in our field. It gives the patient a misleading impression that his or her imbalance is *the* cause of his or her illness, that it needs to be fixed by purely chemical means, that psychotherapy is useless, and that personal efforts and responsibility have no part to play in getting better. . . . To assume . . . that biochemical processes underlie mental activity and behavior does not imply that they are causal agents but rather constitute mediating mechanisms. They are influenced by the information inputs we receive from our body and environment and by the subjective meaning of that information for us. It is that meaning which largely determines what we feel, think, and do. This is not to deny, of course, the importance of . . . biological factors for the way in which we respond to information and how it affects us for better or for worse (p. 252).

The psychopharmacological method has also been criticized for *ex juvantibus* logic (Bignami, 1982) because it argues from the effect of a drug backward to the cause of a condition—a deductive error; no drug has a single site of action. The method of pharmacological challenge has its drawbacks too: disparate drugs can sometimes induce the same condition, as can purely psychological interventions, sometimes without any known hyperfunction occurring. In fine, although certain drugs can induce behavioral symptoms, and certain medications can alleviate behavioral symptoms, it may be grossly improper to reason from pharmacological-response experiments that behavioral symptoms are the consequence of innate biochemical determinants. Lader (1990), a leading authority in the area of pharmacological-response research, has warned the field about reductionism, although he believes valuable clues to etiology can in some instances be gained:

> When pharmacological treatments are deemed effective for a psychiatric condition, a stimulus is given to biological research. Although few are so unsophisticated as to aver that if a condition is helped by drugs, it must be biological *in origin,* most would accept that biological *mechanisms* are involved in some way. Working out how a drug ameliorates a certain condition will not necessarily tell us much about the etiology or even the pathogenesis—but it might! (pp. 150–151)

Pharmacological Challenge

The experimental induction of psychosis in animals or humans has a long history (Munkvad, Fog, & Randrup, 1975). As reported by Munkvad et al. (1975), in 1845, Moreau de Tour described the mental effects of hashish; in 1927 Berger reviewed the literature on mescaline, comparing its effect with symptoms of schizophrenia; and in 1931, De Jong produced experimental catatonia in different animal species by means of mescaline. Bercel (1960) reported on the bizarre web-weaving of spiders who had been exposed to schizophrenic blood serum. More recently, LSD has received considerable attention as a "psychoto-mimetic" drug (Hollister, 1968), as have amphetamine and cocaine (Snyder, 1977). Claims were made that drugs that drive up dopamine levels were repeating the natural action of the brain in schizophrenia, but speculations as to the pharmacological properties of drugs inducing paranoialike symptoms have so far not led to any breakthrough in schizophrenia research. It remains a question as to how relevant "model psychosis" phenomena are to clinical cases. For example, Hollister (1968) showed that clinicians can readily distinguish between drug states and schizophrenic reactions based on mental status examination, and Bleuler (Lipton, 1970) concluded that psychotomimetic agents have contributed to our understanding of organic psychosis, not schizophrenia. A neurotoxic theory of schizophrenia must also deal with the fact that model psychosis can be experimentally induced by sensory deprivation—a purely environmental variable (Schultz, 1965). All that model psychosis research amounts to at this point in time is that toxic substances can cause psychosis, but not that psychosis is caused by toxicity.

Oddly enough, neurosis, not psychosis, has offered an opportunity for the most interesting developments in the area of pharmacological challenge. For example, the experimental induction of panic disorder by administration of sodium lactate will be addressed in some detail in a later section on biochemical correlates of emotion.

Psychopharmacology

Since the advent of the phenothiazines in the 1950s, research has focused on why antipsychotic medications are therapeutically effective. Kety (1975) summarized the early thinking by noting the inverse relation between therapeutic potency of the phenothiazines and the Parkinsonian side effects: it appeared that pharmacotherapy for schizophrenia exacerbated Parkinsonism, and pharmacotherapy for Parkinsonism exacerbated schizophrenia. This observation, however oversimplified, inevitably led to the implication of dopamine in the biochemistry of schizophrenia, and intense investigation has been generated to the point where a dopaminergic hypothesis is now widely regarded within biological psychiatry as an established "finding" in the etiology of schizophrenia. Although it has been shown that phenothiazines block CNS receptor sites activated by dopamine, this still doesn't necessarily mean that schizophrenia is a biochemical disease; no phenothiazine does more than alleviate certain acute symptoms. Psychopharmacological research is intrinsically limited: it can be no more specific than the therapeutic value of its drugs. Hence, the scientific standing of the dopaminergic hypothesis cannot be better than ambiguous at this juncture. It is also clear that even if dopamine is proven to be involved, it is involved as well in every kind of human behavior and is always just part of a very complex neurotransmitter story.

Despite vigorous laboratory investigation, no psychiatric disorder has thus far been "cured" by medication, not even manic disorder where lithium treatment has been so helpful. In the area of depression research, van Praag and Korf (1975) declared the findings concerning antidepressant medication have failed to revolutionize the treatment of depression, despite the information gained on relationships among metabolism, mood, and motor activity. In the metaphor of Akiskal and McKinney (1975), we now know something about the "pharmacological bridge" from metabolic events to behavioral symptoms, but we are still largely ignorant about reverse traffic on that bridge, from metabolism backward in time to precipitating psychosocial stressors.

Research on the efficacy of medications is expected from contemporary psychiatry, and biological psychiatrists have responded by developing an advanced psychopharmacology. But the "fishing expedition" of using response to medication as an index to the biochemical etiology of a disorder is inefficient and, worse yet, can get us lost at sea. The efficacy of a drug does not prove that a particular mental disturbance is biochemically determined. For example, aspirin relieves headaches but no one contends that headache is brought about by "aspirin deficiency." Instead, we classify aspirin as an analgesic, thereby suggesting that the troubles of the day may prompt a headache, but chemical relief only comes via reducing sensitivity to pain. Analogously, an agitated patient may be helped by a drug that renders him or her relatively lethargic; or, more precisely, the staff dealing with an agitated patient may be helped by a drug that renders the patient more manageable, with the patient benefiting secondarily (I have seen thorazine used in this manner). In the final analysis, although there is always a somatic process between stressor and symptom by which a drug intervenes to improve a patient's functioning, the therapeutic effect of a drug can be indirect or even unrelated to the cause of the condition. In other words, pharmacological-response research has a key role to play in biological psychiatry, but it need not create a theory of biochemical imbalance to do so.

NEUROPSYCHOLOGICAL-NEUROPHYSIOLOGICAL FINDINGS

On a visit to America, Bertrand Russell came as a guest to a philosophy class taught by Morris Cohen at the City College of New York. The two men fell into dispute over inductive logic. To make his case, Russell invited the class to disprove the following proposition: There is a rhinoceros in this lecture hall. The students proceeded to turn up desks, peer into closets, and ferret out crevices—but they could not lay their eyes on any rhinoceros. Russell was nonplussed for, according to him, it was not yet certain no rhinoceros was present in the hall; the search must go on. Russell's position was that inductive logic is an endless process that may never finally prove or disprove an inference. Common sense must somehow then intervene to set a limit and force a resolution.

This story may be apocryphal (like the rhinoceros; I can find no substantiation of its existence in the biographies of either Russell or Cohen), but its point is well taken. The philosophy of science must take into account that many a "scientific" hypothesis lies beyond confirmation or refutation, until common sense at last calls a halt to infinite speculation and inconclusive research. In this vein, critics of biological psychiatry can point out that here is a discipline that never seems to question its supposition that each psychiatric disorder has a somatic substrate that at least in part causes it. Medicine may not yet know what it is, but it's looking for it and, by God, *will* find it! The history of biological psychiatry can be depicted as a tale of "promising" leads, closure on slender evidence, hyperbole as initial reception to new work, and ultimately unproductive results. With each failure, however, the faith remains undaunted, simply shifting direction in its quest by optimistic lurches from one new idea to another. Heuristically, a lot of research has been generated but, following about a century of effort, a harsh assessment would be that no substantive results have been tendered for the pathogenesis of any major psychiatric disorder. From this unfriendly perspective, it will appear that the time must soon come to stop a futile hunt for what by now might be presumed to be a nonexistent rhinoceros.

In defense of biological psychiatry, it can be replied that the problems studied are complex and it is reasonable to anticipate delays and setbacks before medicine can identify constitutional mechanisms involved in "mental illness." The lack of definitive answers does not mean that there never will be answers or that the task is a pseudoproblem. Moreover, biological psychiatry will insist that considerable progress has already been made in tracing out the pathogenesis of disorders such as schizophrenia and panic attacks; even more progress can be expected in all areas under investigation if current or future research leads pan out. The herculean labors expended on the totality of projects, both planned and heuristic, will be well worth the effort if we can eventually fix the body as a means to fixing the mind.

All that can be done at present to resolve this quandary in how to evaluate the very foundations of biological psychiatry is to review syndrome-by-syndrome what biological psychiatry has to offer. We will next take a look at psychopathy, alcoholism, and schizophrenia as sample topics in the search for organic factors underlying psychopathology. We will then critique the findings of biological psychiatry from the perspectives of sociology and psychodynamic psychology, to get some sense as to whether such psychosocial approaches can interpret the data more plausibly.

Psychopathy

Antisocial behavior has been the subject of intense medical investigation for some time. As Hare (1970) described the general approach, "Most of the research on psychopathy . . . is based on the assumption that there is a physiological basis to the disorder. . . . If we could establish that psychopaths differ from other individuals on some physiological variable, this variable might be used as one of the defining characteristics" (pp. 27–28). Thus, the attribution of antisocial behavior to some physical abnormality has led to laboratory research on criminal populations; the history of such research is usually dated back to the nineteenth-century work, in Italy, of Cesare Lombroso, who gave the following account of his experiments:

> In 1870 I was carrying on for several months researches in the prisons and asylums of Pavia upon cadavers and living persons in order to determine upon substantial differences between the insane and criminals, without succeeding very well. At last I found in the skull of a brigand a very long series of atavistic anomalies, above all an enormous middle occipital fossa and a hypertrophy of the vermis analogous to those . . . found in inferior vertebrates. At the sight of these strange anomalies the problem of the

nature and of the origin of the criminal seemed to me resolved; the characteristics of primitive men and inferior animals must be reproduced in
our times. (Wilson & Herrnstein, 1985, pp. 72–73)

Lombroso branded about 40% of the criminals he studied as incorri-
gible, ascribing their illegal acts to predisposition based on an irre-
sistible "criminaloid" heritage. He distinguished between these "born"
criminals (distinguished by such stigmata as sloping forehead, long
arms, prognathous jaw, large incisor teeth, and so on) and "occasional"
criminals (normal men driven by desperate or passionate circumstances). Lombroso then developed rating scales for criminal propensities based on his anthropometric calculations, but he also could explain
away any case of criminal behavior that did not fit into his "atavistic"
mold simply be referring to some precipitating situational trauma. By
the turn of the century, Lombroso's data were hailed throughout the
Western world as the first "scientific study of the criminal" (Wilson &
Herrnstein, 1985, p. 74) because physical measurements and norms
were involved!

Ironically, it was precisely the anthropometrics that, in the end,
brought Lombroso's theory down. Critics pointed to the inaccuracy of
his anatomical descriptions and the biases of his sampling methods.
Subsequent research did not show correlations between "primitive"
physical characteristics and criminality. In addition, social criticisms
were telling: the so-called "inborn" inferiority of his criminals ostensibly derived from their constitutional heritage but it was obvious they
were circularly being called inferior because they were criminals. Racist
aspects were also evident in Lombroso's view of criminals as phylogenet-
ically lower creatures similar to aborigines whom he deemed unable to
live up to the standards of civilized Europeans; he proposed to pack
Italy's criminals off to penal colonies in Africa (not only where they
"belonged" but also where their rough ways could be utilized to exploit
natives on behalf of the imperialist mother-country). In addition, Lombroso's findings had a sinister effect on the courts and prisons of Europe
during the late nineteenth and early twentieth centuries. In the 1899
novel *Resurrection,* Tolstoy has one of his characters, a prisoner in Czarist
Russia, ask: "Why and by what right does one class of people lock up,
torture, exile, flog, and kill other people, when they themselves are no
better than those whom they torture, flog, and kill?" (Tolstoy, 1946, p.
403). The questions asked in the novel by officials in the criminal justice
system were of a quite different order: Do some human beings lack the
free will to abstain from crime? Could criminal propensities be detected
by measuring the skull? What part does heredity play in crime? Is there
such a thing as congenital depravity?

Further unproductive efforts to derive criminality from bodily traits were made by Goring (1913), who catalogued physical defects among English prisoners (but dropped "atavistic" implications), and Sheldon (1940), who correlated antisocial personality with "mesomorphic" bodybuild. Eventually, diagnosis based on physical appearance was abandoned, and biological psychiatry used advanced technology to focus on more subtle physiological defects. For example, Hare (1970) presented evidence showing "maturational retardation" in that the EEG readings of psychopaths resembled those of children; he also cited findings of autonomic hypoactivity to account for psychopaths' lack of anxiety, failure to learn from painful experience, and thrill-seeking. However, such ventures into neurophysiological etiology have not led to the specification of any biochemical flaw or even of the brain subsystem involved; instead, these ventures usually retreat to evidence from pedigree studies that some such defect must exist. A somewhat recent reincarnation of Lombrosian theory took the form of a briefly popular hypothesis that an XYY chromosomal anomaly produced "supermales" who could not contain their aggression (Jacobs, Brunton, Melville, Brittain, & McClemont, 1965). The designation of the cytogenetic XYY as a criminal stigma has since been exposed as a myth (Borgoankar & Shah, 1974), and Hare held the same viewpoint—on the grounds that it was not a heritable condition, as his literature review proved psychopathy must be!

Cloninger (1978) summarized the case for psychopathy as a heritable condition, referring to the fact that MZ twins have higher concordance rates than same-sex DZ twins, as well as to a favorable Danish adoption study by Mednick, Gabrielli, and Hutchings (1984), but he too could hardly venture a guess as to just what biological property is genetically transmitted, other than to make a passing reference to the reticular formation as a possible site of defect. Cloninger did not critically evaluate the research that supported his own pro-genetic position, but he did discount a contrary Swedish adoption study because subjects were included whose criminal behavior was deemed secondary to alcoholism. Had Cloninger been more universally critical, he might not have missed a much more damaging flaw in the Danish paper whose conclusions he accepted: Mednick et al. state that only 25% of their criminal sample were adopted immediately after birth, 51% were adopted within 1 year of placement in an orphanage, 13% within 2 years of placement, and 11% after 2 years. In addition to this damaging admission of what appears to be selective adoption in Denmark, the research team reported in a comment located in the "References and Notes" section (p. 894, #11) that a statistically significant association was found between later criminality and length of time waiting for adoption!

They then wondered if this association could be due to the deleterious effect of prolonged institutionalization and whether youngsters from a less desirable family genealogy were harder to place. In short, in a note amid references placed after the conclusion of a paper that argued for genetic etiology in psychopathy, these authors acknowledged that the results of their study could have been produced by a combination of selective adoption and the emotional harm inherent in an extended institutional placement.

Sociological criticism of biological approaches to criminality often bores in on the issue of "classism" in psychiatric diagnosis. For example, Cloninger (1978) declared that although nearly all sociopaths are or become criminals (whether or not legally identified as such), "so-called white-collar criminals seldom if ever suffer from antisocial personalities" (p. 97). As with Lombroso, it appears that there are still two kinds of criminals—shall we say "uncivilized" and "civilized"—and only the former is authentically antisocial in the eyes of biological psychiatry. In contrast, sociologists sneer at the presumption that white-collar criminals, as property owners, will only rarely be psychopathic; the position taken in sociology is that class structure and diagnostic bias, not biological variables, account for the label's use. For example, the "muckraker" movement in America in the late 19th and early 20th centuries depicted the leading businessmen of the day—Gould, Rockefeller, Morgan, and others—as "robber barons" who made their fortunes by illicit means but were able to manipulate the political system to thwart prosecution. In other words, given enough social success and clout, one man's psychopath can be transformed into everyman's financial tycoon. It also appears that even the "uncivilized" type of psychopath may still have a redeeming social function; thus, Cleaver (1967) has contended that the street criminal redistributes wealth, sometimes with a rudimentary revolutionary consciousness.

Another bone of contention for sociology is the claim, often advanced by biological psychiatrists, that genetic "predisposition" exists for many disorders, including psychopathy, which environment only activates. Clinard and Meier (1975), specialists in the sociology of deviance, found assertions of this nature unacceptably ignorant of social factors and even unscientific, declaring:

> Some biologists still believe that crime, alcoholism, certain types of mental illness, and certain sexual deviations can be carried as a specific unit in biological inheritance. . . . Deviant behavior cannot be hereditary . . . since social norms that are directly related to deviant behavior cannot be inherited. Such a theory of inheritance assumes that what constitutes disapproved behavior is

the same in all societies and throughout time. . . . Two leading authorities in the field of criminology [Sutherland & Cressey] stated that it is "obviously impossible for criminality to be inherited as such, for crime is defined by acts of legislature and these vary independently of the biological inheritance of the violators of law." (p. 31)

Psychodynamic interpretations of psychopathy focus on early experience as decisive for character formation. A "superego lacuna" (Johnson & Szurek, 1952) may be the result of identification with antisocial parents who raise their children in accord with their own rather than the community's ethical standards. Social learning theory (Bandura, 1973) points to financial rewards for antisocial behavior, inconsistency in discipline, and, especially, aggression modeled by parents, peers, and mass media. Stierlin (1974) looked at family factors, referring to "delegated" children who are often prematurely thrust out of the home to vicariously act-out their elders' forbidden wishes. Bowlby (1951) has written about the "affectionless psychopath" who is unable to empathize and turns against society because of severe maternal deprivation in early years. In the psychodynamic approach, emphasis is placed on how the immediate family and community have failed the child; biological variables are viewed as not particularly pertinent to the genesis of the condition.

In review of the cross-disciplinary data, it is my opinion that biological psychiatry has not yet sufficiently come to grips with social sciences data according to which "criminality" may have more to do with norms, identifications, and values than with any biological "propensity." Sociology has primarily pointed to the inequalities of economic opportunity as the cause of crime; psychology has stressed crucial socialization experiences with parents and peers. Indeed, an integrated psychological-sociological perspective may well constitute a totally adequate etiological formulation. In connection with the issue of classist bias, the notion that a "biological marker" exists for a diagnosis that turns, in many respects, on a moral or legal judgment, usually made by those more privileged of those less privileged, appears innately implausible. Therefore, it does not surprise me that research results in this particular area of biological psychiatry can be considered negligible thus far.

Alcoholism

Alcohol addiction has long been suspected of having some biological component which, in conjunction with opportunity and cultural pressures, causes a "disease." Jellinek (1960) defined alcoholism as a progressive condition characterized first by psychological and then by physiological dependence; Zwerling derived a typology of alcoholism from the DSM-II psychiatric nosology (Block, 1965). However, the disease model has been attacked because it is not clear whether alcoholism is (a) the disease itself or only a symptom of a personality disorder, or (b) is a mental or a physical defect (Clinard & Meier, 1975). In addition, the voluntary nature of behavior that leads to addiction makes alcoholism nonhomologous to any other medical syndrome.

According to Thio (1978), the search for a biological marker for alcoholism had yielded eight different theories put forth by the American Medical Association:

1. Metabolic disturbance;
2. Abnormal sugar metabolism;
3. Endocrine deficiency;
4. Dietary deficiency;
5. Liver deficiency;
6. Sensitivity to food;
7. Dysfunctional "alcohol appestat" in the hypothalamus;
8. Imbalance of the acetylcholine and receptor sites in the ascending reticular formation.

After reviewing the many different and confusing theories, Madsen (1974) concluded that alcoholism is a stress disease; nevertheless, he too compounded the chaos by speculating that it was caused by some sort of dysfunction in the pineal gland. Krimmel (1971) noted several more inconclusive or contradictory constitutional theories not mentioned by Thio, such as missing chromosomes and lowered blood chloride levels; he then quoted Mark Keller, then editor of the *Quarterly Journal of Studies on Alcohol:*

> [E]vidence for physiological addiction has never been produced. The evidence for cell metabolism has not been produced. A tough-minded pharmacologist . . . has called these notions of altered cell metabolism and physical dependence "exercises in semantics or plain flights of imagination." (Krimmel, 1971, p. 49)

Further, although Keller was fully aware that there are marked physiological complications in alcoholism, he knew of no research data that proved they were present before the onset of heavy drinking. In a similar vein, Thio (1978) observed that biological researchers often tend to confuse cause with effect:

> When they discover that alcoholics are more likely than non-alcoholics to have dietary deficiencies or glandular dysfunction, the researchers assume that these physiological defects are the causes of alcoholism. . . . [But] the frequent and heavy consumption of alcoholic beverages is bound to have a damaging effect on the physical constitution. (p. 334)

A notable recent effort to identify a biological marker has pinpointed slight elevations in acetaldehyde levels in the blood of alcoholics after drinking, as compared to controls (Schuckit & Rayses, 1979). Schuckit (1984) has argued that enzymatic mechanisms controlling ethanol metabolism are hereditary and thereby create a biochemical predisposition: higher concentrations mean that the body breaks down ethanol more slowly, making ingestion more pharmacologically potent, causing more organ damage, and leading the at-risk individual to experience inebriation as less impairing. Schuckit is duly cautious in the light of measurement problems in biochemical research and the complexities of ethanol absorption; notwithstanding, his theory must be considered speculative—the validation of his findings can only come from a *prospective* study based on enzyme samples taken in childhood, predicting who will become alcoholic later on and who will not. But he published long before this could be done, and, so far as I know, it has not yet been done.

Because the pathogenic constitutional agent still remains to be identified, biological psychiatry has in the meantime relied on evidence that alcoholism is a genetically transmitted disease. Some pedigree studies are widely cited as conclusive: Goodwin, Schulsinger, Hermansen, Guze, and Winokur (1973) and Goodwin et al. (1974) and Schuckit, Goodwin, and Winokur (1972). The former is an adoption comparison using the Danish files from the schizophrenia series to identify a cohort of males adopted soon after birth, all of whom had a biological parent hospitalized at some point for alcoholism; a control group consisted of matched adoptees without a biological parent known to be alcoholic. The subjects were interviewed at an average age of 30 by a Danish psychiatrist who was blind as to whether they were probandi or controls; the subjects themselves did not know they were participating in an adoption comparison study and volunteered no information indicating whether they knew their birth parents were alcoholic. As for results, *all* subjects were found to be moderate to heavy drinkers. There was no significant difference between the two groups at any level of drinking, except for the extreme category "alcoholic" (10/55 probandi, 4/78 controls), leading the investigators to conclude that only alcoholism per se (as distinct from "heavy drinking") is heritable. Psychopathology in general was rampant in the series of adoptees, running about two-thirds of both groups based on the clinical impressions of the Danish psychiatrist, so that no difference was observable there. The only other difference was found to be in divorce rates (the probandi were three times more likely to end their marriages). Goodwin et al. (1973) made the following incidental comment: "Divorce and alcoholism have often been associated, but the former has generally been attributed to disruptive effects of the latter. Our data suggests that divorce and alcoholism may perhaps be co-variants of a single or related genetic predisposition" (p. 242). Talk about neo-Lamarckism: it seems even acquired legal status can be inherited these days!

The Danish pedigree study has generally been accepted without demur (Mendelson & Mello, 1979; Rutstein & Veech, 1978). However, in terms of its methodology, the tables in this chapter seem to indicate that 1 or 2 subjects were switched without explanation from the control to the index group, and 4 controls were admittedly added at the end and were not blind to the Danish psychiatrist. This latter procedure is, of course, scientifically unacceptable, especially in view of the fact that the reader is given no information as to what the particular disposition in the study turned out to be. Thus, there is already room for suspicion as to investigator bias and statistical loading. In addition, it is impossible to know just what the probandi heard about their birth parents: they were not asked. Further, if the mother of a proband was the alcoholic parent, there is the possibility of neurological damage in utero and of fetal addiction. And, as always, the question of selective adoption comes up, with "undesirable" children going to less satisfactory foster homes—a possibility the coauthors acknowledged.

Schuckit et al. (1972) compared male probandi diagnosed as alcoholic to their half-siblings, with whom they may or may not have lived. Because most of these subjects came from broken homes, it was also possible to study the relative impact of an alcoholic biological parent vs. an alcoholic surrogate parent (defined as a new spouse with whom the child lived for at least 6 years prior to age 17). The subjects were significantly more likely to be alcoholic if their biological rather than their surrogate parent was alcoholic. Contrasting 32 alcoholic subjects with 132 nonalcoholics, it was reported that 62% of the former had an alcoholic biological parent, compared to only 20% of the latter. Simply living with an alcoholic surrogate parent seemed to have no relationship to the development of alcoholism.

In criticism of this study, the probandi were state hospital patients (thus, in today's parlance, likely to be MICA patients) who came from unstable families acknowledged by the coauthors to be extraordinarily rent by divorce, remarriage, and redivorce. It is difficult to believe that these subjects can be considered representative of alcoholics in general.

Beyond sampling problems, the study's design does not even permit blind interviewing. Information concerning alcoholic elders must come from the subjects themselves, as elicited and evaluated by the interviewer. As a member of the research team, the interviewer can hardly be considered unbiased. This questionable experimental design is credited by the coauthors to, of all people, Rudin! It is a contemporary application of his discredited "science of psychiatric genetics," with the only change being that nowadays we would speak of "genetic predisposition" rather than "taint."

Aside from these troubling issues around Schuckit et al.'s research design, concordance rates for alcoholism are consistently higher for half-siblings raised apart than those raised in the same home, a fact that can be interpreted to mean that half-siblings from a hard-drinking father are more apt to be alcoholic than half-siblings from a nondrinking mother (the fathers were usually the alcoholics and the mothers usually had custody). The data do not include comparison of half-siblings by a common alcoholic parent as opposed to half-siblings by a common nonalcoholic parent, to determine the effect on children when the custodial parent is the alcoholic. Finally, as the authors realized but had no way to control for in the study, the mate of an alcoholic may have alcohologenic qualities that influence both choice of a partner and the way children are raised.

A genetic marker study for alcoholism was reported on the front page of *The New York Times* on April 18, 1990. In an article published in the *Journal of the American Medical Association,* Blum et al. (1990) studied brain samples from 35 deceased alcoholic individuals and 35 nonalcoholic matched controls. They found that the presence of the A1 allele of the dopamine D2 receptor gene correctly classified 77% of alcoholics, and its absence correctly classified 72% of nonalcoholics. They concluded that the gene that confers susceptibility to "virulent alcoholism" is located in the q22–q23 region of chromosome 11. Noble, the second author of the study, was optimistic about replication: he held that (a) the dopamine receptor was a likely candidate because it has been strongly associated with the brain's reward mechanisms, and (b) environmental stresses account for only 30 to 40% of the etiological variance of alcoholism (Adler, 1990). Incidentally, this latter estimate is more generous in terms of environmental causation than that of

Cloninger and Reich (1976), who claimed that the genetic factor in alcoholism accounted for 90% of the variance.

Unlike the enthusiastic reception we have seen accorded to previous genetic marker studies on depression and schizophrenia, the alcohol study drew immediate criticism. In an accompanying editorial in the same journal issue, Gordis, Tabakoff, Goldman, and Berg (1990) expressed skepticism that the results would be replicated, noting that no one gene would likely cause alcoholism, the sample size of the study was too small, and sketchy information was provided on the matching of controls, as well as on how "virulent alcoholism" was defined (the index subjects died of a variety of diseases and were only retrospectively diagnosed as alcoholics). The editorial recalled the recent failures to replicate genetic marker studies in depression and schizophrenia, as well as the Egeland retraction, and warned that validity of conclusions in this type of research often hinged on subtle statistical considerations and the stability of the subjects' diagnoses over time. Although interested in the Blum et al. results and awaiting further findings, the editorial writers even decried biological reductionism in the alcohol study, pointing out that the real research challenge is how genes and environment interact to produce alcoholism in any individual. Such a high level of critical sophistication demonstrates that the field of biological psychiatry is finally learning from the bitter lessons of the past, although there is still unswerving commitment in this editorial to the idea that alcoholism has some genetic component.

Another critique of the Blum et al. study came quickly from Peele (1990). He observed that the article was accompanied by press releases, a highly publicized news conference in Los Angeles, and video interviews with the study's authors, which the American Medical Association arranged to have transmitted by satellite in its weekly television news release. In Peele's estimation, such public relations hype in no way enhanced the scientific value of the study, which still left vague the actual physiological mechanisms involved in alcoholism and which seriously underestimated the importance of social factors. Peele complained that American researchers typically ignore the work of Robin Murray, the leading British expert in the genetics of alcoholism; Murray found no difference in rates of alcoholism for MZ and DZ twins, effectively ruling out a genetic hypothesis if these results are replicated by other researchers.

Gelernter, Goldman, and Risch (1993) reviewed nine studies replicating Blum et al.'s hypothesis linking the A1 allele on the dopamine D2 receptor to alcoholism and found no confirmation—indeed, there was more heterogeneity between studies than between subjects and controls! Thus, on empirical grounds, the spectacular discovery of a gene for alcoholism has been laid to rest.

As for criticism coming from outside the mental health field, sociologists often take umbrage when psychiatric theories posit that organic predisposition is necessary for the development of alcoholism. Clearcut data tie alcoholism to such social variables as sex, class, ethnicity, and occupation; this research can be synthesized to form a concept of social role already sufficient to account for differential rates of alcoholism. For example, Trice (1966) compared Irish and Italian drinking patterns, noting that the former tended to try to outdrink each other in bars, while the latter imbibed mainly in family settings around meals; the outcome of these disparate patterns was far greater alcoholism among the Irish. Pittman and Gordon (1958) held that, in many cases, alcoholism could be considered an "occupational disease." They looked at the communal functions of drinking on certain jobs such that every employee became susceptible to eventual addiction through ritual after-hours competitive drinking with buddies, uncomplicated by food or mixed company:

> The Army, the Navy, the work camp, the railroad gang, and the lake steamer, all are rich in drinking culture. In these groups the harsh, monotonous . . . routines are broken by the nights, weekends, and lay-offs which offer opportunities to drink. Drinking is a preoccupation and conversations are filled with talk of drink. . . . The all-male drinking group [becomes] a symbol of manliness and group cohesion. (p. 67)

World rates vary enormously, creating a nettlesome problem for any predominantly constitutional explanation. Social factors appear to be decisive; for example, immigrant groups coming to America tend to have much higher rates here in their native lands, even when opportunity to drink was available in the old country. Fort (1981) has written that the United States is preeminent among nations as a breeder of addicts, hypocritically pushing a variety of drugs, legal and illegal, for pleasure or relief.

Psychodynamic and family therapists are usually as adamantly opposed to the disease model as is sociology. Fox (1967) pointed out that a biological predisposition to alcoholism was still not demonstrated:

> In spite of the fact that 52% of alcoholics have one or both parents alcoholic we do not yet have proof that there is a genetic disturbance underlying alcoholism. It often "runs in families," but this may merely reflect that a child brought up in an alcoholic home has had a shockingly inadequate family life. (p. vii)

Longitudinal studies of alcoholism, such as that of the McCords (1960), typically show a background of broken homes, economic deprivation, and exposure to heavy drinking. Krimmel (1971) held that alcoholics are vulnerable people by virtue of their disturbed childhood experiences, but this is not to say there is an identifiable "alcoholic personality"; alcohol abuse is viewed by Krimmel as just one more psychopathological reaction to ego damage. Cox (1987) has argued that alcoholism cannot be considered a unitary diagnostic entity; he described two disparate subtypes: (a) primary (stemming from an impulse disorder) and (b) secondary (stemming from stress reduction). Psychoanalytic theories of alcoholism have centered on three themes: (a) oral fixation, (b) repressed homosexuality, and (c) insidious suicide. Research has been notoriously poor in confirming these dynamics, although some findings do show that alcoholics drink to feel powerful (McClelland, Davis, Kalin, & Wanner, 1972), perhaps in reaction-formation to ego-dystonic dependency needs or to compensate for recent narcissistic injury.

Cox (1987) insisted that a total biopsychosocial model of alcoholism would include: (a) biological propensity to alcoholism, plus the effects of drinking on the body before, during, and after addiction; (b) psychological factors, especially counterdependent needs in which alcohol gives the drinker an illusion of strength; and (c) social factors, such as a "culture of drinking" that pushes at-risk individuals to progressively heavier consumption. To date, the most dubious part of this biopsychosocial model is the assertion about "biological propensity." Again, as was said about the multidisciplinary research on psychopathy, an integrated psychological-sociological viewpoint may well provide a sufficient explanation as to etiology. Biological factors have still to be identified as part of the predisposing etiology, and pedigree studies are not conclusive in terms of genetic factors. However, both common sense and clinical findings dictate that biological variables enter into the clinical equation once drinking starts, and ever more saliently so once the stage of addiction is reached.

Schizophrenia

Schizophrenia has long been regarded by biological psychiatry as a brain disease whose arcane nature must eventually succumb to laboratory investigation. But this assertion has admittedly never been buttressed by solid research findings "until recently"—the usual notation by whatever writer is doing the reviewing at the moment. Smythies et al. (1968) can be regarded as illustrative of this tendency:

For the last fifty years research workers have sought diligently for some bio-chemical or physiological disorder in schizophrenia without, however, until very recently, any noticeable results. . . . Since there was no specific hy-pothesis to guide research all that could be done was to measure [somatic] variables in schizophrenics and hope by luck to find something abnor-mal. . . . In this way a great number of investigations were carried out on liver function, carbohydrate metabolism, adrenocortical function, the level of certain cerebral enzymes, the "toxicity" of schizophrenic serum, the mode of reaction to stress, etc. Positive results were claimed from time to time but these were invariably contradicted within a few years. Most of the "positive results" are now known to be due to the fact that the schizophren-ics differed from the normal population in respects other than having the illness. (p. 25)

In chastising the field for "hit or miss" research, Smythies et al. be-lieved that biological psychiatry was finally on the right etiological track. They based their optimism on the then-new research on amphetamine–mescaline psychotomimetic effects. Kety (1975) likewise complained that the field seemed very confused when he entered it, but was at last pursu-ing leads that would provide "light at the end of the tunnel"; the new work he made reference to was the transmethylation studies (which at-tributed the cause of schizophrenia to the accumulation of hallucino-genic substances in the brain) and psychopharmacologic studies related to the dopamine hypothesis. In neuropsychology, Buchsbaum and Inquar (1982) gave a similar rags-to-riches recitation of the field's history:

A biological test for schizophrenia has so far eluded investigators. Each new neurohormone, each new putative neurotransmitter becomes a candidate— could it deficiency or excess be the cause of or at least a marker for schizo-phrenia? Each new electrophysiological test similarly raises the possibilities of the ultimate diagnostic test. The schizotiters and schizowaves are tested on small populations of subjects with excitement, but few receive any wide-spread support. After a time, even their own developers move on to new transmitters and recordings, abandoning the techniques in the storm of neuroscientific progress. (p. 235)

Buchsbaum and Inquar then pointed to the latest work on EEG and PET (positron emission tomography)-scans and had no doubt that sig-nificant breakthroughs would now occur. Be that as it may, it is inter-esting to note how they characterized an essentially trendy and serendipitous approach to research in schizophrenia as a "storm of neuroscientific progress."

Lewontin et al. (1984) panned the assumption within the field of bio-logical psychiatry that schizophrenia must be a biochemical abnormality of the nervous system that will reflect itself in the production of abnormal metabolites in the blood and ultimately be excreted in the urine. This view of schizophrenia engenders "heuristic" studies whereby body materials (urine, blood, cerebrospinal fluid) "from certified schizophrenics are compared with those from 'control' normal people with all the assiduity that the Roman augurs used to apply to the examination of an animal's entrails" (pp. 202–203). They reviewed 30 years of such research:

> Among the claims for causative factors in schizophrenia made since the 1950's we may point to: abnormal substances secreted in the sweat of schizophrenics; injection of the blood serum of schizophrenics into other, normal subjects inducing abnormal behavior; and the presence of abnormal enzymes in red blood cells and blood proteins. . . . Conflicting research reports have claimed that schizophrenia is caused by disorders in serotonin metabolism (1955); noradrenaline metabolism (1971); dopamine metabolism (1972); acetylcholine metabolism (1973); endorphin metabolism (1976); and prostaglandin metabolism (1977). Some molecules, such as the amino acids glutamate and gamma-amino-butyric acid, came into fashion in the late 1950's, fell into neglect, and now, in the 1980's, have come back into fashion once more. (p. 205)

In a recent co-twin control study, Suddath, Christison, Torrey, Casanova, and Weinberger (1990) compared the size of ventricles in discordant MZ twins. In 12 out of 15 pairs, the schizophrenic member had larger ventricles as well as subtle cytoarchitectural decrements in temporal lobe structures; 7 control MZ pairs did not have this difference. The authors theorized that the schizophrenic twin must have suffered some type of tissue loss, leading to greater intracranial ventricular space, which was either primary or secondary to the disease. They then showed that reduction in brain matter did not correlate with duration of illness so that such morphological change was either simultaneous with or predated the onset of psychotic symptoms. This work has already been hailed as a "landmark" (Goleman, 1990) and is indeed worthy of follow-up in view of the well-established clinical observation that organicity is frequently associated with chronic schizophrenia. However, the validity of the present results is not yet clear: 12 out of 15 cases is not quite statistically significant, the study is retrospective, the reduced size of brain structures is small and not outside normal limits, the crucial issue as to whether such anatomical atrophy is primary or secondary to schizophrenia is still unsettled, and schizophrenic brains do not always have this feature, while normal brains sometimes do (a reversal that occurred in one of the discordant pairs in the study).

Furthermore, in using discordant MZ twins to demonstrate neurophysiological etiology in schizophrenia, biological psychiatry is inherently disavowing genetic factors. But it seems you *can* have your cake and eat it too. In a disclaimer, Suddath et al. stipulated that they merely addressed "extragenetic" effects. Despite the fact that they were dealing with genetically identical but nonetheless discordant MZ twins, and found evidence in many cases of postconception morphological damage in the brain of the schizophrenic member, they still refused to consider that their results, if valid, would effectively rule out a hereditary predisposition to schizophrenia. Instead, it appears they believe that there must be first a genetic predisposition, followed by a subsequent morphological change in brain structure for unknown reasons, to bring about a case of schizophrenia—all this rather than drawing far simpler conclusions from two research approaches that stand in plain opposition!

Cannon et al. (1993) studied developmental brain anomalies in the offspring of schizophrenic mothers in order to investigate ventricular enlargement from another angle. After carefully controlling for the effects of age, gender, substance abuse, and history of organic brain syndromes, they found significant, stepwise, linear increases in cortical and ventricular cerebrospinal fluid–brain ratios with increasing level of genetic risk for schizophrenia in the parent–child cohorts they studied. Their data implicated two interacting factors—(a) genetic loading and (b) obstetric complications—as predictive of later schizophrenia in the offspring. Accordingly, they drew the inference that abnormalities in the brains of schizophrenics are neurodevelopmental in origin and may play a role in the etiology of the disorder. However, their experimental sample was selected based on a diagnostic criterion of "schizophrenic spectrum disorder" and so cannot be extended to "schizophrenia." A control group was sorely lacking in this research. Data were presented in aggregate form, so one cannot tell whether there were subjects with prenatal ventricular enlargement who later on did not become schizophrenic, or subjects without the prenatal enlargement who did become schizophrenic. Suddath et al.'s prior work on ventricular enlargement in discordant MZ twins is not mentioned, perhaps because that study raises issues that are not compatible with "genetic" findings in this study. Although the Cannon et al. investigation is indeed suggestive, it still has not been shown that all or most schizophrenics have oversized ventricular space at the expense of brain tissue, or even that morphological changes of this nature lead to psychotic behavior.

The bottom line here is that biological psychiatry still is uncommitted to any definite hypothesis as to the site or mechanism of neuropsychological-neurophysiological dysfunction in relation to schizophrenia. van Praag & Korf (1975) acknowledged that laboratory results have been "meager" and urged that research in schizophrenia should henceforth focus on biological correlates of symptoms rather than diagnosis. Hence, we are left with the conundrum as to whether schizophrenia is essentially a brain disease that medicine will ultimately explain, or whether it may be a psychological condition simultaneously reactive and adaptive to a highly problematic social milieu. At this point, the stance of biological psychiatry is to uphold the diathesis–stress approach, in which a constitutional propensity must be triggered by a noxious environment; as we have seen, this putative "propensity" perforce exists because pedigree studies so indicate.

Sociological criticism of biologically oriented explanations of schizophrenia often has centered on the strong relationship between social class and incidence; a series of investigations, culminating in the work of Hollingshead and Redlich (1958), has demonstrated that poverty is a significant risk factor. Aside from the possibility that diagnosis tends to be more benign when the patient is affluent, the major interpretation of these data is that greater stress faced by the poor contributes to higher rates of mental breakdown. However, Dunham (1977) has reinterpreted the data according to a "downward drift" hypothesis that has been endorsed by many biological psychiatrists (Guggenheim & Nadelson, 1982); Dunham argued that vocational failure by schizophrenics accounts for their relatively disadvantaged socioeconomic standing. Both factors are probably operative, but "downward drift" cannot apply very well to the multitude of schizophrenics who were never "up" to begin with.

Psychodynamic criticism has tended to focus mainly on faulty parenting as a necessary and sufficient cause. The "schizophrenogenic mother" concept was propounded by Fromm-Reichmann (1959, p. 164) and has been supplanted by a more comprehensive theory of family communication deficits that presumably can disorganize and drive the helpless child crazy (Bateson, Jackson, Haley, & Weakland, 1956; Lidz, 1973). Laing (1972) went so far as to suggest that the schizophrenic child may be more sane than the family-of-origin! Clinicians are understandably leery of such an extreme position, but the general approach has been to implicate the parents in the etiology, and even to picture the child as sent on a "mission impossible" to preserve the family, often by remaining with an enmeshing parent. Most of the evidence for the view that family pathology causes schizophrenia comes from clinical casework; however, one can also mention the naturalistic observations of Henry (1971), who lived in the homes of psychiatric patients in order to make anthropological field notes about a milieu he too found very disturbing (but this may have already been his bias). Somewhat firmer data have come from Sobel (1961), who followed 8 cases of children born to parents who were both schizophrenic—4 of these children were raised at home and 4 were immediately placed in foster care. Sobel reported that none of the foster-raised children seemed disturbed after 18 months of observation, but 3 of the parent-reared children were already symptomatic by 14 months. Unfortunately, Sobel did not follow his infant cases to an adult diagnosis, with independent confirmation of his clinical impressions. In a more comprehensive longitudinal study, Tienari et al. (1987) reported that none of the children of schizophrenics who were placed in "good" foster homes became schizophrenic, but most of the children placed in what were previously judged to be "bad" foster homes did develop the disorder in young adulthood. In an unusually detailed study, Greenspan (1987) has shown that children of mothers who were severely impaired by psychiatric disorder were already symptomatic by 3 months of age. Reading Greenspan's account of the developmental consequences for infants receiving some of the worst possible mothering, one feels sure that these youngsters would be either dead or irretrievably crazy if there had been no clinical intervention. Of the three studies cited—Sobel, Tienari, and Greenspan—the latter two investigations assumed that predisposing genetic factors would adversely influence the psychic development of offspring of schizophrenics, but they concluded that placement in a proper foster home (Tienari) or intense psychiatric support for mother and infant (Greenspan) can serve as suppressor variables. Nevertheless, in all three of these studies, a noxious family environment can arguably be seen as cause enough of severe emotional disturbance in the children; an academic tip of the hat to biological psychiatry may just be *pro forma*.

Has biological psychiatry made a strong case for organic etiology in schizophrenia? It is the educated guess, but only a guess, of most clinicians that a constitutional factor probably is involved in schizophrenia, but it is far from clear whether such a factor, if it exists, will prove to be cause or effect, genetic or developmental, neurotransmitter or morphological, and so on. To the credit of biological psychiatry, the research effort to date has been formidable, but theoretical findings remain essentially inchoate, shifting, and speculative, without always admitting this is so. Based on what we currently know, it is still conceivable that a noxious-enough environment could bring about psychotic decompensation without any predisposing bodily vulnerability. As I see it, the current state of evidence in favor of a biological origin of schizophrenia can hardly warrant any dogmatic assertion concerning

genetic transmission, constitutional predisposition, or mode of biological action. An example of such dogmatism is the complaint by Torrey
(1983) that family therapists make parents of schizophrenics feel guilty
for what he describes as the "biochemical disorder" of their child; he
then adds that many families have rallied to his "humane" explanation
of the nature of schizophrenia. But what may represent "humane"
truth to Torrey and his clientele can be to others mere biological reductionism that takes away human agency; what Torrey has done is
effectively take the schizophrenic's social system off the hook of responsibility for a family member's tragedy by blaming an impersonal
and hypothetical defect in the body of the patient. In any event, the
claim that a biological explanation of schizophrenia is more "humane"
than one based on psychodynamics or family-systems theory cannot be
accepted as validation of the former's scientific worth.

Comments on the Three Cross-Disciplinary Comparisons

Given that it is not possible to ever disprove some sort of constitutional
basis for psychopathy, alcoholism, or schizophrenia, the research efforts to find a "biological marker" will go on. Despite substantial social science data indicating that environment alone could cause any of
these conditions, this is as it should be; closure on debate would be premature now. But merely carrying on with biological research does not
automatically mean that we will get closer to definitive answers. The
answer may be that there is no answer. In all three areas, I have noted
the same serendipitous and trendy search to identify some organic factor that presumably causes the condition. A succession of studies then
results in "promising leads" that soon get advertised as the long-
awaited "breakthrough" in a supposed storm of scientific progress.
Thus far, when it comes to organic etiology in biological psychiatry, despite growing sophistication in research methodology, it is, more or
less: *Plus ça change, plus c'est la même chose.* I have also noted many assur-
ances in scholarly language that the elusive constitutional mechanism
must exist and is just awaiting discovery. Such claims are based on genetic studies that are not subjected to sufficient critical examination,
although there may be criticism of contrary findings. Finally, I have
noted unwillingness to consider the contingency that social or psychodynamic variables are adequate unto themselves to account for a given
psychiatric condition; instead, biological psychiatry tends to insist on
an ostensible "biopsychosocial" paradigm in which, as it always seems
to turn out, biological factors are prepotent.

Nevertheless, although I believe that purely psychosocial etiology
may have to be accepted for some diagnostic categories in the long run,

nothing I have said should be construed to mean that any of the three diagnostic groupings just reviewed have already been demonstrated to be psychosocial in origin; any of them might ultimately be shown to have some somatic dimension in its etiology. The present paper cannot dismiss this possibility, no matter how substandard, inconclusive, or contradictory much of the research has been.

BIOCHEMICAL CORRELATES OF EMOTION

The search for biological markers in anxiety or depressive conditions is especially hopeful in that affective phenomena, by their very definition, must be somatically expressed. Nevertheless, research is complicated because more than psychophysiological processes need to be studied. There are also metaphysical (mind–body) questions to resolve, and they have long stymied human inquiry.

The very first issue is semantic: What is "emotion"? Rapoport declared that we cannot clearly say, because we regard emotion as both a phenomenon and a dynamic (Plutchik, 1962). The term may also refer to conscious or unconscious experience; Freud postulated that dysphoric or ego-alien affect may be masked by defense mechanisms so as to be denied. The debate continues as to whether "primary" emotions exist. If they do, which ones are they and what is their total number (Izard, 1972)? Further, there are undoubtedly physiological correlates of emotion, but it is not certain that this implies any physiological *specificity* (i.e., a characteristic, humanly universal neurochemical substrate for each emotion). Still further, controversy has swirled around the causal sequence in emotion: Does a psychological aspect precede and trigger the somatic aspect, or vice versa? The James–Lange theory holds that the body reacts to a perception and this reaction *is* the emotion (in other words, the boy is fearful because he trembles, not trembling because he is fearful). This approach argues that the precipitant is an environmental happening that stimulates the thalamus. "Downward discharge" activates the viscera (ANS) and the muscles (CNS) while "upward discharge" subsequently informs the cortex and gives the "feeling tone" of an emotion (Gellhorn, 1964). Such theory offers a process explanation of emotional consciousness (Mandler, 1984) in which some sort of reflex response sets in motion both molecular and molar behavior; labeling of the emotion is a second-order event arising from feedback as to what the body is already doing. Note how the thalamus has replaced the cortex as the "thinker" in this mind–body equation! Refutation of the James–Lange approach was attempted by Cannon (1929), who maintained that even when neurological damage precluded visceral feedback, emotional behavior still occurred; that ANS reactions are too slow to give the cortex much of a clue as to what is "felt"; that patterns of emotional differentiation are not clear; and that, when visceral reactions are chemically induced, no emotional change may follow. An alternative to the James–Lange account came to be called the Cannon–Bard theory; it suggested that emotions could be experienced without occurrence of bodily changes—all that was necessary was activation of the sympathetic adrenal-medullary system in emergency situations (thereby implicating the cortex as the initiator of the process). Thus, according to Cannon–Bard, cortical functions play a key role in affective states, both in the perception of what becomes exciting and in the interpretation of what the body's response means. In other words, general visceral arousal has to be initiated and structured cognitively to have a distinct emotional experience.

Beyond the semantic problems, the next issue concerns the fact that "emotion" is an evolutionary constituent of the human being; because this is so, we are presented with a phylogenetic puzzle when it comes to "emotional disorder." Is such pathology normal behavior in the face of perceived stress (although thresholds may be low or perceptions disordered), or does some abnormal physiological functioning make the situation stressful? The investigations of biological psychiatry into anxiety and depressive states have mainly concentrated on the latter possibility, with exhaustive research efforts going into the identification of a distinct biochemical anomaly in the index cases studied. However, if the former possibility is the correct one, all that can be demonstrated by research into the latter is that autonomic reactivity correlates with symptoms, but without any premorbid marker common to those who are subject to the disorder. Moreover, even if biochemical abnormalities were to be found, we still wouldn't know that these "cause" emotional disorders; constitution is a mechanism for affective expression, not a determinant. Biology sets a limit on what behavior can be, but is not able to dictate its content (Costello, 1976). If biochemical abnormality is why some people feel what they feel, mind–body dualism is supplanted by biological reductionism in those cases, and by logical extension in all cases.

A third point of contention arises from nosological groupings of anxiety and depressive conditions into discrete types. Does each subcategory have its own distinctive biological workings and thus respond to different medications, or do the various subcategories share a common genotype but not a phenotype? Indeed, are anxiety and depressive reactions themselves differentiable on a neurochemical basis? Current answers are far from conclusive; they range from insisting that research address each subcategory separately because underlying pathophysiology is different (Paul & Skolnick, 1984) to proposing that genetics are the same for anxiety and depression and only environment makes them different (Kendler, Heath, Martin, & Evans, 1987). Consideration must also be given to the research data of Schachter, who proposed a "cognitive labeling theory" of emotional activation (Schachter & Singer, 1962). This work is consonant with the James–Lange approach in that bodily changes are shown to precede the experience of emotion, but parted from the James–Lange approach in that very similar physiological changes are shown to accompany different emotions, with only the context permitting discrimination on a cognitive level.

As can be seen, the biochemical correlates of emotion provide an inviting field of investigation for biological psychiatry, but an especially difficult one as well. We now proceed to an outline of the contemporary status of research into anxiety and depressive disorders.

Anxiety Disorders

Panic attacks are nowadays widely held to be accessible to a biochemical explanation (Sheehan, 1982):

> Until recently panic disorder was viewed almost exclusively in psychological terms. It was believed that the patient was overreacting to a life stress or an "unconscious" conflict. A growing body of evidence now suggests that we reverse this view in favor of a medical-illness model. This model suggests that in contrast to stress-related situational anxiety, panic disorder is associated with a biochemical abnormality in the nervous system, to which there is a genetic vulnerability. (p. 156)

The hereditary aspect of panic disorder is reviewed by Crowe (1984), who summarized research to set a lifetime prevalence rate of 2 to 5%, whereas consanguinity studies showed a morbidity risk in first-degree relatives of up to 61%. Several MZ–DZ twin comparisons indicated much higher concordance in the identical pairs. Thus far, no adoption study has been done in this area. Crowe acknowledged he was unable to proffer definitive data in favor of genetic etiology, although he considered the above-cited statistics as more or less convincing! Torgersen (1983) compared 32 MZ and 53 same-sex DZ twins in Norway and concluded hereditary factors were significant in panic disorder but not in generalized anxiety disorder; however, he applied the "equal environments assumption"—a premise, as we have seen, that is likely not tenable. All told, drawing on only family and twin rates, the genetic investigation of panic disorder is still at a relatively crude stage. As to the importance of genetic factors, Rainer (1976) has cited work that estimated that heredity accounts for 80% of the etiological variance in neurotic conditions, without any evaluation of the experimental procedures.

In the research on specific somatic abnormalities, attention has focused on the chemical provocation of panic disorder through such means as lactate infusion, carbon dioxide inhalation, or administration of yohimbine, caffeine, or isoproterenol, despite many questions as to which of these drugs has effects most closely resembling the natural phenomenon (Roy-Byrne & Cowley, 1988). In the most successful pharmacological-challenge work ever done in biological psychiatry, intriguing results were reported by Pitts and McClure (1967) in their demonstration of the experimental induction of neurosis in a laboratory setting. They provoked very convincing panic attacks in 13 out of 14 anxiety patients, as well as 2 out of 10 normal controls, through bringing the venous lactate level to a range usually only attained with maximum muscular exertion or after administration of adrenalin. Nevertheless, attempts to use lactate level as the biological marker for panic disorder have failed (Tuma & Masser, 1975): metabolism of sodium lactate to bicarbonate is so swift that blood lactate levels do not elevate following infusion (Grosz & Farmer, 1972), nor has it been shown that levels are higher in premorbid panic disorder patients than in others. Because it is now well established that lactate infusion does precipitate panic attacks, particularly in persons who already have a history, Gorman (1984) has speculated that a panic attack is an adaptive mechanism gone awry: laboratory provocation by lactate or other chemical agent may trigger an anoxia detector, with some people being hypersensitive enough to create a perceived need to flee. For Gorman, the question these days is no longer deemed to be: "What is the biochemistry of panic disorder?" but rather "Why does lactate produce panic?" However, Lader (1990) disagrees, showing that lactate produces panic symptoms only if administration is preceded by appropriate tension-arousing instructions and then only in already susceptible individuals. Moreover, if lactate is indeed a factor in the biochemistry of panic disorder, it can only be as a mediator—specific environmental events (the phobic situation) are the agents that incite a fight-or-flight somatic reaction, and lactate infusion is essentially limited to producing panic in those long familiar with such symptoms (i.e., it is their way of dealing with stress). Thus, sketching in the biochemical processes, two phases would be necessary to explain the reported experimental findings:

1. A cognitive perception of threat activates the adrenal system, resulting in a release of lactate and a subsequent interoceptive sense of muscular overexertion and oxygen deprivation (a Cannon–Bard sequence);
2. The visceral reaction of "suffocation" feeds back into the perception of threat (a James–Lange sequence).

This hypothetical account still leaves unsettled the problem as to why some people are more susceptible than others to the perception of threat from nonmalignant sources, and such a theoretical gap can perhaps best be bridged by referring to dire associations from one's past as instrumental in setting in motion a psychosomatic alarm-reaction (a psychodynamic sequence). Lader (1991) has offered a very similar but more detailed perspective in which a stimulus is cognitively appraised as "anxiogenic," arousing normal physiological reactions; but, in patients so disposed, a catastrophic interpretation of the physiological changes quickly occurs which triggers yet more anxiety in a feedback loop until a full-blown panic attack is under way. Lader then shows how cognitive therapy at either the perceptual or catastrophic-interpretation stage can prevent the incipient panic, as well as how each of the various antianxiety drugs blocks different phases of the physiological buildup in the pathological psychosomatic process. The cognitive-visceral interaction is obviously a great deal more intricate than is indicated by Carr and Sheehan's (1984) conclusion that "panic disorder is a biological disease. . . . [It is] but one consequence of a primary brain-stem neuronal dysregulation" (p. 107).

Considerable research has also been done relative to other aspects of the biochemistry of anxiety; this work can be summarized as rounding up the usual neurotransmitter suspects whenever there is an investigation. For example, adrenergic receptors, GABA, and catecholamines have been studied with respect to panic disorder, but without substantial results (Hicks, Okonek, & Davis, 1980). Although sympathetic overstimulation has long been assumed in panic disorder, many findings indicate parasympathetic abnormalities as well, so no simple theory can accommodate all the data (Gorman, 1984). Some work has focused on mitral valve prolapse, but Gorman notes that some panic disorder patients have this defect, although most individuals with this defect do not have panic disorder. To further confuse matters, several books in the "pop psych" literature have categorically attributed anxiety conditions to inner ear dysfunction (Levinson, 1986) or to poor nutritional balance (Marmorstein & Marmorstein, 1979).

Another area for recent research has been obsessive-compulsive disorder. Hollander et al. (1988) used biological challenge in the form of the chemical MCPP (m-chlorophenylpiperazine) on obsessive-compulsive patients, producing an exacerbation of symptoms in the majority; the researchers then hypothesized that such patients have overly sensitive serotonin receptors. The research team also found that intravenous injection of the antihypertensive drug clonidine led to reduction of symptoms, suggesting to them that the neurotransmitter norepinephrine moderates anxiety triggered by the disorder. Some difficulties with these inferences are: in model-neurosis designs, a drug may affect many sites of action; it is not demonstrated that afflicted individuals have a premorbidly higher sensitivity to serotonin; and the question is begged as to what causes excess serotonin production as a possible biochemical determinant of anxiety or what causes an insufficient supply of norepinephrine as a possible moderator of anxiety. It is especially troubling that subjects who respond to biological challenge already have an obsessive-compulsive disorder: this could very likely mean that subjects who respond to stress with obsessive-compulsive symptoms do so in laboratory experiments too, rather than that the laboratory procedure pushes their specific symptom above some putative "biochemical" threshold. Also, it must be remembered that laboratory responses are *not* necessarily tantamount to real-life responses, given that insidious "demand characteristics" are imposed once anyone becomes a subject in someone else's experiment (Orne, 1962).

Depression

Depression has well-known vegetative signs—a fact that already speaks to a constitutional component in the pathogenesis. However, as was mentioned with respect to anxiety, organic factors may mediate rather than cause the condition, in which case a cognition sets off a psychosomatic chain of events, with bodily activity then feeding back to the cortex, alerting and confirming messages about emotional state. In this conceptualization, a cognitive interpretation that the situation is "bad" initiates CNS and ANS reactions that are both an expression of depression and a signal to the self that something is wrong (i.e., one is depressed). Put figuratively, what I behold upsets me, so I cry; there are tears in my eyes, which shows how upset I am. In such a Cannon–Bard/ James–Lange feedback model, a premorbid biological marker for susceptibility is not necessary, although markers may be found subsequent to symptom onset as a result of chronic reaction, sometimes doing physiological damage in due course. The theoretical approach I am presenting is not one that biological psychiatry tends to endorse; investigations into affective disorders are usually based on a search for distinctive somatic signs that are presumed to be etiologically crucial, represent some kind of biological aberration, and may be inborn. Thus, our review can start with the contention held by many biological psychiatrists—that depression has a genetic basis and that patients with an affective diagnosis are viewed as having inherited a "predisposition," a latent tendency just waiting to be evoked by some mildly stressful or even ordinary life event.

Gershon (1983) regarded the genetic transmission of depression as a settled issue. In his account of the evidence for heritability, he prematurely intermixed the next issue: what is the pathophysiological vulnerability and what gene or genes are involved? His manifest bias aside, data in support of this genetic thesis start with consanguinity studies, although Gershon acknowledged these are highly inconsistent in reported rates, partly because of differences in procedures and criteria and partly because of likely cross-cultural differences in prevalence. Although aware there can be no "true" rate of diagnosable affective illness, Gershon still argued heritability because within-study comparisons show that relatives have higher rates than controls—the old "runs in the family" fallacy. He then cited MZ–DZ twin research to show higher concordance rates in the former group—another methodology that cannot control for environment as an extraneous variable. Gershon did refer to an MZ-twins-reared-apart study (comprising no less than 12 pairs from one country!) but he was leery of its findings because of the lack of systematic sampling. Gershon realized that adoption studies would be essential for any demonstration of genetic etiology, but unfortunately he could point to only one such investigation, dealing with bipolar disorder, which he nevertheless found adequate for his purposes. This is the report of Mendlewicz and Rainer (1977) which, parallel to the Danish adoption studies in schizophrenia, was able to get significant results only by creating an "affective spectrum," including bipolar, unipolar, cyclothymic, and schizoaffective diagnoses. Working in Belgium, Mendlewicz and Rainer found 31% of the biological parents of adopted bipolar probandi to have "affective spectrum" disorder, more or less comparable to the 26% rate found in parents of home-raised bipolar patients, but significantly higher than the 12% rate found in the adoptive parents. Gershon did not question the validity of this favorable study, but, as always, interpretation of the data was weakened by failure to give any case history information, so that we never know why or when the children were given up for adoption, or whether there were long stays in temporary shelters or institutions before placement. We also do not know whether the children ever knew their mothers were psychiatrically ill (no fathers in their sample were in the "affective spectrum"), nor whether there was contact with the natural mother after placement. Moreover, the mental health of adoptive parents is apt to be better than that of biological parents who lose custody: adoptive parents are screened for mental health before they can receive custody from a foster care agency, whereas biological parents only have to conceive a child and may even have a major emotional disturbance that led directly or indirectly to the placement of the child.

Gershon wound up his survey of evidence for the genetic point of view by referring to preliminary data on a collaterals adoption study of suicide; using the Danish cohort from the schizophrenia study, significantly higher rates were reported for suicide in the biological relatives of adoptees who committed suicide than for adoptive relatives (3.9% vs. 0.6%). Schulsinger, Kety, Rosenthal, and Wender (1979) concluded that suicide per se was in part a product of genetic transmission, quite apart from mental disorders (e.g., depression, alcoholism) frequently associated with suicide. This bold deduction stemmed from the fact that half of the relatives, biological or adoptive, were not in any kind of psychiatric treatment at the time of their suicide. Clayton (1983) questioned such logic on the grounds that not being in treatment does not preclude having a psychiatric disorder. Kety's (1979) interpretation of the same Danish family data was even more problematic: he regarded suicide as a frank product of brain disease. Kety thought research on suicide parallels that once done on pellagra, which was initially found to follow kinship lines without anything more being known about its etiology until Goldberger, in 1915, showed that the mechanism of transmission was a deficiency in B vitamin niacin. Kety expected neurobiological defects to be discovered for all mental disorders which, for now, can only be said to run in families, without information as to the exact mode of transmission. But Kety's use of pellagra as an analogy for suicide is curious: pellagra has an environmental cause (it "runs in families" because the family eats the same food), whereas Kety insisted that suicide is a hereditary condition. If Goldberger had interpreted family concordance rates for pellagra in the same manner as Kety did for suicide, Goldberger never would have investigated the role of diet! Moving to another dimension of criticism, neither the Kety nor the Schulsinger et al. studies dealt with the theoretical considerations that for suicide to be genetic, a major tenet of evolutionary theory would be violated (survival of the fittest) and the heritability of acquired characteristics upheld (neo-Lamarckism).

As to the biochemical pathology that must underlie depression (and suicide) if the condition is inherited, research has tended to follow the fixed ideas of contemporary biological psychiatry—namely, that abnormalities in neurotransmitters cause behavioral disorders. Although no definite findings have yet been established, extensive research has been done based on pharmacological-response studies because manic-depressive states can often be ameliorated by drug therapy. Schildkraut, Schatzberg, Mooney, and Orsulak (1983) were respectful of the pathophysiological complexities of depression but nevertheless felt confident that the emerging field of "psychiatric chemistry" will discover new medications that will provide clues to the various mechanisms resulting in different forms of depression. These researchers hypothesized that a deficiency in brain catecholamines, particularly norepinephrine, led to depression, whereas an excess led to mania. In recent years, alternative models have held that depressive conditions can be dichotomized as either "noradrenergic" or "serotonergic," and still other researchers have stressed the role of acetylcholine. To complicate matters further, Schildkraut et al. pointed out that depression is a neuroendocrinological metabolic disorder; biological markers may be found in biochemical systems other than neurotransmitters. The problem with current research is not so much the plethora of speculation and the lack of definite findings—it is that most of the work is based on drug efficacy, leading to inferences about the somatic processes by presuming the drugs are supplying a deficiency that causes the psychopathology. This is an unabashed medical-model approach, viewing depression as caused by a specific biochemical dysfunction, distinct for each diagnostic subcategory, and with cognitive as well as situational variables reduced to an epiphenomenon of merely incidental interest.

SUMMARY AND CONCLUSIONS OF THE CRITIQUE

Although all research studies have flaws, the present writer believes the literature of biological psychiatry does not come close to meeting scientific standards in terms of methodology. Biological psychiatry must abide by the same criteria for presenting empirical data and drawing careful inferences as any other medical or social science field. This signifies that any studies that do not meet standards for proper research procedures or interpretation of data must not be accepted for publication, or if already published must be discredited within the professional literature. Some of the most egregious errors in terms of sloppy procedure are: citation of older papers that lack a methodology section, give no case-history information, violate the canon of "blind" diagnosis, change diagnostic criteria at midstream of a study to get significant results, and offer no assurance of good-enough environment in

nature–nurture studies in sampling of subjects. Some of the most egregious errors in terms of sloppy inferences are: including virtually no
critique of favorable previous studies, regarding theories as valid before replications or longitudinal results are available, failing to consider
alternate psychosocial explanations, predicating human action on
grounds of biological determinism alone, and automatically explaining
inconsistent results from several studies by invoking, without any empirical basis, such statistical or conceptual artifacts as "incomplete penetrance" or "polygenetic transmission."

In addition to improving the quality of research methodology, it is
incumbent on biological psychiatry to strictly acknowledge and respect
the limitations inherent in current methodology. We will briefly mention some of the limits we have seen repeatedly trespassed in each of
the four types of methodological approaches.

1. In *pedigree studies*, consanguinity rates and MZ–DZ comparisons
are not capable in principle of establishing genetic etiology, nor are they
"suggestive" in the "right" direction. MZ-twins-reared-apart and adoption research are capable of demonstrating genetic effects, provided that
such extraneous factors as selective adoption, inadequate foster conditions, and subsequent contact with biological relatives are controlled for
in the experimental design (practically speaking, a difficult feat). All
told, when explicit evidence for genetic etiology is lacking, biological
psychiatry tends to fall back on implicit evidence such as what "runs in
families" or presentation of statistics without case history data. A century after the Jukes book, this is scientifically scandalous and shows the
influence of the eugenics movement to this day. As previously noted, we
tend to use the parlance nowadays of "genetic predisposition" as a eu-
phemism for "taint," which makes it harder than before to detect any
classist or racist bias.

Furthermore, it is alarming just how preposterous biological research
can be in accounting for human social behavior on genetic grounds without any questioning of its own methodology precisely because implausible positive findings are reported. For example, consider the use of the
co-twin control method by Eaves, Eysenck, and Martin (1989) to investigate the extent to which social attitudes are inherited:

> Our study . . . suggests that genetic factors play a surprising role in main-
> taining human diversity. Even within families, it is clear that dizygotic
> twins hold religious and political views that are significantly more diverse
> than monozygotic twins. Given a "religious" home environment, it may still
> be partly a matter of genotypic predisposition whether one child or another

remains faithful to the beliefs of his parents or chooses a more secular philosophy. Many social and accidental effects may intervene between the individual genotype and the final expression in a particular attitude or belief. In our present Western society, however, the probabilities along the way may be biased as much by the genotype of the individual as they are by the social and educational environment to which he is exposed. If this is a good model of human development then we expect a correlation between genotype and social attitudes. If social attitudes play any part in the behavior of one person towards another then we may find that genetic differences between people are partly responsible for the distinction between godly and ungodly and between liberal and conservative . . . . (pp. 375–58)

Eaves et al. go on to show that ". . . 40% of the variation in [scores on a conservatism scale] is apparently due to additive genetic factors, 30% due to environmental differences within families, and 30% due to . . . differences between families" (p. 360). Beyond the questionable validity of the equal environments assumption in this type of research, common sense (plus a bit of knowledge about sociology) might suggest that a co-twin control methodology that leads to such a conclusion about the genetic transmission of political values must have dubious credentials.

The case is no better with the Plomin, Corley, DeFries, and Fulker (1990) study of the genetics of childhood television-watching habits, based on the method of adoption comparisons. They found that biological, adoptive, and control (nonadoptive) parents looked at television an average of 5 to 10 hours per week and were not significantly different, although the biological parents soon to give up custody, based on self-report during the last trimester of pregnancy, watched somewhat less. However, the viewing habits of biological parents who lost custody significantly correlated with their adopted-away children's viewing habits at ages 4 and 5 (but not at age 3), so that genetic variance is calculated by Plomin et al. at 34% for age 4 and 30% for age 5. Parent–child correlations were significant but at a higher level in the control families, and significant but at a lower level in the adoptive families. These authors concluded that "individual differences in children's television viewing are significantly affected by genetic factors as well as shared environmental influence" (p. 376), but with only about 20% of the variance accounted for by the environment! Despite impressive statistical analysis and research design in the study, one cannot help but wonder about the validity of these inferences from rather ambiguous data, as well as about what ideological purpose is being served in the course of regarding human habits in genetic terms and thereby generating this particular line of research.

2. *Pharmacological-response studies* assume a neurophysiological imbalance causes a condition; they attempt to provoke the condition by chemical challenge or relieve the condition by medication. The trouble is that sundry drugs can induce the same condition, and the condition may also be induced without any drug. There are other questions: Is the induced condition quite the same as the naturally occurring psychopathology? Are there "demand characteristics" in the experimental induction of neurosis or psychosis for the subject to produce such symptoms? As for medications, even when psychotropic agents work (and they only do to some extent), we do not ordinarily know the site of action of the drug, nor whether the drug acts directly or indirectly on the condition. In summary, although pharmacological-response research is pragmatically extremely useful, its theoretical value in relation to etiology is circumscribed in that administration of a chemical may stimulate or inhibit the somatic processes involved in mediating the expression of a behavioral disorder, but without either causing or curing the behavioral disorder.

3. The *search for organic causes* of each type of psychopathology is a "fishing expedition" that generates enormous research and a literature all its own, but without discovering the constitutional basis for any functional disorder thus far. In general, genetic studies are uncritically relied on to ensure that an as-yet-unknown constitutional defect must be *there*. However, in this manner, the possibility is discounted that there may be no *there* there! A research approach committed to find some organic dysfunction to account for psychological disorder has a limitation: if environment should be the cause of the disorder, such research will go on *ad infinitum* in a fruitless search because no means exists to check its own assumptions. What's more, such self-perpetuating research will insist all along the way that there is imminent "light at the end of the tunnel"! Only knowledge of alternative social science explanations can make possible an evaluation of biological theories vis-à-vis environmental theories.

Biological psychiatry has been fixated on the premise that a neurophysiological abnormality accounts for nonadaptive emotional reactions. In so doing, somatic processes are seen as causing rather than mediating behavioral events (as is also the case in pharmacological-response research). Further, short shrift is given to the possibility that emotional experience may be physiologically nonspecific (just representing a state of autonomic arousal that is differentiated at a cortical level according to context), leading to pitfalls in research methodology. If each emotion is not physiologically distinctive, there can be no biological marker for each type or subtype of emotional pathology, and thus most current research in this area would be inappropriate in design. Insofar as "panicogenic" compounds that can experimentally induce anxiety are concerned, it must be remembered that several quite different drugs can provoke panic attacks, and then mainly when anticipatory set has been established in vulnerable subjects (i.e., subjects who have a history of responding to even slight stress or bodily discomfort with severe and disabling anxiety symptoms).

4. Some of the problems of biological psychiatry derive from *general ideological premises* not associated with any particular research methodology. In this venue, there is the fantastic conceit that psychiatric diagnosis, based on a historically evolved descriptive clinical phenomenology, actually coincides with biological parameters that underlie and cause the behavior. van Praag (1993) vehemently warned fellow biological researchers that diagnosis in psychiatry is too unclear and unreliable to be a satisfactory correlate in research; instead, he recommended only the investigation of somatic aspects of well-defined symptoms. Moreover, the system of psychiatric classification we now use has been created by generations of brilliant clinicians, as well as the consensus vote of their professional colleagues on the successive DSM committees, but it is a system much too subjective, debatable, and culture-bound to be taken literally as representing biological truth. Dumont (1984) has been eloquent on this point:

> Modern medicine has been guilty of what Alfred North Whitehead termed "the fallacy of misplaced concreteness." Nowhere is this more true than with mental, intellectual, or behavioral disorders. Contemporary psychiatry is going through a paroxysm of line-drawing. It is attempting to divide all human behavior into discrete categories of "illness" decided by a consensus. . . . The schizophrenic label provides the best example of an arbitrary and fluid designation wreaking havoc in its efforts to assume the authority of a "disease." Schizophrenia is a German invention (it could not have been called a "discovery"). (pp. 327–328)

Unfortunately, the preponderance of research contributed by biological psychiatry up to the present is rendered questionable or even invalidated by the criticisms just presented. A harsh judgment perhaps, but it remains a puzzlement how a field with so many distinguished practitioners could be so susceptible to being thus rebuked. Sad to say, much of the work reviewed in the course of this chapter can be characterized in the same fashion as the evaluation of genetic research in schizophrenia by Cassou, Schiff, & Stewart (1980): "Garbage in, garbage out" (p. 124).

A survey of the field of biological psychiatry should not end on such a dour note; there *are* some achievements to applaud. The quality of clinical methodology and inference is improving at last, with the result that recent studies are far more sophisticated. For example, the Kendler et al. Roscommon study (1993a) does not interpret its family history data as showing genetic causation of schizophrenia; instead, it refers more cautiously to some admixture of genetic and environmental causation. The Gordis et al. (1990) review of the alcoholism gene study is a masterpiece of critical acumen. Some researchers now carefully avoid any reductionistic thinking and view somatic mechanisms as mediators, not determinants; indeed, van der Kolk (1988) has suggested that traumatic psychosocial experiences, especially in early life, influence and change neurological functioning. This represents an alternative biological paradigm to the reductionist models that have been so pervasive in psychiatry in the last two decades of the twentieth century.

REFERENCES

Abood, L. (1960). A chemical approach to the problem of mental disease. In D. Jackson (Ed.), *The etiology of schizophrenia* (pp. 99–119). New York: Basic Books.

Adler, T. (1990). Alcoholism gene study is controversial. *The American Psychological Association Monitor, 21*, 8.

Akiskal, H., & McKinney, W. (1975). Overview of depression: Integration of ten conceptual models into a comprehensive clinical frame. *Archives of General Psychiatry, 32*, 285–305.

Akiskal, H., & Webb, W. (1978). *Psychiatric diagnosis: Exploration of biological predictors.* New York: SP Medical & Scientific Books.

Angier, N. (1993, January 13). Scientists now say they can't find a gene for manic-depressive illness. *New York Times*, C1.

Bader, M. J. (1990). A response to Reginald E. Zelnick. *Tikkun, 5*, 48–50.

Bandura, A. (1973). *Aggression: A social learning approach.* Englewood Cliffs, NJ: Prentice-Hall.

Bassett, A., McGillivray, B., Jones, B., & Pantzar, J. (1988, April 9). Partial trisomy chromosome 5 cosegregating with schizophrenia. *Lancet, I*, 799–800.

Bateson, G., Jackson, D., Haley, J., & Weakland, J. (1956). Towards a theory of schizophrenia. *Behavioral Science, 1*, 251–264.

Benjamin, L. (1976). A reconsideration of the Kety and associates study of genetic factors in the transmission of schizophrenia. *American Journal of Psychiatry, 133*, 1129–1137.

Bercel, N. (1960). A study of the influence of schizophrenic serum on the behavior of the spider: Zilla-X-Notata. In D. Jackson (Ed.), *The etiology of schizophrenia* (pp. 159–174). New York: Basic Books.

Bignami, G. (1982). Disease models and reductionist thinking in the bio-medical sciences. In S. Rose (Ed.), *Against biological determinism* (pp. 94–110). London: Allison & Busby.

Block, M. (1965). *Alcoholism: Its facets and phases.* New York: John Day.

Blum, K., Noble, E., Sheridan, P., Montgomery, A., Ritchie, T., Jagadeeswaran, P., Nogami, H., Briggs, A., & Cohn, J. (1990). Allelic association of human dopamine D2 receptor gene in alcoholism. *Journal of the American Medical Association, 263,* 2055–2060.

Borgoankar, D., & Shah, S. (1974). The XYY chromosome male—or syndrome? *Progress in Medical Genetics, 10,* 135–222.

Bowlby, J. (1951). Maternal care and mental health. *Bulletin of the World Health Organization, 3,* 355–534.

Buchsbaum, M., & Inquar, D. (1982). New visions of the schizophrenic brain: Regional differences in electrophysiology, blood flow, and cerebral glucose use. In F. Henn & H. Nasrallah (Eds.), *Schizophrenia as a brain disease* (pp. 235–252). New York: Oxford University Press.

Cannon, T. D., Mednick, S., Parnas, J., Schulsinger, F., Praestholm, J., & Vestergaard, A. (1993). Developmental brain abnormalities in the offspring of schizophrenic mothers. Part I: Contributions of genetic and perinatal factors. *Archives of General Psychiatry, 50,* 551–564.

Cannon, W. (1929). *Bodily changes in pain, hunger, fear, and rage: An account of recent researches into the function of emotional excitement.* New York: Appleton.

Carr, D., & Sheehan, D. (1984). Evidence that panic disorder has a metabolic cause. In J. Ballenger (Ed.), *Biology of agoraphobia* (pp. 100–107). Washington, DC: American Psychiatric Press.

Carson, R. C., & Sanislow, C. A. (1993). The schizophrenias. In P. B. Sutker & H. E. Adams (Eds.), *Comprehensive handbook of psychopathology* (pp. 295–298). New York: Plenum.

Cassou, B., Schiff, M., & Stewart, J. (1980). Génétique et schizophrenie: Réevaluation d'un consensus. *Psychiatrie de l'Enfant, 23,* 87–201.

Chase, A. (1977). *The legacy of Malthus: The new scientific racism.* New York: Knopf.

Clayton, P. (1983). Epidemiologic and risk factors in suicide. *Psychiatric Update, 2,* 428–434.

Cleaver, E. (1967). *Soul on ice.* New York: McGraw-Hill.

Clinard, M., & Meier, R. (1975). *Sociology of deviant behavior* (5th ed.). New York: Holt, Rinehart & Winston.

Cloninger, C. (1978). The antisocial personality. *Hospital Practice, 13,* 97–106.

Cloninger, C., & Reich, T. (1976). Genetic heterogeneity in alcoholism and sociopathy. In M. Sperber & L. Jarvik (Eds.), *Psychiatry and genetics* (pp. 56–65). New York: Basic Books.

Conrad, P. (1980). On the medicalization of deviance and social control. In D. Ingleby (Ed.), *Critical psychiatry: The politics of mental health* (pp. 102–119). New York: Pantheon.

Costello, C. (1976). *Anxiety and depression: The adaptive emotions.* Montreal: McGill-Queen's University Press.

Cox, W. (1987). Alcoholism: Personality theory and research. In H. Blane & K. Leonard (Eds.), *Psychological theories of drinking and alcoholism* (pp. 55–89). New York: Guilford Press.

Craike, W., & Slater, E. (1945). *Folie à deux* in uniovular twins reared apart. *Brain, 68,* 213–221.

Crowe, R. (1982). Recent genetic research in schizophrenia. In F. Henn & H. Nasrallah (Eds.), *Schizophrenia as a brain disease* (pp. 235–252). New York: Oxford University Press.

Crowe, R. (1984). The role of genetics in the etiology of panic disorder. *Psychiatric Update, 3,* 402–410.

Dugdale, R. (1887). *The Jukes: A study of crime, pauperism, disease, and heredity.* New York: Putnam.

Dumont, M. P. (1984). The nonspecificity of mental illness. *American Journal of Orthopsychiatry, 54,* 326–334.

Dunham, H. (1977). Schizophrenia: The impact of sociocultural factors. *Hospital Practice, 12,* 61–68.

Eaves, L. J., Eysenck, H. J., & Martin, N. G. (1989). *Genes, culture, and personality: An empirical approach.* London: Academic Press.

Egeland, J., Gerhard, D., Pauls, D., Sussex, J., Kidd, K., Allen, C., Hostetter, A., & Housman, D. (1987). Bipolar affective disorders linked to DNA markers in chromosome 11. *Nature, 325,* 783–787.

Ford, B. D. (1993). Emergenesis: An alternative and a confound. *American Psychologist, 48,* 1294.

Fort, J. (1981). *The addicted society.* New York: Grove.

Fox, R. (1967). Introduction. In R. Maickel (Ed.), *Biochemical factors in alcoholism* (pp. vii–xi). London: Pergamon Press.

Fromm-Reichmann, F. (1959). *Psychoanalysis and psychotherapy.* Chicago: University of Chicago Press.

Gelernter, J., Goldman, D., & Risch, N. (1993). The A1 allele at the D2 dopamine receptor gene and alcoholism. *Journal of the American Medical Association, 269,* 1673–1677.

Gellhorn, E. (1964). Recent investigation of the physiological basis of emotions. In P. Hoch & J. Zubin (Eds.), *Anxiety* (pp. 205–217). New York: Hofner.

Gershon, E. (1983). The genetics of affective disorder. *Psychiatric Update, 2,* 434–457.

Goddard, H. (1912). *The Kallikak family: A study in the heredity of feeble-mindedness.* New York: Macmillan.

Goleman, D. (1990, March 22). Brain structure differences linked to schizophrenia in study of twins. *New York Times,* B15.

Goodwin, D., Schulsinger, F., Hermansen, L., Guze, S., & Winokur, G. (1973). Alcohol problems in adoptees raised apart from alcoholic parents. *Archives of General Psychiatry, 28,* 238–243.

Goodwin, D., Schulsinger, F., Moller, N., Hermansen, L., Winokur, G., & Guze, S. (1974). Drinking problems in adopted and nonadopted sons of alcoholics. *Archives of General Psychiatry, 30,* 164–169.

Gordis, E., Tabakoff, B., Goldman, D., & Berg, K. (1990). Editorials: Finding the gene(s) for alcoholism. *Journal of the American Medical Association, 263,* 2094–2095.

Goring, C. (1913). *The English convict: A statistical study.* London: Darling & Son.

Gorman, J. (1984). The biology of anxiety. *Psychiatric Update, 3,* 467–482.

Gottesman, I., & Erlenmeyer-Kimling, L. (1971). Prologue: A foundation for informed eugenics. *Social Biology, 18* (Suppl.), S1–S8.

Gottesman, I., & Shields, J. (1972). *Schizophrenia and genetics: A twin study vantage point.* New York: Academic Press.

Gottesman, I., & Shields, J. (1982). *Schizophrenia—the epigenetic puzzle.* Cambridge, England: Cambridge University Press.

Gould, S. J. (1981). *The mismeasure of man.* New York: Norton.

Greenspan, S. (1987). *Infants in multi-risk families.* Madison: International Universities Press.

Grosz, H., & Farmer, B. (1972). Pitts and McClure's lactate-anxiety study revisited. *British Journal of Psychiatry, 120,* 415–418.

Guggenheim, F., & Nadelson, C. (1982). *Major psychiatric disorders.* New York: Elsevier.

Hare, R. (1970). *Psychopathy: Theory and research.* New York: Wiley.

Henig, R. (1988, September 11). Chosen and given. *New York Times Magazine,* 70–72.

Henry, J. (1971). *Pathways to madness.* New York: Random House.

Heston, L. (1966). Psychiatric disorders in foster home-reared children of schizophrenic mothers. *British Journal of Psychiatry, 112,* 819–825.

Heston, L. (1970). The genetics of schizophrenia and schizoid disease. *Science, 167,* 249–256.

Heston, L., Denney, D., & Pauly, I. (1966). The adult adjustment of persons institutionalized as children. *British Journal of Psychiatry, 112,* 1103–1110.

Hicks, R., Okonek, A., & Davis, J. (1980). The pharmacologic approach. In I. L. Kutash, L. B. Schlesinger, & Associates (Eds.), *Handbook on stress and anxiety* (pp. 428–450). San Francisco: Jossey-Bass.

Hodgkinson, S., Sherrington, R., Gurling, H., Marchbanks, R., Reeders, S., Mallet, J., McInnis, M., Petursson, H., & Brynjolfsson, J. (1987). Molecular genetic evidence in manic depression. *Nature, 325,* 805–806.

Hollander, E., Fay, M., Cohen, B., Campeas, R., Gorman, J., & Liebowitz, M. (1988). Serotonergic and noradrenergic sensitivity in obsessive-compulsive disorder: Behavioral findings. *American Journal of Psychiatry, 145,* 1015–1017.

Hollingshead, A., & Redlich, F. (1958). *Social class and mental illness: A community study.* New York: Wiley.

Hollister, L. (1968). *Chemical psychoses: LSD and related drugs.* Springfield, IL: Thomas.

Hutchings, B., & Mednick, S. (1975). Registered criminality in the adoptive and biological parents of registered male criminal adoptees. In R. Fieve, D. Rosenthal, & H. Brill (Eds.), *Genetic research in psychiatry* (pp. 105–116). Baltimore: Johns Hopkins University Press.

Ingleby, D. (1980). Understanding "mental illness." In D. Ingleby (Ed.), *Critical psychiatry: The politics of mental health* (pp. 23–71). New York: Pantheon.

Ingleby, D. (1981). The politics of psychology: Review of a decade. *Psychology and Social Theory, 2,* 4–18.

Izard, C. (1972). *Patterns of emotion: A new analysis of anxiety and depression.* New York: Academic Press.

Jackson, D. (1960). A critique of the literature on the genetics of schizophrenia. In D. Jackson (Ed.), *The etiology of schizophrenia* (pp. 37–87). New York: Basic Books.

Jacobs, P., Brunton, M., Melville, M., Brittain, R., & McClemont, W. (1965). Aggressive behavior, mental subnormality, and the XYY male. *Nature, 208,* 1351–1352.

Jellinek, E. M. (1960). *The disease concept of alcoholism.* New Haven, CT: Hillhouse Press.

Johnson, A., & Szurek, S. (1952). The genesis of antisocial acting out in children and adults. *Psychoanalytic Quarterly, 21,* 323–343.

Juel-Nielsen, N. (1965). Individual and environment: A psychiatric-psychological investigation of MZ twins reared apart. *Acta Psychiatrica Scandinavica, 183* (Suppl.), Ad volumen 40, 1964, Suppl. 183.

Kallmann, F. (1938). *The genetics of schizophrenia.* New York: Augustin.

Kallmann, F. (1946). The genetic theory of schizophrenia. *American Journal of Psychiatry, 103,* 309–322.

Kallmann, F., & Roth, B. (1956). Genetic aspects of preadolescent schizophrenia. *American Journal of Psychiatry, 112,* 599–606.

Kamin, L. (1974). *The science and politics of IQ.* Potomac, MD: Erlbaum.

Kendler, K. (1987). Genetics of schizophrenia. *Psychiatric Update, 6,* 25–41.

Kendler, K., Heath, A., Martin, M., & Evans, L. (1987). Symptoms of anxiety and symptoms of depression: Same genes, different environments? *Archives of General Psychiatry, 44,* 451–457.

Kendler, K., McGuire, M., Gruenberg, A., O'Hare, E., Spellman, M., & Walsh, D. (1993a). The Roscommon family study. Part I: Methods, diagnosis of probands, and risk of schizophrenia in relatives. *Archives of General Psychiatry, 50,* 527–540.

Kendler, K., McGuire, M., Gruenberg, A., O'Hare, E., Spellman, M., & Walsh, D. (1993b). The Roscommon family study. Part II: The risk of non-schizophrenic, non-affective psychosis in relatives. *Archives of General Psychiatry, 50,* 645–652.

Kendler, K. S., Neale, M. C., Kessler, R. C., Heath, A. C., & Eaves, L. J. (1993). A test of the equal-environment assumption in twin studies of psychiatric illness. *Behavior Genetics, 23,* 21–27.

Kennedy, J., Giuffra, N., Moises, H., Cavalli-Sforza, L., Pakstis, A., Kidd, J., Castiglione, C., Sjogren, B., Wetterberg, L., & Kidd, K. (1988). Evidence against linkage of schizophrenia to markers on chromosome 5 in a northern Swedish pedigree. *Nature, 336,* 167–170.

Kety, S. (1975). Progress toward an understanding of the biological substrates of schizophrenia. In R. Fieve, D. Rosenthal, & H. Brill (Eds.), *Genetic research in psychiatry* (pp. 15–26). Baltimore: Johns Hopkins University Press.

Kety, S. (1979). Disorders of the human brain. *Scientific American, 241,* 202–214.

Kety, S. (1983). Observations on genetic and environmental influences in the etiology of mental disorder from studies on adoptees and their relatives. In *Genetics of neurological and psychiatric disorders,* (pp. 105–114). [Research Publications: Association for Research in Nervous and Mental Disease, Vol. 60,] New York: Raven Press.

Kety, S., Rosenthal, D., Wender, P., & Schulsinger, F. (1968). The types and prevalence of mental illness in the biological and adoptive families of schizophrenics. In D. Rosenthal & S. Kety (Eds.), *The transmission of schizophrenia* (pp. 345–362). Oxford, England: Pergamon Press.

Kevles, D. (1985). *In the name of eugenics.* New York: Knopf.

Konner, M. (1982). *The tangled wing: Biological constraints on the human spirit.* New York: Holt, Rinehart & Winston.

Krimmel, H. (1971). *Alcoholism.* New York: New York Council for Social Work Education.

Lader, M. (1990). The biology of panic disorder: A long-term view and critique. In J. Walker, G. Norton, & C. A. Ross (Eds.), *Panic disorder and agoraphobia* (pp. 150–174). Pacific Grove, CA: Brooks/Cole.

Lader, M. (1991). Bio-psycho-social interactions in anxiety and panic disorders: A speculative perspective. *Irish Journal of Psychological Medicine, 8,* 154–159.

Laing, R. (1972). *The politics of the family.* New York: Vintage Books.

Lander, E. (1988). News and views: Splitting schizophrenia. *Nature, 336,* 105–106.

Levinson, H. (1986). *Phobia-free: A medical breakthrough linking ninety percent of all phobias and panic attacks to a hidden physical problem.* New York: Evans.

Lewontin, R., Rose, S., & Kamin, L. (1984). *Not in our genes: Biology, ideology, and human nature.* New York: Pantheon.

Lidz, T. (1973). *The origin and treatment of schizophrenic disorders.* New York: Basic Books.

Lidz, T., & Blatt, S. (1983). Critique of the Danish-American studies of the biological and adaptive relatives of adoptees who became schizophrenic. *American Journal of Psychiatry, 140,* 426–434.

Lidz, T., Blatt, S., & Cook, B. (1981). Critique of the Danish-American studies of the adopted-away offspring of schizophrenic parents. *American Journal of Psychiatry, 138,* 1063–1068.

Lipowski, Z. J. (1989). Psychiatry: Mindless or brainless, both or neither? *Canadian Journal of Psychiatry, 34,* 249–254.

Lipton, M. (1970). The relevance of chemically induced psychoses to schizophrenia. In D. Efron (Ed.), *Psychotomimetic Drugs* (pp. 231–240). New York: Raven Press.

Liston, E., & Jarvik, L. (1976). Genetics of schizophrenia. In M. A. Sperber & L. Jarvik (Eds.), *Psychiatry and Genetics* (pp. 76–94). New York: Basic Books.

Livesley, W. J., Jang, K. L., Jackson, D. N., & Vernon, P. A. (1993). Genetic and environmental contributions to dimensions of personality disorder. *American Journal of Psychiatry, 150,* 1826–1831.

Madsen, W. (1974). *The American alcoholic: The nature–nurture controversy in alcohol research and therapy.* Springfield, IL: Thomas.

Magid, K., & McKelvey, C. (1987). *High risk: Children without a conscience.* Toronto: Bantam Books.

Mandler, G. (1984). *Mind and body.* New York: Norton.

Marmorstein, J., & Marmorstein, N. (1979). *The psychometabolic blues.* Santa Barbara, CA: Woodbridge Press.

McClelland, D., Davis, W., Kalin, R., & Wanner, E. (1972). *The drinking man: A theory of human motivation.* New York: Free Press.

McCord, W., & McCord, J. (1960). *Origins of alcoholism.* Stanford, CA: Stanford University Press.

Mednick, S. (1970). Breakdown in individuals at high risk for schizophrenia: Possible predispositional perinatal factors. *Mental Hygiene, 54,* 50–63.

Mednick, S., Gabrielli, W., & Hutchings, B. (1984). Genetic influences in criminal convictions: Evidence from an adoption cohort. *Science, 224,* 891-894.

Meehl, P. (1972). A critical afterword. In I. Gottesman & J. Shields (Eds.), *Schizophrenia and genetics: A twin study vantage point* (pp. 367–415). New York: Academic Press.

Mendelson, J., & Mello, N. (1979). Biologic concomitants of alcoholism. *New England Journal of Medicine, 301,* 912–921.

Mendlewicz, J., & Rainer, J. (1977). Adoption study supporting genetic transmission in manic-depressive illness. *Nature, 268,* 327–329.

Morris-Yates, A., Andrews, G., Howie, P., & Henderson, S. (1990). Twins: A test of the equal environments assumption. *Acta Psychiatrica Scandinavica, 81,* 322–326.

Munkvad, I., Fog, R., & Randrup, A. (1975). Amphetamine psychosis: A useful model of schizophrenia? In H. van Praag (Ed.), *On the origin of the schizophrenic psychoses* (pp. 50–57). Amsterdam: De Erven Bohn DV.

Neale, J., & Oltmanns, T. (1980). *Schizophrenia.* New York: Wiley.

Newman, H., Freeman, F., & Holzinger, K. (1937). *Twins: A study of heredity and environment.* Chicago: University of Chicago Press.

Orne, M. (1962). On the social psychology of the psychological experiment. *American Psychologist, 17,* 776–783.

Paul, S., & Skolnick, P. (1984). The biochemistry of anxiety: From pharmacotherapy to pathophysiology. *Psychiatric Update, 3,* 482–490.

Peele, S. (1990, August). Second thoughts about a gene for alcoholism. *The Atlantic Monthly,* 52–58.

Pittman, D., & Gordon, C. (1958). *The revolving door.* New York: Free Press.

Pitts, F., & McClure, J. (1967). Lactate metabolism in anxiety neurosis. *New England Journal of Medicine, 277,* 1329–1336.

Plomin, R., Corley, R., DeFries, J. C., & Fulker, D. W. (1990). Individual differences in television viewing in early childhood: Nature as well as nurture. *Psychological Science, 1,* 371–377.

Plomin, R., DeFries, J. C., & McClearn, G. K. (1980). *Behavior genetics: A primer.* San Francisco: Freeman.

Plutchik, R. (1962). *The emotions: Facts, theory, and a new model.* New York: Random House.

Rainer, J. (1976). Genetics of neurosis and personality disorder. In M. Sperber & L. Jarvik (Eds.), *Psychiatry and genetics* (pp. 56–65). New York: Basic Books.

Robertson, M. (1987). News and views: Molecular genetics of the mind. *Nature, 325,* 755.

Rosenthal, D. (1970). *Genetic theory and abnormal behavior.* New York: McGraw-Hill.

Rosenthal, D. (1971). *Genetics of psychopathology.* New York: McGraw-Hill.

Rosenthal, D., Wender, P., Kety, S., Schulsinger, F., Welner, J., & Ostegaard, L. (1968). Schizophrenics' offspring reared in adoptive homes. In D. Rosenthal & S. Kety (Eds.), *The transmission of schizophrenia* (pp. 377–391). Oxford, England: Pergamon Press.

Rosenthal, D., Wender, P., Kety, S., Welner, J., & Schulsinger, F. (1971). The adopted-away offspring of schizophrenics. *American Journal of Psychiatry, 128,* 307–311.

Ross, C. A. (1986). Biological tests for mental illness—their use and misuse. *Biological Psychiatry, 21,* 431–435.

Roy-Byrne, P., & Cowley, D. (1988). Panic disorder: Biological aspects. *Psychiatric Annals, 18*, 457–463.

Rutstein, D., & Veech, R. (1978). Genetics and addiction to alcohol. *New England Journal of Medicine, 298*, 1140–1141.

Sacks, O. (1985). *The man who mistook his wife for a hat and other clinical tales.* London: Duckworth.

Scarr, S., & Carter-Saltzman, L. (1979). Twin method: Defense of a critical assumption. *Behavior Genetics, 9*, 527–542.

Schachter, S., & Singer, J. E. (1962). Cognitive, social, and physiological determinants of emotional state. *Psychological Review, 69*, 379–399.

Scheinfeld, A. (1939). *You and heredity.* New York: Frederick Stokes.

Schildkraut, J., Schatzberg, A., Mooney, J., & Orsulak, P. (1983). Depressive disorders and the emerging field of psychiatric chemistry. *Psychiatric Update, 2*, 457–471.

Schmeck, H. (1989, November 7). Scientists now doubt they found faulty gene linked to mental illness. *New York Times,* Science Section, C3.

Schuckit, M. (1984). Genetic and biochemical factors in the etiology of alcoholism. *Psychiatric Update, 3*, 320–328.

Schuckit, M., Goodwin, D., & Winokur, G. (1972). A study of alcoholism in half-siblings. *American Journal of Psychiatry, 128*, 1131–1136.

Schuckit, M., & Rayses, V. (1979). Ethanol ingestion: Differences in blood acetaldehyde concentration in relatives of alcoholics and controls. *Science, 203*, 54–55.

Schulsinger, F., Kety, S., Rosenthal, D., & Wender, P. (1979). A family study of suicide. In M. Schou & E. Stromgren (Eds.), *Origin, prevention, and treatment of affective disorders* (pp. 277–287). London: Academic Press.

Schultz, R. I. (1965). *Sensory restriction: Its effects on behavior.* New York: Academic Press.

Scott, K. G., & Carran, D. T. (1987). The epidemiology and prevention of mental retardation. *American Psychologist, 42*, 801–804.

Sheehan, D. (1982). Panic attacks and phobias. *New England Journal of Medicine, 307*, 156–158.

Sheldon, W. (1940). *The varieties of human physique: An introduction to constitutional psychology.* New York: Harper & Brothers.

Sherrington, R., Brynjolfsson, J., Petursson, H., Potter, M., Duddleston, K., Barraclough, B., Wasmuth, J., Dobbs, M., & Gurling, H. (1988). Localization of a susceptibility locus for schizophrenia on chromosome 5. *Nature, 336*, 164–167.

Shields, J. (1962). *MZ twins brought up apart and brought up together.* London: Oxford University Press.

Slater, E. (1961). Hysteria 311. *The Journal of Mental Science, 107*, 359–371.

Slater, E. (1968). A review of earlier evidence on genetic factors in schizophrenia. In D. Rosenthal & S. Kety (Eds.), *The transmission of schizophrenia* (pp. 15–26). Oxford, England: Pergamon Press.

Smith, J. D. (1985). *Minds made feeble: The myth and legacy of the Kallikaks.* Rockville, MD: Aspen Publications.

Smythies, J., Coppen, A., & Kreitman, N. (1968). *Biological psychiatry: A review of recent advances.* New York: Springer Verlag.

Snyder, S. (1976, May 17). *Medical World News,* 24.

Snyder, S. (1977). Biochemical factors in schizophrenia. *Hospital Practice, 12,* 133–140.

Sobel, D. (1961). Children of schizophrenic parents: Preliminary observations on early development. *American Journal of Psychiatry, 118,* 512–517.

Stierlin, H. (1974). *Separating parents and adolescents: A perspective on running away, schizophrenia and waywardness.* New York: Quadrangle.

Suddath, R., Christison, G., Torrey, E. F., Casanova, M., & Weinberger, D. (1990). Anatomical abnormalities in the brains of monozygotic twins discordant for schizophrenia. *New England Journal of Medicine, 332,* 789–794.

Thio, A. (1978). *Deviant behavior.* New York: Harper & Row.

Tienari, P. (1991). Interaction between genetic vulnerability and family environment: the Finnish adoptive study of schizophrenia. *Acta Psychiatrica Scandinavica, 84,* 460–465.

Tolstoy, L. (1946). *Resurrection* (R. Edmonds, Trans.) London: Penguin Books. (Original work published 1899)

Torgersen, S. (1983). Genetic factors in anxiety disorders. *Archives of General Psychiatry, 40,* 1085–1089.

Torrey, E. F. (1983). *Surviving schizophrenia: A family manual.* New York: Harper & Row.

Trice, H. (1966). *Alcoholism in America.* New York: McGraw-Hill.

Tuma, A., & Masser, J. (1975). *Anxiety and the anxiety disorders.* Hillsdale, NJ: Erlbaum.

van der Kolk, B. A. (1988). The trauma spectrum: The interaction of biological and social events in the genesis of the trauma response. *Journal of Traumatic Stress, 1,* 273–290.

van Praag, H. M. (1977). The significance of dopamine for the mode of action of neuroleptics and the pathogenesis of schizophrenia. *British Journal of Psychiatry, 130,* 463–474.

van Praag, H. M. (1993). *"Make-believes" in psychiatry, or the perils of progress.* New York: Brunner/Mazel.

van Praag, H. M., & Korf, J. (1975). The dopamine hypothesis: Some direct observations. In H. van Praag (Ed.), *On the origin of the schizophrenic psychoses* (pp. 81–98). Amsterdam: De Erven Bohn BV.

Wallace, M. (1986). *The silent twins.* New York: Ballantine.

Wender, P. (1976, May 17). *Medical World News,* 23.

Wender, P., & Klein, D. (1981, February). The promise of biological psychiatry. *Psychology Today,* 25–41.

Wender, P., Rosenthal, D., Kety, S., Schulsinger, F., & Welner, J. (1974). Cross-fostering: A research strategy for clarifying the role of genetic and experiential factors in the etiology of schizophrenia. *Archives of General Psychiatry, 30,* 121–128.

Wilson, J., & Herrnstein, R. (1985). *Crimes and human nature.* New York: Simon & Schuster.

Zerbin-Rudin, E. (1972). Genetic research and the theory of schizophrenia. *International Journal of Mental Health, 1,* 42–62.

2

ERRORS OF LOGIC IN BIOLOGICAL PSYCHIATRY

Colin A. Ross

When I entered my psychiatry residency, I believed that research had demonstrated the genetic foundation of schizophrenia and had shown that schizophrenia is primarily a biomedical brain disease. This view was almost universally accepted at my medical school, and I never heard serious criticism of it while in training. It was by a gradual process that I began to become more and more aware of the cognitive errors pervading clinical psychiatry—unwittingly demonstrated to me by my residency supervisors. As I became more acquainted with the psychiatric literature, I learned that these cognitive errors are ubiquitous in the profession and are rarely challenged.

I also observed that challenging either of the dominant paradigms in psychiatry—psychoanalysis and biomedical reductionism—could lead to a charge of "antipsychiatry," and I was surprised at the ease with which the complex ideas of Thomas Szasz (1974) were casually dismissed as antipsychiatry, as if they did not demand careful and reasoned refutation. When I read Szasz myself, I was not convinced at all by his thesis that schizophrenia is a myth of psychiatric construction, and I still am not, but much of his writing is civil-libertarian, psychological in nature, and no different from the accepted wisdom of my supervisors who called him an antipsychiatrist.

In the first year of my residency, I listened carefully to staff psychiatrists who made discontinuous switches back and forth between the two dominant paradigms in discussion of a single case, within the same spoken paragraph, and I realized that psychiatry does not have a coherent, unified model or doctrine. In one instance, a psychiatrist was discussing a young man with schizophrenia from a biomedical case management point of view. Suddenly, he lurched into a discussion of projection as the underlying mechanism for some of the man's symptoms; then, after a couple of sentences, he as suddenly returned to his biomedical mode and vocabulary. Although this might be heralded as an eclectic approach, it was simply unintegrated. Psychiatry suffers from an identity disorder, which it is currently trying to solve by forcing the adoption of a bioreductionist paradigm.

I was taught that psychiatry has become much more modern and scientific since the introduction of neuroleptics in the 1950s, and the enthusiasm of psychiatrists for biological explanations of mental illness was presented as being based on a solid scientific foundation. It was therefore somewhat surprising to notice in the *Comprehensive Textbook of Psychiatry/III* (Kaplan, Freedman, & Sadock, 1980) that in a meta-analysis of double-blind chlorpromazine studies in schizophrenia, the drug was found to be superior to placebo in 55 trials but equal to placebo in 11 (p. 2258). This meant that in 17% of trials, chlorpromazine is no better than placebo in treatment of schizophrenia.

Additionally, a graph on page 2259 showed schizophrenics treated with placebo differing from those treated with chlorpromazine by only one point on a seven-point scale of severity of illness at the end of a large study. Although this was statistically significant, it appeared that the clinical efficacy of chlorpromazine in schizophrenia was far less than the confident, dogmatic statements I was hearing from my supervisors. I did not hear any serious discussion of the possibility that the overall cost–benefit of neuroleptics in schizophrenia may be only modestly positive, although the data in the major textbook pointed directly to this possibility.

I also saw how badly biological psychiatrists want to be regarded as doctors, and accepted by the rest of the medical profession. In their desire to be accepted as real clinical scientists, these psychiatrists were building far too dogmatic an edifice on a very meager scientific foundation, and in fact were undermining the scientific basis of psychiatry by pushing their certainty far beyond what the data could support. A chief example of this process was the enthusiasm for the use of the dexamethasone suppression test (DST) as a routine clinical diagnostic test for depression, which peaked during my residency years (1981 to 1985).

Another observation forced on me early in my residency was the universal disavowal of biomedical reductionism upon direct challenge. It was almost as if there was an unconscious program of plausible denial in place. Any direct challenge to the cognitive errors of biomedical reductionism was always met with the response that the biopsychosocial model was accepted throughout biological psychiatry. Once lip service was paid to the biopsychosocial approach, however, and the challenge forgotten, the logical fallacies rose to the conversational surface immediately.

One of the most disturbing effects of the errors of logic in biological psychiatry I witnessed in ten years as a resident and academic psychiatrist, from 1981 to 1991, was their influence on medical students. Already intensively socialized into biomedical reductionism by the time they arrived on the psychiatry wards, many medical students accepted the folklore and logical errors of biological psychiatry as scientific fact. I would hear them parroting the teaching that psychiatry has become more scientific recently, has many effective drugs, has demonstrated the genetic foundation of schizophrenia, and is moving ever-forward into more specific psychopharmacology. The problem was not that all these propositions were completely false; rather, it was the uncritical acceptance of the dogma that alarmed me.

It was not surprising that medical students accepted the dogma of biomedical reductionism in psychiatry uncritically: they had no time to read and analyze the original literature. What took me a while to understand, as I moved through my residency, was that psychiatrists rarely do the critical reading either. The dogma that the genetic foundation of schizophrenia has been scientifically established is by and large accepted without serious question in contemporary psychiatry, although, as Dr. Pam has shown irrefutably in Chapter 1, the data are subscientific in standard.

In this chapter, I discuss errors of logic in biological psychiatry. The errors overlap and intertwine with each other, and some are included for purposes of exposition, when they could be treated as variants of other errors without being listed separately. I do not provide herein references illustrating each error because (a) that is, in part, my task in the next chapter, and (b) finding isolated examples of each error in the literature would not establish the pervasive, tacit nature of the errors, which are similar to the automatic negative thoughts analyzed in cognitive therapy (Beck, Rush, Shaw, & Emery, 1979). The errors are not listed in any particular order; they are interrelated in a complex net, although some are stated explicitly more often than others.

On direct challenge, a biomedical reductionist psychiatrist will disavow adherence to the errors, describe them as oversimplifications or stereotypes, and emphasize that all biological psychiatrists recognize the importance of psychosocial factors in mental illness. This is actually true of some biological psychiatrists, especially the most creative ones, but many are, in fact, pure reductionists in a way that pervades their bedside manner, clinical practice, time management, treatment modalities, diagnostic habits, and even their dress (only bioreductionist psychiatrists wear white lab coats). None of this would necessarily be objectionable if the psychiatrists were internists of the brain; but they aren't, because psychiatry has not acquired even a tiny fraction of the scientific foundation of internal medicine.

It is self-evident that there must be a biological component to mental illness, because without brains patients could not produce symptoms or behaviors, and there could be no psychiatry. There is nothing anti-biological about my analysis of these cognitive errors.

IF IT RUNS IN FAMILIES, IT MUST BE GENETIC

During the third year of my residency, I spent a year on a teaching fellowship devising the first scientifically reliable method of teaching and evaluating biopsychosocial psychiatric case formulations (Ross & Leichner, 1986; Ross, Leichner, Matas, & Anderson, 1990). At this stage in my career, I was still uncritically accepting the dictum that a family history of a given psychiatric disorder is evidence of a genetic component to the illness. I taught residents and students to make such statements in listing biological factors in their cases, and these declarations of biological etiology were accepted without criticism every time they were made—by myself and all other members of the department. This is how pervasive the logical error was, and still is, in much psychiatric practice.

Scientifically, a pattern of family transmission is neutral with respect to genetic versus environmental etiology. The fact that other family members have been depressed, schizophrenic, alcoholic, or bulimic, does not to the smallest degree support the conclusion that there is a genetic component to the illness. In a psychiatry dominated by dogmatic environmentalism, one hostile to biology, the existence of relatives with the same diagnosis would be uncritically accepted as convincing evidence that the disorder was *learned*.

This central dogma in biological psychiatry is adhered to solely because of ideology, an intellectual distortion that can occur only when there is a pervasive suspension of critical, scientific thinking. Scientifically, the only conclusion that can be reached from studying the pattern of occurrence of a disorder in a pedigree is an inversion of biological psychiatry's logical error: *If there is no familial pattern, one can rule out an inherited cause.* If there is a pattern of family transmission, on the other hand, there may be a purely inherited cause, a purely environmental cause, or a mixture of the two.

A simple example will illustrate the point. Let's assume that, going back for four generations, every single member of a pedigree who had schizophrenia also had a characteristic abnormality of the fingernails, and no nonschizophrenics had the nail abnormality. According to the logical error of bioreductionist psychiatry, the nail abnormality would be regarded as a marker for schizophrenia, and someone would search the nail physiology literature for information about the role of peripheral dopamine in nail physiology. This would seem reasonable, but it is not. The error of the bioreductionist is the degree of dogmatic certainty that a genetic conclusion can be reached and that the nail abnormality is linked to the schizophrenia. The certainty results in decisions about what kind of research gets funded, who gets full professorship, and how psychiatry is marketed to politicians and insurance companies.

I have deliberately chosen a fingernail abnormality as an example because the link between the fingernails and schizophrenia is not intuitively obvious, and therefore the fallacy in the thinking is more apparent. However, the same logic applies when the abnormality is in the brain, or on a specific chromosome: within biological psychiatry, a dogmatic jump to a high level of certainty of direct etiological linkage is made, at both genetic and pathophysiological levels, and the new finding is prematurely heralded as a breakthrough and as further proof of the biological nature of schizophrenia. In the pedigree in question, it may be that cultural factors result in schizophrenics varying their diets in a specific fashion that affects nail growth, and it may be that schizophrenic-pedigree children adopted out of this culture at birth never display the nail abnormality, while those adopted in do. The pattern of transmission of schizophrenia and fingernail abnormalities could get heralded as further proof of the anthropologically determined nature of schizophrenia in a psychiatry dominated by a different ideology.

Consider another pedigree in which a characteristic eyefold co-occurs with speaking Chinese. Would we conclude that speaking Chinese is genetically determined and that the eyefold gene is closely linked to the gene for speaking Chinese? That conclusion is preposterous. But the logic is no different from that of biomedical psychiatry, except that biological psychiatrists talk about mental disorders and abnormalities in the brain.

When I was teaching formulation, it was obvious to all that very few specific biological factors could ever be identified in psychiatric cases, other than the fallacious family pedigree argument. In fact, in hundreds of cases formulated and discussed, the only specific biological factor ever identified was discontinuing medications against medical advice, the paradox being that this was a *behavior*, and would be understood in purely nonbiological terms by many psychologists and social scientists. Even here, there was not an exclusive biological factor. At the present time, there is no proof that biology causes schizophrenia, bipolar mood disorder, or any other functional mental disorder.

IF IT RESPONDS TO MEDICATION, IT MUST HAVE A BIOLOGICAL CAUSE

I have heard this cognitive error—and its variants—countless times. The chief variant is the belief that clinical response to medications can be used as a factor in the differential diagnosis of psychiatric disorders. As a coeditor of a textbook on panic disorder (Walker, Norton, & Ross, 1991), I consider myself fairly up-to-date on the subject, so I will use it as an example without further referencing.

The phenomenology of panic attacks is well documented, and there are a number of reliable measures for recording and describing them. A classical pattern of clear panic disorder is unmistakable, can be diagnosed with a high degree of interrater reliability (kappa above 0.90), and has major treatment validity in terms of specific response to specific treatments. What do we know about the biopsychosocial matrix of panic disorder?

A classical panic attack in someone with a specific phobia can be set off by a specific environmental trigger such as an elevator, but this same trigger will have no effect on someone without the phobic panic attack. I am referring to someone with panic disorder who has both spontaneous and situational panic attacks, not to someone with a pure simple phobia. We also know that the panic attacks can be triggered in the laboratory by a variety of biological challenges including caffeine, carbon dioxide, sodium lactate, and other agents, while individuals without panic disorder almost always have unremarkable reactions. This observation is placebo-controlled. The phenomenology of psychologically and biologically triggered panic attacks is indistinguishable, except perhaps for a few fine points at most.

Both environmentally cued and biologically induced panic attacks can be blocked by drugs like imipramine, which are effective in the treatment of panic disorder. Panic disorder can also be effectively treated by cognitive-behavioral therapy. The only remaining cell in this matrix is the ability of cognitive-behavioral therapy to block the panic response to biological challenges in individuals with panic disorder. If we assume for the moment and for the purpose of the argument that this is a scientific reality, although the data on this point are not yet conclusive, what can we conclude?

We know that panic disorder tends to run in families and is a strong candidate for the first cognitive error discussed above. We also know that panic attacks can be induced and blocked in all possible combinations at biological and psychosocial levels. Therefore, we cannot conclude that the responsiveness of panic disorder to imipramine and alprazolam is evidence that it must have a biological cause, because other data of equally good quality would support a psychosocial cause. It is a logical fallacy to conclude that treatment response at one level of organization within the organism implies primary causation at that level.

In a biopsychosocial model of panic disorder, one could postulate an inherited predisposition to autonomic hyperarousal, although this could equally as well be environmentally induced by family transactional patterns and cognitive errors. Setting aside whether the hyperarousal is inherited or culturally induced, we can postulate the existence of such hyperarousal. For panic attacks to occur, characteristic psychodynamics, catastrophizing cognitive errors, and errors in learning need to be present. It is therefore possible to intervene by prescribing drugs that dampen down the arousal to a subthreshold level at which the cognitions cannot trigger panic, or to treat the cognitive errors such that the subclinical autonomic instability is of no clinical consequence.

Whether the putative biological abnormality in panic disorder is inherited or not cannot be inferred from any of the above findings or reasoning, yet dogmatic statements that panic disorder is an inherited biomedical brain disease localized in the locus coeruleus can be found within biological psychiatry. This is a locus of control error.

The same logic applies to all medications prescribed for all psychiatric disorders. Panic disorder is a more compelling example than schizophrenia because most cells of the matrix have been filled by data for panic disorder, whereas the situation with schizophrenia is much more muddled.

I have heard many times that response to medication can also be used in differential diagnosis within psychiatry. The pseudomedical nature of this belief is evident if one makes a comparison to internal medicine. An infectious disease may respond with initial symptom suppression to rehydration, steroids, aspirin, or antibiotics, but no internist draws etiological conclusions from these observations or uses the drug response in differential diagnosis. Within psychiatry, such observations are used to support preconceived biomedical reductionist ideology in a way that occurs far less often in other areas of medicine. It is as if the psychiatrists are trying so hard to be doctors that they are overshooting the mark.

Many times, I have heard that a patient's response to lithium, antidepressants, or neuroleptics can be used in differential diagnosis of bipolar mood disorder versus schizoaffective disorder, versus schizophrenia. Although there is some informal, rough truth to this proposition at the level of an individual patient, the diagnostic conclusions are reached with a far greater degree of certainty than is scientifically warranted. Problems glossed over in reaching such conclusions include the substantial placebo-responsiveness of all three conditions in double-blind trials, the differential-diagnostic nonspecificity of many psychotic symptoms targeted by neuroleptics, the nonspecific actions of neuroleptics such as anxiolysis and behavioral calming, and the impossibility of differentiating pure mood disorder from schizoaffective disorder by lithium response. This impossibility arises from the same logical problems with false positives and negatives as apply to the diagnostic use of the dexamethasone suppression test, to be discussed below.

In actual clinical practice, in biological psychiatry, what often occurs is a forcing of diagnosis prior to a trial of medication. I observed this repeatedly, and I mention it although it is not strictly a cognitive error. If a given patient has not responded to lithium, the psychiatrist may begin to selectively ignore symptoms that support a diagnosis of bipolar mood disorder, and give augmented weight to symptoms supporting schizophrenia, prior to initiating a trial of a neuroleptic (in actual practice, this process more often occurs in the reverse direction). In another case, or at another time in the same patient, the weighting of symptoms may go in reverse or there may be a shift toward a trial of an anticonvulsant based on sudden observation of symptoms suggestive of temporal lobe epilepsy, which are usually actually dissociative symptoms.

Concurrent with an increase in the degree of confidence in the pseudoscientific conclusion that the genetic basis of mental disorders has been demonstrated, a paradoxical observation within psychopharmacology is also being made regarding the efficacy of certain medications in a wide variety of different disorders. For instance, serotonin reuptake blockers like fluoxetine can be effective in depression, bulimia, obsessive-compulsive disorder, posttraumatic stress disorder, and other conditions that are supposed to be unrelated to each other.

Alprazolam, first developed as an anxiolytic, is effective in panic disorder and generalized anxiety disorder, but may have antidepressant properties; imipramine, first developed as an antidepressant, is effective in panic disorder. How has biological psychiatry reacted to this development?

One conclusion biological psychiatrists could draw from the fact that one medication works for many different disorders is that there is no biological specificity to different psychiatric disorders. Because this threatens the one gene–one illness model of biomedical reductionism, that conclusion is disallowed. What inference is made in its place? There are several strategies, the first of which is simply not to address the problem, and to keep searching for specific genes for specific illnesses while psychopharmacological research further demonstrates the biological nonspecificity of psychiatric disorders. This allows both the genetic research and the drug company contracts to remain in place.

The second strategy is to argue that the disorders responding to a given medication are all variants of a single disorder, usually depression. This occurred for bulimia, in which the response of bulimia to imipramine was used to argue that bulimia was a variant of depression. This argument was purely artifactual: it depended on the historical accident that imipramine was first shown to be effective for depression, and therefore was classified as an antidepressant. If it had first been shown to be effective for panic disorder and its antidepressant properties had not yet been discovered, then the argument would have to be that bulimia is a variant of panic disorder (perhaps bulimics self-medicate with food to prevent panic attacks, someone would suggest).

The depressive-spectrum argument can only be pushed so far before it threatens the genetic specificity of psychiatric disorders, and the one gene–one illness model can only be softened so far to accommodate the pharmacological data before it collapses. Complicated but nevertheless pseudoscientific efforts so salvage the genetic hypothesis with polygenetic loci, partial penetrance, and other genetic mechanisms will eventually undo themselves because they will lead to a conclusion that one can speak at most of a polygenetic predisposition to psychopathology in general. If there is no specific relationship between the mechanism of action of many effective drugs and diagnostic category, then the only way to maintain the genetic hypothesis would be to dismantle and entirely reorganize the DSM-IV diagnostic system, eliminating the concept of separate categories of mental illness. This would feed back on the genetic hypothesis to undermine its specificity, because there would be no specific clinical disorders if the system was based on family studies, drug responses, and genetic findings alone, rather than on clinical symptoms. There would be no separate mental disorders and no separate genes to find in nature. This reorganization will never happen politically; besides, there is psychotherapeutic treatment outcome specificity to many of the separate diagnostic categories, which will block their unification. The specificity of distinct psychotherapies for different mental disorders could prove to be more rooted in the differential biology of the disorders than the comparatively nonspecific response to medications.

Biological psychiatry has trapped itself in a logic box that will self-destruct.

PROVING A MENTAL ILLNESS IS BIOLOGICAL WILL REDUCE THE STIGMA

One of the humanitarian cognitive errors of biological psychiatry is the belief that establishing the genetic and/or biological nature of mental illness will reduce the stigma of psychiatric disorders. This is false reasoning, both politically and logically. Leprosy is a biological illness, but understanding its infectious etiology has done nothing to reduce the stigma of the disorder. Some parents restrict their children from playing with other children who have cancer because they fear infection of their children. These parents demonstrate that establishing the biological nature of a condition does not necessarily reduce stigma, nor does it necessarily result in more informed responses and attitudes.

The reasoning is politically false for several reasons in addition to those just listed. One hope is that a biomedical definition of psychiatric disorders will increase the lobbying power of psychiatry, the effectiveness of consumer lobbies, and the funding of psychiatric treatment and research by making psychiatry more of an equal partner in medicine. To achieve this goal, biological psychiatry goes overboard in emphasizing the biogenetic model, beyond the level observable in the rest of medicine. Cardiovascular disease is not talked about within internal medicine the way biological psychiatrists talk about the gene or genes for schizophrenia, for instance. Of the risk factors for coronary artery disease, a family history is only one; the others are predominately psychosocial in nature—smoking, inadequate exercise, low-nutrition diet, failure to control cholesterol, obesity, and hypertension. Hypertension is almost always idiosyncratic with no defined etiology, and the risk it contributes for coronary artery disease is substantially due to medication noncompliance and failure to modify life-style. Coronary artery disease is universally understood within medicine as the final common pathway of many different combinations of factors, with genetics accounting for a small proportion of the variance in the overall population. Pedigrees with specific biomedical risk factors like hyperlipidoses are a small subset of the general population's morbidity and mortality, yet biological psychiatry behaves as if most or all cases of schizophrenia, by analogy, are due to genetically specific lipid metabolism disorders.

The financial and political success of the cardiovascular lobby depends to a very small degree on the endogenous genetic foundation of such illness, therefore one might conclude that emphasizing the psychosocial and public health factors in major mental illness would be a better political strategy. Similar logic applies to cancer and AIDS research, in which environmental variables are key to all public health efforts and preventive measures.

One cannot speak of a gene for lung cancer as such, given the data on smoking, because there would be no clinical cancer in many individuals if they had not smoked heavily for years. One can speak of a set of genes for the oncogenic reaction to cigarette smoke in such individuals, but there is no gene for the disease as such. There is a location in the human genome controlling the interaction of the organism with the cigarette smoke, undoubtedly, but a complex sequence of promoters and cofactors is required to create the clinical illness. Scientifically, it is necessary to talk about multifactorial etiologies even at the genetic level, none of which by itself can be regarded as a "gene for lung cancer." Although I am out of my league on the genetic details here, the point I am making is that the discussion of genetics within biological psychiatry is often simplistic and ideologically driven in a way that doesn't occur elsewhere in medicine to the same degree.

The biogenetic model dominating psychiatry today is too much like that for Huntington's chorea, or Tay–Sachs disease, which have well-established modes of inheritance. The hope is that schizophrenia can be shown to be another Huntington's chorea. Within medicine, though, from a public health point of view, such Mendelian illnesses account for a tiny proportion of the severe morbidity and mortality in the general population, and a tiny proportion of the total clinical time of all physicians. The behavior of biological psychiatrists is too often a caricature of the medical approach to serious human illness, driven by reductionist ideology, and fostered by a paucity of serious scientific thinking.

ALCOHOLISM IS A DISEASE

This doctrine has been adopted throughout the chemical dependency field including Alcoholics Anonymous (AA), despite the fact that it has no scientific foundation and is logically incorrect. The search for the gene for alcoholism is heavily funded currently, and the cognitive error that if it runs in families, it must be genetic, is strongly adhered to in the alcoholism field. This is also true of the cognitive error that a genetic etiology will reduce stigma, because this error has had its most profound influence in the alcoholism field. The idea that alcoholism is inherited is viewed as a scientific fact at many levels in our society, not just within biological psychiatry. The idea that alcoholism is genetic is the leading example of the effective marketing of psuedoscience by biological psychiatry.

There is a paradox here, as in previously analyzed errors of logic: AA workers and biological psychiatrists who view alcoholism as an inherited medical condition simultaneously promulgate the doctrine that the alcoholic has to *decide* to recover before any serious attempt at recovery is possible. Alcoholics who continue to drink heavily are viewed as not yet having made the *choice* to recover, and the inefficacy of treatment efforts is attributed to lack of willpower, personal fiber, and surrender to a higher power on the part of the alcoholic, with no attribution of causality to the model or the treatment method. The alcoholism field is dominated by a tautology in which treatment failure is due to not working the steps hard enough, a conclusion that rules out the possibility of lack of efficacy of the treatment package in subpopulations.

There cannot be a gene for alcoholism, and alcoholism cannot be a biomedical illness, for logical reasons; therefore, no empirical study of the question is required, and the search for the gene can be abandoned. Scarce research funds can be much better utilized elsewhere. Why is this true? I will analyze the simplest form of the model, because the same logic applies to all genetic models of alcoholism, no matter how sophisticated or polygenetic. I will postulate the existence of a single gene for alcoholism, then demonstrate the logical self-contradictions and fallacies inherent in the hypothesis.

One statement that is made about the biological foundations of alcoholism is that alcoholics are born with a reduced tolerance to alcohol, and therefore get drunk more easily than nonalcoholics, resulting in their drinking to intoxication more readily and more often. This concept has been applied in a racist way to findings that Native Americans have different levels of alcohol dehydrogenase than other people, although none of the findings, to my knowledge, has controlled for numerous other factors including lifetime total alcohol dose. The idea that those who get drunk more easily have a *disease* called alcoholism, which places them in a separate category from those who do not have the disease, is untenable for several reasons. For one thing, as the disease progresses, tolerance rises, which should initiate a feedback loop limiting the development of alcoholism, according to sensitivity models, because the alcoholic's sensitivity becomes less than that of nonalcoholics.

To use alcohol dehydrogenase levels as an example of sensitivity models, this biological variable is distributed in a continuous fashion in the general population, with a range of normal, not in discrete categories. This is a completely different picture from that which occurs in Lesch–Nyan syndrome, a biologically specific inherited deficiency of hypoxanthine, guanine-phosphoribosyl transferase, or other truly genetic enzymatic abnormalities that produce specific clinical syndromes. Alcohol consumption is also distributed in a continuous fashion in the general population, with no valid scientific threshold for case definition, although severe alcoholics can easily be differentiated from teetotalers. This is completely different from Lesch–Nyan syndrome, which one either has or does not have: there is no continuous distribution. In alcoholism, there are many grey-zone cases in which it is a matter of judgment whether the individual is an alcoholic or just someone who likes to drink more than average. This never occurs in truly Mendelian diseases. The fact that specific genetic disorders like Huntington's chorea may be difficult to diagnose in their early stages is irrelevant to this analysis, as are arguments about partial penetrance.

All theories about differential enzyme levels, or inherited biological sensitivity levels, are scientifically erroneous for another reason: they are basically dose-response curve models in which a shift in the curve defines the presence of the illness. This is fallacious because the shift of the curve occurs in a continuous fashion within a normal range, as stated above. A more important fallacy is the fact that the only effect of the curve shift is to reduce the number of drinks required to get drunk. This could be a significant factor in the development of alcoholism only if many people failed to experience full expression of their alcoholic gene due to financial or time constraints, which is a necessary postulate of the model. Anyone who has been to a pub or bar should understand the absurdity of this concept.

To scientifically demonstrate the reality of a dose-response model, one would have to demonstrate that a significant number of nonalcoholics will become clinical alcoholics if they earn more or have more time to spend in bars getting drunk. Otherwise, differential enzyme levels in alcoholics are of no relevance to development of the disorder of alcoholism. What defines the alcoholic must be another factor having to do with experiencing intoxication as reinforcing, pleasant, and a reward. It is more accurate to speak of a gene for perceiving intoxication as desirable than to speak of a gene for alcoholism as such.

If intoxication was perceived as unpleasant because of the existence of another enzyme genetically unrelated to the genes for "alcoholism," then the existence of the intoxication gene, and the promoter gene resulting in valuing intoxication, would be biologically meaningless, because of the overriding effect of the dysphoric response gene. There would then be no such thing as alcoholism. If intoxication was experienced as unpleasant, then it would be in effect a psychological diarrhea, and alcohol would be avoided, despite the presence of all the other genetic machinery for alcoholism. Alternatively, if Ex-Lax was psychoactive, reductionists would postulate the existence of a gene for Ex-Laxism. The presence or absence of an addictive reaction to a food or drink may be accidentally related to its primary biological processing, to the genetics of that processing, and to its primary psychological effect. If there was no gene for suffering, there would be no addictions.

There are other problems with the hypothesis that there is a single gene or group of genes for alcoholism. The prevalence of alcoholism in our culture is far too high, given its survival disadvantage, for it to be inherited the way truly genetic diseases are. Additionally, the expression of the gene, if it exists, is *entirely* dependent on the existence of alcohol. If man had never discovered alcohol, there would be no alcoholics, and no one would be talking about the disease of alcoholism or its gene. This simple fact is always overlooked in endogenous biomedical reductionist models of alcoholism; it has to be, because the fact destroys the model. Alcoholism cannot be a primarily genetically driven condition like Huntington's chorea because Huntington's chorea occurs no matter what human beings are doing culturally, as do Tay–Sachs disease and Lesch–Nyan syndrome. Once one has the gene for one of these illnesses, it will inevitably be expressed as a full disease syndrome.

There cannot be a gene for alcoholism because there would be no way for such a gene to evolve prior to the invention of alcohol. In the absence of alcohol on the planet, it couldn't be a gene for *alcoholism*. Biological reductionists might respond that (a) the gene was always there, it simply wasn't activated in the absence of the environmental promoter, and (b) without the gene, the availability of alcohol does not cause alcoholism. This is to miss the point.

All human beings would die if the nitrogen content of the atmosphere rose to 98%. From this scientific fact, does one conclude that there is a gene for nitrogen toxicity, one that awaits the appearance of the promoter, and that there is an inherited illness called nitrogen toxicity? No; that conclusion is patently absurd. Alternatively, would the logic be less erroneous if one modified the definition of the illness to call it oxygen deprivation disease? The biological requirement of mammals for oxygen is genetically based, and all mammals die in the absence of oxygen, so why isn't suffocation defined as a genetic illness? What is the difference in logic between oxygen deprivation disease and alcoholism?

For political, financial, and ideological reasons, not because of logic or science, alcoholism is placed in the category of biomedical illness while oxygen deprivation disease is viewed as an obviously absurd construct. There cannot be a gene for alcoholism in the simplistic way postulated by biological psychiatry. Alcoholism is the behavioral outcome of an accidentally related set of circumstances: (a) the invention of alcohol, (b) the fact that alcohol causes intoxication, and (c) the fact that intoxication is highly valued by some human beings. The first cause is purely environmental, and second is biologically true of all human beings, and the third is the only possible genetically specific factor. Yet the third factor is the only one that is clearly psychosocially and culturally determined, as demonstrated by extensive evidence from the social sciences and by common sense. Do traveling salesmen drink more and eat more french fries than control groups because of genetic illnesses called alcoholism and french frieism, which drive them into this occupation? Isn't it likely a scientific fact that more people die from the long-term biomedical consequences of eating fast food than of alcoholism in North America? Why is there no inherited disease of fast food consumption? This does not occur because decisions about what gets conceptualized as a biomedical illness within psychiatry are entirely socially determined.

LABORATORY TESTS CAN IMPROVE THE ACCURACY OF PSYCHIATRIC DIAGNOSES

Early in my residency, which lasted from 1981 to 1985, supervisors were frequently ordering dexamethasone suppression tests (DSTs) as part of their diagnostic workup of clinical patients, in the belief that a positive result would support a diagnostic conclusion of a mood disorder. I would guess that throughout North America tens of millions of dollars must have been spent on clinically useless, pseudoscientific DSTs in the first half of the 1980s. The test, heralded as psychiatry's first blood test for mental illness, was regarded as a window into the pathophysiology of depression—depression, in turn, being conceptualized as a genetically based biomedical illness.

Analysis of the logical fallacies inherent in this pseudoscientific enthusiasm led me to publish an editorial in *Biological Psychiatry* (Ross, 1986) pointing out the cognitive errors inherent in this misuse of the DST. I was surprised at the minimal reaction this paper generated, even though it struck at the heart of pseudoscience in biological psychiatry, and I cannot gauge its influence in the complete disappearance of clinical use of the DST in psychiatry by the early 1990s. A sociologist ought to conduct a detailed inquiry into the rise and fall of the DST, a history that reveals a great deal about the ideology and politics of reductionist psychiatry.

A simple analysis can demonstrate that the DST cannot have clinical utility as a diagnostic test for depression. Three diagnostic groups have to be considered in the analysis: (a) clearly clinically depressed, (b) intermediate cases such as schizoaffective disorder, and (c) clearly not clinically depressed. For each of these three cells there are two subcells, positive DST and negative DST, making a total of six cells.

For individuals who are showing no signs of depression, not even pseudodementia or masked depression, the DST can be of no clinical utility because no treatment for depression will be instituted regardless of the results. A positive result will be defined as a false positive (rate about 5%), and a negative result as a true negative. Neither result can influence diagnosis or treatment. In individuals who are unequivocally clinically depressed, the DST will not affect treatment because they will get an antidepressant, cognitive therapy, or some other treatment for depression regardless of test results. Positive DSTs will be defined as true positives (about 66%) and negative results as false negatives.

This leaves only the intermediate, clinically ambiguous group. In this group, a negative DST cannot be interpreted because there is no way to determine whether it is a true or false negative, therefore a negative result cannot influence either diagnosis or treatment. This leaves only one cell out of six in which the DST has possible clinical utility, the diagnostically uncertain group with a positive test.

It is precisely in this group that a positive result cannot be used without undermining the scientific foundation of the DST. If a positive result is regarded as a true positive, then there is no way to determine the false positive rate for the DST, and the reliability and validity of the test as a diagnostic tool for depression are destroyed. This means that the DST cannot be used in the only clinical group for whom it might be useful, and therefore it has no clinical utility.

I began to mentally catalog the errors of logic in biological psychiatry as I heard them from supervisors, encountered them at meetings, and read them in the literature. I learned that a complex network of interlocking cognitive errors is active in biological psychiatry, the totality of which supported the pseudoscientific use of the DST in the 1980s. Also, I observed that the enthusiasm for the DST disappeared from clinical psychiatry very quickly, while the underlying errors of thinking continued unchallenged. The rise and fall of the DST was never discussed; enthusiasm moved from the DST to PET scans.

This logic concerning the DST applies to all biological tests for all mental illnesses. The dream of biological psychiatrists is that an "objective" laboratory test for one of the major mental illnesses will be discovered, and that this will place psychiatry on equal footing with internal medicine, while eliminating the vagaries of syndromic, phenomenological psychiatric diagnosis. This dream is logically unsound and can never be realized. Although biological psychiatrists speak of *external validation* of psychiatric diagnoses by laboratory findings and specific markers, this can never happen. Why?

One problem has to do with signal detection and systems theory. An individual, let us say, suffers from the biomedical illness of schizophrenia. How does the psychiatrist know this? The only possible way to notice that a person suffers from schizophrenia is to observe behaviors and signs and listen to the report of symptoms, which support the diagnosis. The only standard by which it is possible to decide that an individual has schizophrenia is clinical, therefore the reliability of the concept of schizophrenia is limited by the kappa value for the clinical or structured interview diagnosis, which is in the range of 0.65–0.70.

Biological psychiatrists talk as if a blood test or brain scan could increase the kappa for schizophrenia to 0.95, but this is scientifically impossible. They believe that a specific abnormality in a brain scan, cerebrospinal fluid value, or blood test could provide an *external, objective* measure that is more precise than clinical diagnosis. This is not possible because the biological signal emitted by the system and detected in the lab test is no more external to the system or "objective" than the behavioral signals. There is a fallacy that if a machine measures a biological signal emitted by a system, that is a more scientific and precise measure than direct observation of behavior. This is an ascientific reductionist cognitive error; it is not true methodologically or statistically. The error is caused in part by a scientifically naive faith in gadgetry.

Imagine that one tried to use a brain scan for diagnosing schizophrenia; the same problem would arise as in use of the DST: how could one decide which results are true positives and which are false positives? The only way to do this is by clinically assigning subjects to the categories of schizophrenic or nonschizophrenic. Once the scan results are used to make these assignments, the reliability, and therefore the validity of the laboratory test is destroyed. The lab test can never increase the kappa for the diagnosis because of this problem with false positives.

The only solution to this problem, from a bioreductionist perspective, is to propose that the lab values be the diagnostic criteria—by this logic, everyone with an abnormal test result has schizophrenia, regardless of clinical findings. If the lab test detects an abnormality that can be corrected with drugs, then the normalization of the lab value becomes the measure of successful treatment outcome, again regardless of clinical findings. According to this logic, it would be possible to be diagnosed and treated successfully for schizophrenia without ever having had any psychiatric symptoms. The potential for political abuse of such a psychiatric system is considerable.

The use of such lab tests would be impractical because it would be a waste of finite biomedical resources to screen for and treat a "disease" in a population with no symptoms. There would be no meaningful way to decide whom to test other than making clinical diagnoses, which returns us to the problem of false positives. The dream is analogous to the treatment of hypokalemia by internists, except that internists don't attempt to remove the clinical findings from the loop, and they have a better grasp of the concept of clinically spurious false positive findings.

Another tack proposed within biological psychiatry is to find biological markers for mental illnesses that can be detected prior to the onset of clinical symptoms and therefore can be used for preventive interventions in childhood or, the ultimate dream, in utero through abortion or genetic engineering. This potential use of laboratory tests in psychiatry is confounded by the same problem with false positives, except that the question is who will develop the category of schizophrenia in the future, rather than who has it in the present.

A destructive impact on the scientific quality of clinical psychiatry might occur if enthusiasm for the pursuit of markers and lab tests draws too much energy away from research on reliable phenomenological diagnosis, because this could potentially result in a drop in the kappas of diagnoses made in the clinic, which would in turn reduce the ceiling value for the reliability of any blood test. Biological psychiatry is absolutely dependent on the scientific rigor and precision of clinical diagnosis, and there is no way around this. Advances in biological psychiatry cannot occur without reliable diagnoses. The dream that there can be a genetic analysis or lab test with a perfect 1:1 fit with psychiatric clinical disease is actually a nightmare, and it cannot be pursued in the full waking state. The logical outcome of this sociology, if it was pushed to its extreme, would be psychiatrists functioning as totalitarian mind-control police, screening the population for "illnesses" and "treating" them with drugs and genetic engineering, irrespective of clinical reality.

THE PHYSICIAN'S ROLE IS TO TREAT BIOLOGICAL ILLNESSES

Reductionist biomedical psychiatry is supported by a network of tautologies, of which the dogma about the physician's role is one. Here we have not just philosophical or ideological issues at stake, but major variations in the actual clinical behavior of psychiatrists. The point is best illustrated if we take two polarized extremes within psychiatry: (a) the private practice psychoanalyst, and (b) the state-employed biological psychiatrist. I will deliberately use extreme examples. The psychoanalyst has a caseload of 20 or fewer patients, each of whom is seen for an hour per contact, and many of whom are seen five times per week. The biological psychiatrist, on the other hand, has an average face-to-face encounter time of five to ten minutes, and sees 30 to 50 patients a day. These appointments are medication followups with schizophrenics, manic-depressives, and other patients with major mental illnesses.

The appointment book of the biological psychiatrist looks like that of the average family physician, who sees about 40 patients a day; the appointment book of the psychoanalyst appears to represent a completely different profession. Part of the purpose of the reductionist ideology is to provide a rationale for the average appointment duration of the biological psychiatrist. If psychiatrists provide primarily psychotherapy for psychosocial problems, it makes no sense to see 40 people for ten minutes each in a single day, because the patients cannot possibly derive any benefit from such encounters. For such an appointment book to make sense, psychiatric disorders *must* be defined as primarily biological in nature, with the psychiatrist's adjustment of medications as the only necessary, meaningful, or effective intervention he or she makes—"supportive counseling" can be done by devalued paraprofessionals such as social workers.

Although the reductionist psychiatrist may pay lip service to the value of psychotherapy when pressed, and may claim to do psychotherapy, in reality psychotherapy is reduced to common-sense-based counseling, psychoeducation about mental illness and medication side effects, and reassurance.

Further, the psychiatrist's superior status in the mental health hierarchy depends on the dogma that the most serious illnesses are biological in nature, which helps maintain the income differential between psychiatrist and social worker. If the physician's role in our society was to treat spiritual problems with shamanic interventions, the ideological platform of the biological psychiatrist would be severely endangered and would not be able to borrow from the prestige of medicine.

Because psychiatrists are the only mental health professionals who are physicians, they have greater expertise in diagnosis and treatment of biomedical mental illnesses, but this is not how the greater expertise of psychiatrists is actually marketed. The marketing is done through allegiance to a biopsychosocial model, and the claim is that psychiatrists have the most *comprehensive* expertise and are therefore best qualified to head the mental health team. In practice, what actually happens is different, however: the bioreductionist psychiatrist restricts his or her activity to diagnosis and prescribing medication, and implicitly (or explicitly, at times) belittles the rest of the team as dealing with minor matters. This would not be possible if the physician's role was not defined as treating biological illnesses.

A related logical error in biological psychiatry is the idea that psychosis is more biological than neurosis. The sociological component of the error serves a turf-definition function within the mental health field, and helps to identify certain disorders as predominantly medical in nature and therefore requiring the unique skills of the psychiatrist. The key disorders are schizophrenia and the mood disorders, especially bipolar mood disorder and psychotic or endogenous depressions. These are the psychiatric turf *par excellence,* and therefore are most targeted for biomedical reductionist definition. The neuroses, on the other hand, tend to be regarded as less severe, less biological in nature, and therefore more suitable for the treatment efforts of psychologists and social workers. The criterion by which these illnesses were selected as the primary property of psychiatry had nothing to do with any scientific data about biological etiology; it was solely one of symptom severity. The responsiveness of these disorders to neuroleptics, lithium, and antidepressant medication only reinforced the already established selection of them as the intrinsically psychiatric illnesses.

A profound and disparaging psychiatric chauvinism is inherent in biological psychiatry, because all other mental health professionals are implicitly defined as junior in status and expertise. The neuroses are reduced to *problems in living* and are not included in the category of *disease,* which belittles them as constructs and belittles those who suffer from them. Alternatively, when any bioreductionist attention is paid to the neuroses, the ideological bias can be reversed, and the neuroses can be regarded as minor biological illnesses, although this is not the predominant implicit stance of biological psychiatry.

The corrective cognition is that mildness of symptoms and/or impairment does not in any way imply a less biological etiology. The severity-implies-biology error of biological psychiatry would be viewed as a preposterous doctrine if proposed anywhere else in medicine. The common cold is a biomedical illness with a specific etiology (this is true despite the fact that a number of different viruses can cause the common cold). The common cold is no less biological in nature than cancer of the pancreas. To stretch the point somewhat, one might argue that the basic etiology of a fatal gunshot wound is entirely psychosocial in nature, because the prevalence of this cause of death is profoundly affected by the availability of firearms in a given population. One might mount a similar argument about motor vehicle fatalities caused by drunk drivers, none of which would occur if either alcohol or cars were absent in a culture. Immediate causes of death may be far less biomedical in nature than the common cold.

Another related cognitive error is the belief that biological psychiatry is closer to medicine than psychological psychiatry. This error serves a particular, focused purpose—the exclusion of psychologists, psychiatrists' main competitors, from senior rank in the mental health field. The division created within psychiatry between biological and psychological psychiatry is in part an artifact of the effort to exclude psychologists form the social, political, and financial advantages of physician status.

Psychologists, in turn, have made strategic end runs around psychiatry in the past two decades, and have begun developing direct consultation relationships with internists and surgeons. Part of their strategy has been to use terms like *behavioral medicine* and to offer expertise in behavioral analysis and therapy, which psychiatrists tend to lack. These maneuvers and counter-maneuvers are all political in nature, on both sides.

Defining biological psychiatry as closer to medicine has had a major impact on the distribution of research money within psychiatry. A clear hierarchy is in place, with psychiatry at the bottom of the totem pole within medicine, biological psychiatry at the top of the totem pole within psychiatry, and psychosocial psychiatry at the bottom overall. Defining biological psychiatry as closer to medicine depends on a prior reductionist definition of medicine, which takes us to the model currently dominant within medicine as a whole.

The medical model, as the term is currently used in our culture, actually means the bioreductionist model of medicine, which is only one of many possible models. Others include ancient Chinese, Greek, and shamanic medical models. By calling the bioreductionist model *the* medical model, reductionists imply that all medical models other than their own are not medical. They call their own particular model of medicine *the medical model,* then define all other models as superstitious, primitive, prescientific, or otherwise unworthy. With this sleight of hand, the prestige of thousands of years of medicine is appropriated by the bioreductionists, and everyone else becomes a fringe practitioner.

The political power of biological psychiatry depends on its cultural context and is rooted in the dominant ideology of industrialized medicine. Depending on the perspective of the analyst, modern medicine could be characterized as atheistic, male chauvinist, or mechanistic-reductionist. If the dogma that biology is more real than psychology did not dominate medicine at large, biological psychiatry could not borrow the prestige of medicine to bolster its ideology, because doing so would weaken its position.

THE GENETIC BASIS OF SCHIZOPHRENIA IS SCIENTIFICALLY ESTABLISHED

Dr. Pam demonstrated, in Chapter 1, that research into the genetic foundation of schizophrenia is inconclusive. The genetic basis of schizophrenia has not been scientifically established, even at a preliminary level. In fact, some key findings in schizophrenia studies are the opposite of those predicted by a genetic model, such as a greater incidence of schizophrenia in second-degree than in first-degree relatives. It would be difficult to find a clearer example, at anytime in the twentieth century, of substandard pseudoscience dominating the ideology of a field.

The concordance of monozygotic versus dizygotic twins for schizophrenia is a chief example of how preconceived ideology drives the interpretation of findings: these results argue as strongly for environmental as for genetic etiology. Yet the results are always cited by bioreductionists as evidence supporting the heritability of schizophrenia. This skewed interpretation can be disavowed, on challenge, which is another example of the plausible denial-like organization of the reductionist conceptual system. In practice, the reductionist cites the twin studies as conclusive evidence of the heritability of schizophrenia and reduces psychosocial factors to pathoplastic influence only.

This argument is made by bioreductionists in sequential steps. First, the fact that the lifetime prevalence of schizophrenia is about 1% worldwide is interpreted as evidence that schizophrenia is a biomedical, genetically driven disease evenly distributed throughout the human race. This epidemiological fact could as easily be interpreted as evidence of the universal impact of certain basic characteristics of human culture. Having noted the 1% incidence and mentioned the twin and adoption studies, the reductionist will go on to acknowledge that culture plays a role in affecting the *content* of delusions and hallucinations; for example, schizophrenic African tribesmen tend not to have delusions about the CIA or about being controlled by gyroscopes implanted in their brains. The reductionist will then emphasize that the *structure* or *form* of the delusions is constant across cultures, because structure is a direct expression of the biomedical foundation of the disease. The bioreductionist thus maintains the illusion of a biopsychosocial approach while reducing psychosocial factors to the content level. Content, however, is no more important in biomedical schizophrenia than in delirium, and the same drugs are prescribed no matter what the content. The psychosocial domain is acknowledged, then robbed of any clinical importance. The draining of clinical significance out of the psychosocial realm is the reciprocal strategy of its diversion into the biological and is evidence of the pseudoscientific nature of biological psychiatry. Undermining the psychosocial would not be necessary if the biological actually had a solid scientific foundation. If there actually was a scientifically established genetic basis to schizophrenia, there would be nothing for biological psychiatrists to be defensive about, and therefore no need to belittle psychosocial variables.

The ideological war within psychiatry about the dogma of biological psychiatry is itself evidence of the pseudoscientific nature of biological psychiatry. Within internal medicine, in comparison, there is no ideological conflict about the etiology of Tay–Sachs disease, because its genetic basis has been conclusively established.

There is another confound in the reductionist argument—the fact that bioreductionist psychiatrists cannot differentiate schizophrenia from dissociative identity disorder, clinically or in their research. The 1% prevalence of schizophrenia worldwide is probably not a fact, because the prevalence of false-positive schizophrenia probably varies proportionally to the prevalence of false-negative dissociative identity disorder. If this is shown to be the case by epidemiological studies that take dissociative disorders into account, bioreductionists will be undisturbed, because they will then argue that schizophrenia is a genetic illness *unevenly* distributed around the world. This would be the only possible reactive position for them to take.

THE DOPAMINE THEORY OF SCHIZOPHRENIA DESERVES TO BE CALLED A THEORY

The dopamine theory of schizophrenia is a point of pride in biological psychiatry. It is not a theory, for several reasons. In my experience, nonmedical mental health professionals are usually surprised when I explain to them that the dopamine theory of schizophrenia was arrived at in reverse. What do I mean by this? The dopamine theory was built up in the following sequence of steps. First, it was serendipitously noticed that the phenothiazines have antipsychotic properties in humans, and they were used clinically with dramatic results.

Second, it was established in rat brain preparations that the antipsychotic drugs are postsynaptic dopamine receptor blockers. They block the neurotransmitter effects of the brain's dopamine. In the third step, it was concluded that because neuroleptics reduce psychosis and block the effect of dopamine, psychosis must be caused by an overactivity of the dopamine system. This reasoning was then given the title, the dopamine theory of schizophrenia.

This is a different process from the development of the theory of relativity, and it belongs to a different category of intellectual function. The theory of relativity and the dopamine theory of schizophrenia cannot meaningfully be placed in the same category, with both called scientific theories.

The bioreductionist response might be that I am proposing an elitist definition of a scientific theory, attainable only by rare geniuses. That is untrue. If I reviewed several books on the history of science, I could enumerate dozens of examples of scientific theories, major and minor. I am saying that the dopamine theory of schizophrenia does not belong to that *category*.

The naming of the dopamine theory of schizophrenia is a political strategy. One could not so easily obtain a grant to study the *dopamine idea of schizophrenia* or even the *dopamine model of schizophrenia*. Calling it a theory makes it, and the field, sound more high-falutin' and scientific but is really a semantic sleight of hand. Psychiatry does not have an adequate theory of any kind. It has various biological ideas, but no biological theories.

The dopamine hypothesis in schizophrenia is scientifically interesting and is worthy of serious scientific study. To call it a theory, though, is a cognitive error. Current interest in psychiatry is focused on presynaptic serotonin uptake blockers and the serotonin hypotheses that flow from them. The actual phrase *serotonin theory* is not used, however, partly because this class of medication is effective for so many different categories of mental illness. The *serotonin theory of depression, obsessive-compulsive disorder, posttraumatic stress disorder, some aspects of borderline personality disorder, trichotillomania, and other disorders,* does not have a good ring to it, and if used would threaten to expose the cognitive errors in the conceptual system. Drug companies market new psychotropic medications on the basis of the serotonergic action of their products, but they too have avoided the phrase *serotonin theory.*

DEPRESSION IS BASED ON A BIOLOGICAL DEFICIT, LIKELY OF SEROTONIN OR NORADRENALIN FUNCTION

The history of noradrenalin and serotonin models of depression is interesting and is related to the dopamine theory of schizophrenia. The idea that depression is based on a biological deficit comes from the observation that depressed people are low on energy, plus bioreductionism. A severely depressed person is like a record playing at slow speed, with reduced energy, slowed movements, a reduced range of body movement, slowed thinking, a reduced range of facial expression, and little interest in things. The intuitively obvious conclusion is that the depressed person is low on something: the thinking that led to biological deficit theories of depression is no more sophisticated than this. Combined with the deficit theory of depression is an excess theory of mania, because mania is the clinical opposite of depression. The fact that antidepressants sometimes switch a depressed bipolar patient into mania is consistent with this model.

Biological excess models of mania are not emphasized to anywhere near the degree of deficit theories of depression, however. One reason is that neuroleptics, which block dopamine, are effective for treating mania but do not induce depression in bipolar patients. The same is true of lithium, which brings a person down out of mania, but not up from depression: lithium holds a responsive bipolar patient in a normal mood state on a long-term basis. Lithium does not interact with receptors and so does not fit into the receptor–transmitter models that dominate biological psychiatry. Additionally, cognitive therapy of depression is as effective for the treatment of nonpsychotic unipolar depression as antidepressants. These clinical facts do not fit into a simple model. It is logically possible that depression results from an excess of something that slows you down, and mania from a deficit, but these models are rarely if ever mentioned in biological psychiatry.

When I was a resident, during the DST era, the focus in biological psychiatry was on noradrenergic deficiency states as the cause of depression, with the DST tied into the neurotransmitter regulation of the hypothalamic-pituitary-adrenal axis. Then it was discovered that serotonergic antidepressants are also effective in depression, so there was excited discussion about the possibility of noradrenergic and serotonergic subtypes of depression. Researchers measured levels of noradrenalin, serotonin, and their metabolites in the blood, urine, and cerebrospinal fluid of depressed patients, and tried to predict response to one or the other type of antidepressant based on the results. The results were contradictory, inconclusive, and all over the map.

One could have normal levels of noradrenalin, high levels of noradrenalin metabolite, and respond to a serotonergic antidepressant; or high levels of serotonin, low levels of serotonin metabolite, and respond to a noradrenergic antidepressant. For some years, supervisors identified the really first-rate residents by which ones had the antidepressants memorized according to whether they were noradrenergic or serotonergic, but this rating system quietly disappeared when the data failed to support it.

This would appear to be an example of proper scientific hypothesis making and testing, but it is not. Ideological enthusiasm for serotonin has far outstripped the interest in noradrenalin, with the development of fluoxetine and other serotonin reuptake blockers, which have a broad spectrum of action and a low side-effect profile. The fact that these drugs block serotonin presynpatically is clinically incidental.

If noradrenalin and serotonin were really being looked at dispassionately within biological psychiatry, rather than on the basis of hype and marketing buzz, there would be more comment on the fact that noradrenergic antidepressants are equally effective as serotonergic ones for many disorders in the affective spectrum, thereby destroying the specificity of serotonin hypotheses. The enthusiasm is driven by drug company marketing tactics and by the fact that the new serotonergic agents are more specific for serotonin receptors than noradrenergic drugs are for noradrenalin receptors, and therefore have fewer side effects. This is an accident of pharmacological history and has nothing to do with the biology of mental illness.

The marketing of buspirone is a good example of drug company strategies and their acceptance by biological psychiatry. When I was involved with buspirone in Phase III drug trials in 1984, the drug company's predominant emphasis was on the dopaminergic actions of the drug, with little mention of its serotonergic properties. Two things caused this emphasis to flip 180 degrees: (a) clinicians became worried about possible neuromuscular side effects of buspirone because of their experience with neuroleptics, and (b) serotonergic drugs like fluoxetine began to take a major market share in future projections. In reaction to these two developments, the dopaminergic properties of buspirone were completely dropped from discussion by the drug company, and the serotonergic properties were emphasized exclusively. This had nothing to do with any discoveries about the biology of mental illness; it was a clever marketing strategy leading to biological psychiatry's ignoring the dopaminergic properties of the drug and speaking only about its serotonergic actions.

Someone who had not been on the inside of this history would see only the progression of normal science, not realizing that the biological deficit model of depression is based on simple reasoning, drug company marketing, and no good data. There is no scientific evidence whatsoever that clinical depression is due to any kind of biological deficit state. Yet, like the heritability of schizophrenia, the deficit model of depression is regarded as established—a given, within biological psychiatry, unless directly challenged.

THE PLACEBO RESPONSE IS AN ARTIFACT OF NO INTRINSIC INTEREST

I recall being present at a drug company-sponsored marketing consultant dinner for which I and the other psychiatrists attending were paid $500 each (and given a free meal). The drug company was presenting video and brochure material for the marketing of a new product, and wanted consumer feedback from the psychiatrists. The company also presented slides of the multicenter, double-blind, randomized, placebo-controlled trial showing that their product was as effective for the target disorder as the standard medication already on the market. Symptom response curves for the two drugs showed a visually dramatic drop in symptom levels on a standardized measure. It was a typical drug company protocol with no methodological problems, and there was animated discussion of the pros and cons of the glossy brochures and computer-generated animation on the video.

During the latter part of the evening, I raised my hand and earned my $500. I suggested that, because the curve for placebo also took the same degree of dramatic drop on the slide of treatment response, they might want to consider de-emphasizing that slide in their marketing, and focus instead on the equivalent efficacy of their product compared to the other medication; anyone who noticed the placebo curve would be unlikely to be impressed by the need to prescribe a medication no more effective than placebo. The drug company representatives were polite and thankful for my feedback, both publicly, and privately afterward, because they have good marketing skills.

In biological psychiatry, the placebo response is a major anomaly that is almost entirely ignored, although it poses a fundamental biological problem. When I say "ignored," I mean ignored as a serious scientific puzzle of paradigm-threatening proportions. The placebo-responsiveness of major depressive episode illustrates the major role of the placebo effect in biological psychiatry. Placebo is a powerful psychotropic medication, and causes considerable side effects in double-blind trials. Not everyone realizes that placebo causes a measurable number of side effects—I have had subjects drop out of double-blind studies because of placebo side effects, and I have had subjects randomized to placebo experience a 90% drop in symptom levels. This is a common experience in drug trials.

During my residency, a major rationale for prescribing the antidepressants that I was taught to give patients was that the natural history of depression is that it tends to last six, nine, or more months before it remits spontaneously. By taking an antidepressant, it would be possible to be better in a few weeks, thereby avoiding the many months the patient, if untreated, would have to wait for spontaneous remission. At the same time, I learned that in a six-week drug study for depression, 70% of people would respond to a standard antidepressant and 30% would respond to placebo. Nobody ever pointed out the problem with the arithmetic: far too many people get better on placebo within the first two to three weeks of drug trials for spontaneous remission to get all the credit.

If major depressive episode is a biological illness, how can it so often be cured by placebo? This problem is simply ignored by biological psychiatry. The percentage of subjects who do not respond to the "active" antidepressant is about the same as the percentage who respond to placebo, in any large antidepressant drug trial. This is a well-established fact. One might conclude from these data that 30% of clinically depressed individuals have a nonbiological form of depression unresponsive to antidepressant medication.

More importantly, it is always said in psychiatry that 70% of depressed people will get better if given an antidepressant. This is true but deceptive. Of the people who get better on an active antidepressant, 30% are actually doing so because of a placebo response, not because of the chemical properties of the medication. This means that, overall, only 50% of clinically depressed patients get better when given an antidepressant drug because of the chemical effects of the drug, and 30% would get better on placebo. This is not so impressive a gap. If one defined antidepressant nonresponders as suffering from nonbiological depressions, this would be half of all patients. Doing so would be as logical and reasonable as the inverse assumption made by biological psychiatry: that response to medications is an indication of biological etiology.

If one did a cost–benefit analysis of medication versus placebo based on the 50% to 30% differential, taking into account the side effects and the deaths from overdose, the cost benefit for tricyclic antidepressants would be very modest. Such calculations are never made by bioreductionists, because they are ideologically unfavorable. The cost benefit for the newer serotonin uptake blockers would be more positive because of their lower side-effect profile.

Thirty percent of every treatment response obtained by biological psychiatry is due to the placebo effect. Yet the placebo effect receives virtually no research funding in and of itself within psychiatry. This does not make scientific sense.

I learned about the clinical power of the placebo effect as a second-year medical student, when I was learning how to start I.V.s and draw blood gases. I was doing rounds with the technologist, who advised me that the next patient was the most difficult person to draw gases from in the hospital. The patient was a six-year-old asthmatic girl in an oxygen tent who became very upset, frightened, and uncooperative every time blood was drawn, which was daily. Because of her size, the blood had to be drawn from the femoral artery.

I told the girl that I had a special anesthetic with me that I would rub on her before I stuck the needle in, and this would completely take away the pain, so that she would feel nothing. The agent worked perfectly—the little girl was completely calm, felt no pain, said thank you, and smiled when I was finished. The anesthetic agent was an alcohol swab. The failure to systematically study and augment the placebo response, because it does not fit with reductionist ideology, is depriving many people of symptom reduction they could otherwise receive. This is not good medicine.

If the placebo response was carefully studied and was augmented to the maximum possible level, the gap between antidepressants and placebo might narrow to nothing. This would happen if the placebo response rate was 40%, because the specific drug effect would then also be 40%, given that only 60% of the 70% of subjects responding to medication would be experiencing a pharmacologically based effect. Systematic study and augmentation of the placebo effect by only 25% would eliminate the difference between placebo and antidepressants in the treatment of depression.

BIOLOGICAL PSYCHIATRISTS TREAT CHEMICAL IMBALANCES IN THEIR PATIENTS' BRAINS

I have listed this cognitive error separately because the phrase *chemical imbalance* is so widely used by biological psychiatrists and their patients. On many occasions, I have listened to a patient tell me that his or her doctor is treating him for a chemical imbalance.

Patients with reductionist, chemical-imbalance models of their psychiatric disorders seldom want to do any psychotherapeutic work, because the reductionist model has reinforced their denial and has led them to conclude, "It's not my fault." Such patients often take a passive role in treatment and are difficult to engage in any kind of working partnership. They want to be told what to do and what pills to take, and they believe the doctor knows best. Paradoxically, receiving a reductionist countertransference response of this sort may actually be the best thing for such patients, and the cognitive errors of biological psychiatry may actually help hold them together, although the effect is attributed to the irrational polypharmacy, through an attributional error.

The chemical imbalance model may be quite appropriate and helpful for a pure lithium-responsive, bipolar mood disorder patient, but the model gets overgeneralized to patients with borderline personality disorder, eating disorders, dissociative disorders, gender identity disorders, and a wide range of other psychiatric difficulties. These people need to be active participants in their treatment, in a way that is very different from the requirement to take lithium regularly, and they must take psychological responsibility for their problems in order to get better (this is true of successfully surgically reassigned transsexuals, for instance, when reassignment is defined as recovery). The most medical treatment in psychiatry is the chemical and surgical reassignment of transsexuals, yet biological psychiatry as such has contributed nothing to this treatment, which is done primarily by endocrinologists and surgeons. It is ironic that the one psychiatric disorder that is actually treated by rebalancing chemicals in a medically rational manner, is of minor interest to biological psychiatry.

FINDING A BIOLOGICAL FACTOR IN A MENTAL ILLNESS WILL MAKE IT MORE REAL AND VALID

The dogma in biological psychiatry is that biology is more real than psychology. From this follows the cognitive error that any biological findings specific for a mental illness will make it more real. This cognitive error mirrors the professional chauvinism of the relationship between physics and biology: biologists are dismissed by reductionist physicists as dealing in the soft epiphenomena of underlying physical processes. In reaction to this, biologists feel inadequate, dream of eventually tagging biology to observations at the level of quantum physics, and do not share in the prestige of physics within the Faculty of Science. The same chauvinist division exists between experimental and theoretical physicists, with the experimental physicists being viewed as engineers and lab technicians by the theoreticians.

The search for a biological component to mental illness also occurs in a hierarchy of levels. The most fundamental and sought-after prize is a gene, because in the reductionist hierarchy, the gene is the ground floor of psychology. Less valued is a *marker*, which means any biological abnormality specifically related to a given psychiatric disorder. Markers are in turn divided into those that are intrinsically related to the core pathophysiology of the illness, and those that are more accidentally related. At a psychiatry conference, the speaker with incomprehensible slides and vocabulary from genetics is most intimidating to the audience.

A real biological finding in psychiatry would not necessarily be of any fundamental interest. It might consist of no more than filling in a blank. For instance, it is obvious that there must be a brain neurotransmitter that regulates pain. Before the endorphins were isolated (which was not done by a psychiatrist), the transmitter could have been called *pain regulatron*, without any knowledge of its structure of receptor. It has made no difference to clinical psychiatry that we can now use the word *endorphin* instead: for psychiatry, this is merely a semantic substitution. We don't understand pain any better within psychiatry because we now know that the pain regulatron is an endorphin; we have no new treatments, and nothing has changed in the life of any psychiatric patient.

To many, this will seem like a preposterous argument or an indication that I oppose scientific progress. But those reactions would be mistaken. It is a good thing that the endorphins were discovered, and the discovery was part of the desirable and proper progression of normal science.

Imagine that the genetics and physiology of the brain had been completely described from a biomechanical point of view, leaving no work to be done on the biology of the brain. We would be no further ahead in understanding the mind–body problem. We would not understand *pain*. We would understand all the biological correlates of pain, and could manipulate pain clinically with greater precision, but we would not understand where the subjective perception of pain comes from, because we would not have located the connection between mind and body.

Reductionist science deals with this problem by dismissing the mind as an unreal epiphenomena and defining the problem as a nonproblem, which is the only possible strategy open to reductionism. Where in the biological machinery does the *pain* come from? Does the pain spring into the mind from the receptor, from the axonal transport molecules, from the electrical charge in the neuron, from the vesicles, or from the synaptic cleft? This is an absurd question with no answer; it is absurd because the connection between mind and body cannot be localized in Newtonian space. The mapping of Newtonian space, which is the program of reductionist science, can never result in an understanding of the mind.

The truth is the other way around: only clinical psychiatric findings can make biological factors real in psychiatry. A biological finding is by itself meaningless unless it correlates with a problem in the *mind,* which is the domain of study of psychiatry. Without the mind, without clinical symptoms and human suffering, there could be no field called psychiatry. There would be only mammalian brain physiology and mechanistic neurology. The drive of reductionist biomedical psychiatry is to destroy psychiatry by making the mind irrelevant. Psychiatry is being taken over by other mental health professionals, because psychiatrists are focusing on biological pseudoscience and the pursuit of the impossible. A map of the brain is worth nothing without a map of the mind. If it were not for the subjective perception of pain, there would be no reason to even look for the endorphins, and if isolated, they would be biologically meaningless.

BIOLOGICAL PSYCHIATRISTS HAVE MADE IMPORTANT DISCOVERIES ABOUT MENTAL ILLNESS IN THE PAST TEN YEARS

Biological psychiatry has not made a single discovery of clinical relevance in the past ten years, despite hundreds of millions of dollars of research funding. The argument in this section can be conducted by placing the burden of proof on biological psychiatry to describe a single finding derived from the bioscientific work of psychiatrists that has had any direct clinical utility or application.

Bioreductionist psychiatry maintains its funding position based on hype and the promise of future results. Claims that we are in the decade of the brain, that major discoveries are just around the corner, or that the latest brain scan or blood test is of fundamental interest, have been highly successful marketing strategies for biological psychiatry, but are cognitive errors. Biological psychiatry has conducted by far the most successful marketing campaign, in terms of research dollars, political power, and prestige, ever mounted by psychiatry, yet most bioreductionists would probably disavow participation in any kind of marketing scheme and would claim to be scientists and academics. This claim is itself part of the marketing strategy.

Bioreductionist psychiatry has adopted the position that it is closely allied with mushrooming developments in the brain sciences, nuclear medicine, molecular biology, and other sciences. However, none of the fundamental developments in these other fields has been due to the work of psychiatrists, and biological psychiatry has borrowed the techniques and methods of other fields for application to psychiatric patients. For instance, the MRI scan was developed entirely outside psychiatry, then psychiatrists used it to scan the brains of individuals they had placed in different DSM-IV categories, looking to see if the computer would find any differences. Such research does not require any creative scientific thinking; it simply involves running psychiatric subjects through preexisting technologies and protocols. One has to look far and hard to find original, creative, scientific thinking conducted within the boundaries of biological psychiatry by psychiatrists, a situation radically different from that in molecular biology, where ingenious experiments abound.

As far as the development of new psychiatric medications is concerned, biological psychiatry can take little credit for the advances made. I have been a drug company contractor in a number of different Phase III multicenter, double-blind, randomized, placebo-controlled trials, have been to Europe twice at drug company expense, have published the results of drug trials as first author, have been a paid speaker for drug companies in four different cities, and have been on about ten drug company-sponsored trips within North America. I have participated in trials of neuroleptics, antidepressants, and anxiolytics, and have published an original neuroanatomical and neurotransmitter model for the use of buspirone in tardive dyskinesia. Based on this experience, I conclude that psychiatrists are contract technicians in new drug development, not creative scientists.

The development of a new psychiatric medication takes at least ten years and $100 million. The selection of drugs for study in humans follows the synthesis of new agents by chemists, who use a procedure called *chemical roulette*. This involves making minor chemical modifications to known drugs or simply trying out new molecules based on educated speculation. Once these chemicals are synthesized and purified, they are tested in animals to see whether they affect the animals in the way known antidepressants, neuroleptics, or anxiolytics do. Standardized animal models have been developed by chemists and rat psychologists for this purpose; none of the models has anything to do with the research findings of biological psychiatrists. Biological psychiatry as such has no role in the development of drugs up to the point of testing in humans.

Once human studies are initiated, no creative thinking is required from biological psychiatry. The protocols are drawn up in a highly standardized fashion based on the requirements of the Federal Drug Administration (FDA) and its equivalents around the world. Although some psychiatrists are in the loop at this point, no creative thinking of a scientific nature is required from them. After the protocols are set, psychiatrists are recruited through industry contacts to conduct the trials. The psychiatrists, at most, contribute a few minor modifications of the protocols.

Why are psychiatrists required at all? The reasons are technical, logistical, and political. *Scientifically,* there is no need for biological psychiatry in the development of new psychotropic medications. The drug companies need academic psychiatrists by decree of regulatory agencies, which insist that there be a contractual, arm's-length relationship between the physicians conducting the trials and the company with the patent. This is a proper and necessary arrangement. Additionally, psychiatrists are required logistically, but not scientifically, for patient recruitment. This is also a good financial arrangement: physicians can be employed contractually on an as-needed basis, without being company employees. The contractual arrangement reduces research and development costs for psychiatrists to zero during periods in which no drugs of a given class are under development.

Drug company contracts, now a major source of research income for medical schools and biological psychiatrists, are used to finance a large amount of other research. There is nothing wrong with this, and I used such contracts to finance my own research. There is a pressing need for new drug development. The new serotonin reuptake blockers are a major and highly beneficial development for psychiatric patients, and I prescribe them regularly—for dissociative identity disorder patients, among others. There is no disputing the fact that these medications are more effective than placebo.

The medications do not come from biological psychiatry, however; they come from drug companies that employ psychiatrists as contract technicians. Psychiatrists are a politically and logistically indispensable part of the loop, as they should be, but their contribution to the process is not that of creative scientist. The advances in psychopharmacology during the second half of the twentieth century cannot be attributed to a scientific effort by biological psychiatry, although biological psychiatry should get full credit for its technical achievements.

A possible objection to this reasoning would be that biological psychiatrists have been responsible for innovative applications of medications in psychiatry, such as the use of anticonvulsants like valproic acid and carbamazepine in certain psychiatric conditions. This argument would actually reinforce my position, rather than provide a counterargument. Borrowing drugs from neighboring disciplines and trying them out on different DSM-IV categories is the clinical equivalent of chemical roulette, requires no creative scientific thinking, and is a secondary industrial application of an already manufactured product.

Overlooking the distinction between secondary technical applications and original scientific discovery has been a key strategy in the marketing of biological psychiatry.

THE ASCENDANCE OF BIOLOGICAL PSYCHIATRY IN THE 1980S HAS RESULTED IN A MORE SCIENTIFIC AND EFFECTIVE PSYCHIATRY

Biological psychiatry depends on an ahistorical perspective, which it fosters in psychiatry residents. A not uncommon attitude is to regard anything written before 1970, or even 1985, as antiquated and prescientific. Even when that attitude is softened and a hat is tipped to Kraepelin, it is still said that over 90% of the serious writing in the field has been published since 1980. This is a manifestation of the grandiosity that pervades the field: bioreductionists think of their field as exploding scientifically like molecular biology, with major advances in the understanding of brain physiology, fundamental new findings arising from brain scan research, and revolutionary new clinical applications due shortly, especially in genetic engineering. They view the field as having taken off exponentially since 1980, with most developments before that being of "historical" interest only. In reductionist language, "historical" is a condescending and dismissive term, like the popular phrase "of academic interest only." Both phrases mean that the problem under discussion is of no real importance and can be consigned to the ivory tower.

A dogma of biological psychiatry is that symptoms of serious mental illness are a direct expression of primary physical pathology in the brain. Even in an illness with a predominantly endogenous-biological etiology, this need not necessarily be the case. The depression of Cushing's syndrome when the problem originates in the adrenal glands, the anxiety of hyperthyroidism, and mental status changes in paraneoplastic syndromes are good examples of biomedical psychiatric disorders accompanied by normal brain physiology. This is the case in the sense that changes in brain physiology in these disorders are secondary to pathophysiology elsewhere in the body: given the abnormality elsewhere in the body, the brain's response is biologically normal and the genetics of the brain are normal. It is theoretically possible that the primary abnormality in schizophrenia is in the gastrointestinal tract, and that the abnormality causes absorption of a protein, which in turn produces psychosis. The emphasis on primary brain pathophysiology is not a necessary postulate of bioreductionist psychiatry.

The second aspect of this cognitive error is that causality within the brain–mind field is unidirectional in reductionist psychiatry. The third is the directness of the causality, even in instances in which the direction of the arrow is correct. Given the complexity of the brain, the number of transductions of signal that occur between the primary biological defect and the symptoms is likely considerable. Production of a psychiatric disorder by the brain is probably like the production of a commercial airline disaster, in that multiple unrelated factors must come together to produce the final outcome. These factors may be no more directly related to each other in the brain, biologically speaking, than wind shear, metal fatigue, and pilot error are intrinsically related to each other in nature.

The linear model of scientific development, as readers of Thomas Kuhn (1962) know, ignores the widely accepted thesis that scientific progress occurs through discontinuous paradigm shifts. Here we find another paradox in the conceptual system of biological psychiatry: biological psychiatry acts as if it has initiated a paradigm shift, when actually it is an example of "normal pseudoscience," a term I just coined. In normal science, an established paradigm dominates a given field, and researchers within the field work comfortably within the paradigm. Minor discrepancies in research findings are easily explained away as artifacts or errors until, gradually, enough anomalous data accumulate that the entire paradigm is threatened.

At this point, a discontinuous intellectual and creative leap is taken by the leaders of a new school of thought, and there is a paradigm shift. The new paradigm gradually takes over the field, and established adherents of the old school have to literally die out before this can occur. During the transition period, there is ideological warfare. A key feature of the new paradigm is that it can account for all the data and observations understood within the old perspective, while also encompassing the anomalous data that drove the shift. The classic example of a paradigm shift is the transition from Newtonian to relativistic physics.

Once serious mental illness is defined as always biological in nature, the cognitive error that biological research offers the only real hope for victims of major mental illness becomes a tautology and is regarded as self-evident. The tautology feeds back on other reinforcers of the differential flow of research money, prestige, and academic appointments to bioreductionists, and maintains the pseudoscientific paradigm intact.

Dissociative identity disorder is a major piece of anomalous data threatening this cognitive error. At this point in the history of psychiatry, the dissociative disorders have the status of anomalous data, and a paradigm shift to a trauma model of psychopathology has not occurred. Dissociative identity disorder is a major mental illness by all criteria for that category, including severity of symptoms, morbidity, impact on psychosocial function, economic cost to society, and, probably, mortality. The paradigm shift has not occurred yet because an insufficient quantity of anomalous data has accumulated to date.

Dissociative identity disorder is the only major mental illness about which we can make any of the following statements:

We understand its etiology, which is the dissociative response to chronic childhood trauma;

We understand at a microdetailed level the relationship between the etiology and the phenomenology, and we can relate the signs and symptoms of the disorder to a detailed understanding of structure within the organism;

We have a microdetailed understanding of the specific relationship between the phenomenology and the treatment interventions;

The disorder can be cured with currently available methods;

We understand all the requirements for primary, secondary, and tertiary prevention (although we lack the political will).

All of these statements are true at a psychosocial level of analysis. The pathophysiology of dissociative identity disorder is not understood in anything but the most speculative, preliminary fashion, which is not surprising, given that bioreductionist researchers do not acknowledge the reality or importance of the disorder and do not devote research resources to it.

From a public health point of view, I believe the contribution of diagnostically specific genes for mental illness, even if they exist, occurs in a small number of pedigrees and accounts for a minute fraction of psychiatric morbidity and mortality. Comparatively, serious chronic childhood trauma is the overwhelming major driver of psychopathology in Western civilization. This estimation can be tested with currently available structured interviews and epidemiological methods. The bulk of psychopathology in our culture represents the normal human response to chronic childhood trauma, based on a normal genetic endowment. This is entirely analogous to evidence in what used to be Yugoslavia: the bulk of current morbidity and mentality is due to physical trauma and is based on normal genetic endowment and the normal response of the human organism to environmental insult.

If my viewpoint (which is not unique to me) is correct, then biological psychiatry in its current form is a major diversion of resources in the wrong direction, and these resources need to be redirected to the normal psychobiology of trauma. Here, they would quite quickly yield biologically and clinically meaningful findings rooted in mammalian physiology, within a biopsychosocial paradigm. Reductionist biological psychiatry cannot study the normal biology of psychosocial trauma without destroying itself; therefore, it does not do so.

BIOLOGICAL PSYCHIATRISTS ARE GOOD DIAGNOSTICIANS

Many biological psychiatrists are poor diagnosticians either because of (a) poor application of DSM-IV rules or (b) proper application of the diagnostic rules, which themselves are full of contradictions and cognitive errors. The DSM-IV system is one of the truly important achievements of twentieth-century psychiatry, and it far outweighs the contribution of biological research. I am a firm believer in the necessity for operationalized diagnostic criteria. Nevertheless, the DSM-IV diagnostic system arises from the reductionist philosophy of late twentieth-century North American psychiatry, although it takes the position of being aphilosophical and phenomenological, not realizing that the decision to be phenomenologically based is itself a philosophical decision.

In the DSM-IV system, psychiatric disorders are largely treated as separate entities, consistent with the hypothesis that there is a gene for schizophrenia, a gene for depression, and another separate gene for alcoholism. Although there are groupings of disorders, and various exclusion rules based on the presence of other disorders, the main purpose of the system is to sort patients out into discrete categories. The way in which diagnoses are placed in categories, rather than being phenomenologically based, is highly determined by historical artifacts, the residual effects of Freudian theory, and political turf disputes among different subcommittees.

For instance, in DSM-IV, conversion disorder is classified as a somatoform disorder and is grouped with hypochondriasis and body dysmorphic disorder, with which it has no natural relationship. This reflects the influence of Freudian ideas about somatization and conversion, and the simple fact that all disorders in the somatoform section have something to do with the body. In the *International Classification of Diseases-10* (ICD-10), however, conversion disorder is classified as a dissociative disorder and is grouped with psychogenic amnesia, which is a much more logical, naturalistic, and phenomenologically based location for it. For some reason, European nosologists have grasped the dissociative nature of conversion disorder and have not been politically trapped into grouping conversion disorder with hypochondriasis.

In DSM-IV, dissociative identity disorder (DID) is an exclusion criterion for dissociative disorder not otherwise specified (DDNOS): one can receive a diagnosis of DDNOS only if one does not meet criteria for one of the other defined dissociative disorders. However, in ICD-10, which comes from Europe, where there is far less acceptance of the concept of DID, DID is still called multiple personality disorder and is listed as a form of DDNOS. These differences in classification are entirely ideologically based and have nothing to do with any scientific data or phenomenological approach to nosology.

The history of brief reactive dissociative disorder, a diagnosis invented during the DSM-IV process, is also instructive. This entity was constructed primarily by Robert Spitzer and David Spiegel to capture trauma-induced dissociative disorders of short duration, and was accepted favorably by the DSM-IV committee examining the dissociative disorders, of which I was a member. Where does this diagnosis appear in DSM-IV? If the anxiety disorders section, with its name changed to *acute stress disorder.* How did this happen?

The first problem with brief reactive dissociative disorder was that, after a month's duration, if it had not remitted, the diagnosis changed to posttraumatic stress disorder (PTSD), which is classified as an anxiety disorder. This would mean that a patient would switch *categories* of mental illness at the end of a month, which made no sense. If brief reactive dissociative disorder was to be preserved, and the switch to PTSD after one month was to be preserved, there were only two possible solutions to the problem: (a) move PTSD to the dissociative disorders or (b) move brief reactive dissociative disorder to the anxiety disorders. The decision to move brief reactive dissociative disorder to the anxiety disorders was based solely on the greater political power of the anxiety disorders group compared to the dissociative disorders group. Once the switch was made, it was necessary to change the name of the disorder, because one cannot have an anxiety disorder called brief reactive dissociative disorder. This was done.

How is acute stress disorder defined in DSM-IV? Criterion A is the experience of a trauma. Criterion B lists five dissociative symptoms, of which one must have three:

1. Subjective sense of numbing, detachment, or absence of emotional responsiveness;
2. Reduction in awareness of one's surroundings;
3. Derealization;
4. Depersonalization;
5. Dissociative amnesia, that is, an inability to recall an important aspect of the trauma.

Criterion H is a generally worded exclusion criterion: "Not due to the direct effects of a substance (e.g., drugs of abuse, medication) or a general medical condition, and is not merely an exacerbation of a preexisting Axis I or II disorder." The other criteria include avoidance behavior, a duration criterion, and intrusion and hyperarousal criteria; the intrusion symptoms are dissociative in nature.

There are no specific diagnostic rules for how to differentiate acute stress disorder from dissociative amnesia disorder, depersonalization disorder, and DDNOS. What we have is a dissociative disorder placed in the anxiety disorders section for political reasons, then defined as if the dissociative disorders section did not exist. This is also true of PTSD, which is much more logically grouped with the dissociative disorders than with simple phobia and obsessive-compulsive disorder. The *phenomenology* of PTSD, as defined in the DSM-IV diagnostic criteria, is far more like that of the dissociative disorders than the other anxiety disorders. The pretense to a purely phenomenologically based diagnostic system is transparently false.

There is a similar problem with the DSM-IV rules for diagnosing schizophrenia: they are designed as if DID doesn't exist. There are five criteria for schizophrenia. Criterion A is the presence, for at least a month or two, of the following:

1. Delusions;
2. Hallucinations;
3. Disorganized speech (e.g., frequent derailment or incoherence);
4. Grossly disorganized or catatonic behavior;
5. Negative symptoms (i.e., affective flattening, alogia, or avolition).

Note: Only one A symptom is required if delusions are bizarre or hallucinations consist of a voice keeping up a running commentary on the person's behavior or thoughts, or two or more voices are conversing with each other.

The other four criteria involve social/occupational deterioration, presence of the illness for at least six months, and ruling out schizoaffective disorder, mood disorder with psychotic features, substance abuse, and general medical conditions as causes of the symptoms.

Clinically, every DID patient I have ever met meets criterion A, most meet criterion B (the dysfunction criterion), all meet criterion C (the duration criterion), and all meet the exclusion criteria. The diagnostic rules of biological psychiatry result in a false positive diagnosis of schizophrenia in 100% of DID cases in which there is social/occupational deterioration. If DID affects 1% of the general population (Ross, 1991) and at least 5% of general adult psychiatric inpatients (Ross, Anderson, Fleisher, & Norton, 1991; Saxe et al., 1993), then the DSM-V schizophrenia group will have only two responses open to it: act as if DID doesn't exist, or radically modify the diagnostic criteria for schizophrenia in DSM-V, and include DID in the exclusion criteria and the text.

I have included these examples of political decisions in DSM-IV because they refute the proposition that biological psychiatrists are good, scientific diagnosticians, because I know the history firsthand, and because the politics illustrate the paradigm-threatening nature of dissociative identity disorder. It might be objected that the DSM-IV system and biological psychiatry are two separate things, and that problems with DSM-IV cannot necessarily be blamed on bioreductionists. Although this is true in theory, in reality the system is driven by bioreductionist assumptions and ideology.

As I mentioned previously, DID is a test case demonstrating that bioreductionist psychiatrists cannot differentiate a disorder they consider to be hysterical and artifactual from a disorder (schizophrenia) they consider to be a biomedical brain disease. This differential diagnostic inadequacy has had a direct and major impact on the lives of hundreds of thousands of people in North America.

BIOLOGICAL PSYCHIATRY IS BRINGING MORE RESPECT TO PSYCHIATRY

This cognitive error has depended on a dissociation of biological psychiatry from other sectors of the mental health field, with disavowal of culpability for the dissociation by biological psychiatry, and a substantial degree of amnesia for it. In certain sectors of the mental health field, bioreductionism is creating scorn and loss of business for psychiatry. This is best illustrated by feminist, community-based master's level therapists who treat sexual abuse survivors with psychotherapy. The scorn is militant and mutual.

The bioreductionists take the stance of being rational and scientific, and they denigrate the psychotherapists for being impressionistic, hysterical, and poorly trained. The therapists, on the other hand, deal daily with the effects of hostile and sadistic countertransference toward their clients, sexual exploitation of them, rude behavior, minimally helpful polypharmacy with numerous side effects, and condescending attitudes toward the therapists. Not all biological psychiatrists are like this, but many are. The therapists complain about the great difficulty they have finding psychiatrists who will prescribe rationally for their clients, not interfere destructively in their cases, and support their clients' recovery. Most of the therapists are female, and most of the biological psychiatrists are male.

During my residency, I didn't realize the size of the chasm between academic psychiatry and the rest of the mental health field. As part of my residency, I had virtually no contact with nonacademic mental health professionals based outside the teaching hospital system, except for case workers on child and adolescent cases. I had no idea how towered the ivory tower actually is, and I had a vague impression of community-based therapists being feminist, antiscientific, and poorly trained. When, as a staff psychiatrist, I started to work predominantly with sexual abuse survivors (they comprised over half the clientele of the department, but there was no teaching on sexual abuse in my residency), I began to work closely with community-based therapists, and found the bioreductionist stereotype to be confirmed in some instances. I met female therapists who were antimale, antihospital, antiscientific, antimedical, antimedication, anti-DSM, and antime, and I could not work with them.

However, I found a majority of skilled, conscientious, well-educated therapists who were keenly interested in supervision, consultation, and continuing education. They had infinitely more expertise in the long-term sequelae and treatment of childhood sexual abuse than biological psychiatrists, and were doing excellent work for low wages with few resources. These therapists were inundated with the treatment failures and casualties of bioreductionist psychiatry.

As a strategic plan for the next ten years, investment in bioreductionism by psychiatry, I predict, will further alienate psychologists and master's-level therapists from psychiatry, will reduce the domain of psychiatry, will divert resources away from psychiatry into the trauma model, and will bring psychiatry into further disrepute. This is a prediction I would never have made had I stayed insulated in academia. Because it is a sociopolitical prediction, it cannot be a compelling argument. Time will tell.

CONCLUSION

These errors of logic in biological psychiatry can all be corrected, and none is essential to a scientific psychiatry. I have enumerated them in the hope that the destructive influence of reductionism and pseudoscience within psychiatry will thereby be modulated. Biological psychiatry could be a fascinating and important field, if it was shorn of its pervasive cognitive errors and if its academic standards were higher.

As a logic system, the conceptual system of biological psychiatry is organized in a fashion similar to the personality systems of patients with dissociative identity disorder. The tautologies, positive feedback loops, closure to alternative hypotheses, pervasive overgeneralization, use of dissociation to eliminate cognitive dissonance, and other structural and functional properties of the system maintain it in a dysfunctional homeostasis. Given that this system responds to cognitive and systemic interventions in the individual dissociative identity disorder patient, one can be hopeful that it will do so within bioreductionist psychiatry. The main factor that militates against this possibility is the massive amount of secondary gain experienced by biological psychiatry in North America in the late twentieth century.

REFERENCES

Beck, A. T., Rush, A. J., Shaw, B. F., & Emery, G. (1979). *Cognitive therapy of depression.* New York: Guilford Press.

Kaplan, H. I., Freedman, A. M., & Sadock, B. J. (1980). *Comprehensive textbook of psychiatry/III.* Baltimore: Williams & Wilkins.

Kuhn, T. (1962). *The structure of scientific revolutions.* Chicago: University of Chicago Press.

Ross, C. A. (1986). Biological tests for mental illness: Their use and misuse. *Biological Psychiatry, 21,* 431–435.

Ross, C. A. (1991). Epidemiology of multiple personality disorder and dissociation. *Psychiatric Clinics of North America, 14,* 503–517.

Ross, C. A., Anderson, G., Fleisher, W. P., & Norton, G. R. (1991). Frequency of multiple personality disorder among psychiatric inpatients. *American Journal of Psychiatry, 148,* 1717–1720.

Ross, C. A., & Leichner, P. (1986). Canadian and British opinion on formulation. *Annals of the Royal College of Physicians and Surgeons of Canada, 19,* 49–52.

Ross, C. A., Leichner, P., Matas, M., & Anderson, D. (1990). A method of teaching and evaluating formulation. *Academic Psychiatry, 14,* 99–105.

Saxe, G. N., van der Kolk, B. A., Berkowitz, R., Chinman, G., Hall, K., Lieberg, G., & Schwartz, J. (1993). Dissociative disorders in psychiatric inpatients. *American Journal of Psychiatry, 150,* 1037–1042.

Szasz, T. (1974). *The myth of mental illness.* New York: Harper & Row.

Walker, J., Norton, G. R., & Ross, C. A. (1991). *Panic disorder and agoraphobia: A comprehensive guide for the practitioner.* Pacific Grove, CA: Brooks/Cole.

3

PSEUDOSCIENCE IN
THE AMERICAN JOURNAL OF PSYCHIATRY

Colin A. Ross

The American Journal of Psychiatry, the Official Journal of the American Psychiatric Association, has been published continuously since 1844. It is now under the editorship of Nancy C. Andreasen, M.D., Ph.D., who is the eleventh editor of the journal; the immediate past editor, from 1978 to 1993, was John C. Nemiah, M.D. The *Journal* appears monthly, and a full annual volume occupies about 1,800 pages. Each issue contains a variety of Special Articles, Editorials, Regular Articles, Brief Reports, Letters to the Editor, Book Reviews, and other material. The *Journal* is the flagship publication of American Psychiatry and is one of a handful of top psychiatric journals in the world. It is broad in scope and includes research, clinical, and review papers on all areas of psychiatry.

I coauthored four papers in the *Journal* from 1990 to 1993 (Ross, Miller et al., 1990; Ross, Joshi, & Currie, 1990; Ross, Anderson, Fleisher, & Norton, 1991; Carlson et al., 1993), and consider it to be the preferred place to publish psychiatric papers. I mention this to demonstrate that I am not in any way hostile to *The American Journal of Psychiatry*. I have chosen it for review in this chapter precisely because the *Journal* is eclectic, authoritative, and prestigious. Psychiatrists, including myself, mention with pride papers they have published in "The Green Journal."

My task in this chapter began with a review of all issues of the *Journal* for 1990 through 1993. I have drawn from this substantial body of literature illustrative examples of the logical errors, methodological flaws, and ideological biases of biological psychiatry. These illustrate the points made by Dr. Pam and myself in the previous chapters. For convenience, I have grouped papers into categories that illustrate each of these intellectual weaknesses. I have made no attempt to do anything other than provide examples of cognitive errors, and have not commented on sound papers. My purpose is to show that pseudoscience is endemic in biological psychiatry.

STATEMENTS OF BIOREDUCTIONIST IDEOLOGICAL BIAS

I include this category to demonstrate that direct statements of reductionist ideology can be found in the psychiatric literature. If this were not so, the thesis of this book would have to be that the bias is pervasive but entirely covert.

> *Wu, J. C., & Bunney, W. E. (1990). The biological basis of an antidepressant response to sleep deprivation and relapse: Review and hypothesis. 147, 14–21.*

The cognitive error that biology underlies psychology, and is the level of primary etiology, is evident in this sentence, "An intensive review of the phenomenology and mechanisms of action of sleep deprivation may provide important clues for understanding the underlying biological substrate of depressive illness and for the future development of rapidly acting antidepressant treatments or drugs."

In their quite lengthy review article, the authors make passing note of the methodological limitations of this literature:

> None of the 61 studies used a double-blind, placebo-controlled design because of the difficulty in ensuring that the subjects and the experimenters are blind to a manipulation such as sleep deprivation and in part because of the difficulty of finding a suitable placebo control. It is possible that the antidepressant response could be due to experimental bias expectations or the nonspecific effects of attention by the raters.

Sixty-one studies is a large amount of effort to expend without ever developing a research design that meets minimum scientific criteria. It is doubtful that a literature this low in methodology would support a long review article in a top journal in a rigorous scientific field.

> *Raine, A., Venables, P. H., & Williams, M. (1990). Autonomic orienting responses in 15-year-old male subjects and criminal behavior at age 24. 147, 933–937.*

In this study, skin conductance and heart rate measures of orienting were obtained in 101 noninstitutionalized 15-year-old boys, and criminal status was determined 9 years later at age 24 (17 had a criminal record by age 24). The two groups differed significantly on the measures, leading the authors to conclude: "Given the strong evidence for the role of genetic factors in criminal behavior and the fact that the psychophysiological variables in this study are in part genetically determined, it seems possible that the genetic predisposition to criminal behavior finds its expression to some degree through these autonomic nervous system factors."

No such conclusions are warranted logically or scientifically; one would want to examine the cognitive errors leading to the conclusion that the measures have a demonstrated genetic component. This study will be referenced in other studies as evidence supporting the genetic foundation of criminal behavior, which is how the bioreductionist literature works: erroneous conclusions in one paper are used to support erroneous conclusions in others, and a network of confirmatory pseudoscience is constructed.

> *Pardes, H. (1990). Presidential address: Defending humanistic values. 147, 1113–1119.*

The following paragraphs convey both the pervasive cognitive errors and the feeling tone of biomedical psychiatry, with lip service paid to the psychosocial:

> Humanistic values are at the very heart of our profession. The study of the mind, and the healing of the mental anguish that can rob people of the fulfillment of their humanity, is our life's work. To this work we bring both our own humanity and the force of modern science.
>
> The rewards can be enormous. In the past decade, especially, we have been dazzled by advances in brain imaging, molecular genetics, psychopharmacology, and other fields of study that have revolutionized neuroscience. The most exciting aspect of these advances is what they promise for our capacity as physicians. Because of this panoply of research—encompassing high-tech findings about the brain, evaluation of the psychotherapies, linkage studies, epidemiology and the refinement of diagnostic

criteria, the discovery of effective medications, and the development of effective rehabilitation—we can see and begin to deliver new kinds of relief for mental suffering. Few of us would have dreamed that these advances were possible in the days when we entered the field. It has been very moving to find that our progress is understood by our patients, their families, and our friends in the citizens' movement, who are now devoting their own considerable vitality and talents to the fight against mental illness.

In contradistinction to this rhetoric, the purposes of the present book are: to reduce the degree of dazzle in the contemporary mind, and to being the force of modern science to bear on biological psychiatry.

Sabshin, M. (1990). Turning points in twentieth-century American psychiatry. 147, 1267–1274.

This paper was delivered as the Adolph Meyer Lecture at the American Psychiatric Association Meeting in 1989. It contains a rare glimmer of critical thinking about the costs and excesses of bioreductionist ideological enthusiasm, while remaining uncritical of the pseudoscientific nature of the "best stories" in psychiatry:

> During this past decade, the best stories about psychiatry in print and electronic media have involved the scientific advances in the field. As these stories have increased, they have begun to offset the continuing negative stories and may be moving to a point where they will go beyond offsetting. The need to change the public image of psychiatry has also played a key role in producing the current turning point. For some of my research colleagues, this effect is passionately denied as if it meant that their work is designed to influence the public. Just the opposite is true; high quality work affects the public because it is high quality. But we must want to seek public support while reducing the stigma against patients and practitioners. In this process, a tendency to overcorrect for previous errors is inevitable. A focus on genetic markers for manic-depressive illness gets much more attention than stories about the less fashionable reports of successful psychotherapy. This attention and the resultant allocation of resources affect many segments of our training programs, certification procedures, and accreditation processes. The overreaction certainly has many practical consequences.

Faraone, S. V., Biederman, J., Keenan, K., & Tsuang, M. T. (1991). A family-genetic study of girls with DSM-III attention deficit disorder. 148, 112–117.

This excellent paper is almost free of ideological bias; yet, even here, acquiescence to biomedical reductionism appears. The authors commit the cognitive error of *if it runs in families it must be genetic* in their title and in this sentence: "The familial transmission of attention deficit disorder among families with a son who has the disorder provides external validation for the diagnosis in boys and suggests genetic influences in the disorder." Such data suggest environmental influences just as much, but that is not the authors' bias. Nor can such data provide external validation for a disorder: lying, malingering, and factitious disorders could all run in families.

Zorumski, C. F., & Isenberg, K. E. (1991). Insights into the structure and function of GABA-benzodiazepine receptors: Ion channels and psychiatry. 148, 162–173.

This is a comprehensive and scholarly paper, and its solidity is derived largely from review of research done by nonpsychiatric biologists. In the final paragraph, the authors caution psychiatry (in sentences that do not follow each other logically) against simpleminded biological theories, but they are nevertheless committed to a bioreductionist model of serious mental illness, one tied to receptor subunits rather than neurotransmitters:

> Simple notions of increases or decreases in transmitter levels, metabolites, or receptors in a disease state will need to be tempered by an understanding of how such changes may affect each of the receptor subtypes in a given region. It is possible that specific disorders may reflect abnormalities of only a single receptor subtype. Thus, crude measurements of transmitter levels offer little hope of shedding light on pathophysiology. In addition, molecular genetic studies offer the opportunity of directly considering receptor subunit gene involvement in psychiatric disorders.

Winchel, R. M., & Stanley, M. (1991). Self-injurious behavior: A review of the behavior and biology of self-mutilation. 148, 306–317.

This paper contains 116 references of which 2 are on childhood sexual abuse, a major driver of self-mutilative behavior. Even when an overwhelming environmental factor is identified, however, the reductionist can invert it into evidence of primary etiology lying in the genetic domain:

> Although the importance and grave traumatic effects of childhood sexual abuse should not be underestimated, a cause-and-effect relationship between abuse and self-injurious behavior should not be automatically assumed. Sexual abuse may serve to elicit symptoms in an individual already at risk, but frequent histories of such trauma may also reflect a familial predisposition to impulsive—and perhaps violent—behaviors. An interplay of

both factors suggests the unfortunate possibility that those who are biologically endowed with a vulnerability to self-injurious behavior may also have
a greater probability of being raised in a familial environment where the
stresses that might elicit such behavior—such as childhood sexual behavior—are more likely to occur.

The authors, without quite being direct, are proposing a genetically
driven category of impulse control disorders, with the gene expressing
itself as perpetration in the parental generation and wrist slashing in
the victim generation. The gene causes the victim to become a perpetrator of her children, who also carry the gene, and who will cut themselves as a result. This spectrum could be treated with selective
sterilization.

**Russell, J. L., Kushner, M. G., Beitman, B. D., & Bartels, K. M.
(1991). Nonfearful panic disorder in neurology patients
validated by lactate challenge. 148, 361–364.**

This would be a good paper if the authors had not emphasized the cognitive error about external validation by biological tests in their title
and their discussion: "Positive responses to lactate by these patients
lend substantial credence to the nosological validity of nonfearful
panic disorder as a panic disorder subdiagnosis." Positive responses to
psychosocial triggers of panic would be no less validating, but would
not be as likely to result in the paper's being accepted at *The American
Journal of Psychiatry.*

**Volkow, N. D., & Tancredi, L. R. (1991). Biological correlates of
mental activity studies with PET. 148, 439–443.**

These are the only authors, in the four years of the *Journal* reviewed,
who displayed any evidence of an ability to differentiate their bioreductionist ideology from scientific method and logical analysis: "In
interpreting these findings, one should also keep in mind the reductionism of this approach."

**Swift, R. G., Perkins, D. O., Chase, C. L., Sadler, D. B., & Swift,
M. (1991). Psychiatric disorders in 36 families with Wolfram
syndrome. 148, 775–779.**

The authors believe: "Identifying genes that predispose individuals to
psychiatric disorders and understanding their metabolic basis will lead,
in many instances, to effective prevention or treatment measures for
these disorders." Although *prevention* is usually supposed to imply some
unknown but humane form of genetic engineering to be perfected in the
next few decades, in fact it means abortion and sterilization.

| Samson, J. A., Mirin, S. M., Hauser, S. T., Fenton, B. T., &
| Schildkraut, J. J. (1992). Learned helplessness and urinary
| MHPG levels in unipolar depression. 149, 806–809.

I include this paper because the authors propose that a biological measure, urinary MHPG levels, could be used to differentially triage depressed clinical patients into psychopharmacology or cognitive-behavioral therapy. The authors demonstrate that bioreductionist bias is not intrinsic to biological psychiatry, and their proposal is a concrete example of how such bias would limit and restrict such research, because a reductionist would never make this suggestion. From a bioreductionist research team, we would expect instead speculation about different genetic subtypes of depression based on the same data.

| Freedman, D. X. (1992). The search: Body, mind, and human
| purpose. 149, 858–866.

This paper was delivered as the 1991 Adolph Meyer Lecture at the American Psychiatric Association Meeting. It communicates the bedazzled state of contemporary psychiatrists, as did Pardes (1990) in his Presidential address, discussed above:

> In all of medicine, for the bedazzled clinician the sweep and promise of modern science is, in fact, breathtaking. We should be appreciative but not mesmerized. For, in sobriety, we will have to determine which of the plethora of science leads to apply practically in the clinic and clinical research. The gap between visions of what may be and application is still huge but narrowing.

In another paragraph, Freedman combines correct caution and humility, on behalf of psychiatry, with the characteristic tone of biological reductionism:

> Thus, for all our power to understand synaptic regulations, we are still calibrating precisely where and how brain substances and mechanisms are relevant to the manifestations of disease. We want to know whether brain receptors are different in the diseased patient—as they ought to be. We have truly enticing starts, some secondary pathophysiology, and a high index of suspicion as to genetics, but to be clear: clinically diagnostically specific, etiopathological definitions of our diseases remain an ultimate goal.

By the end of this chapter, the reader may wish to consider whether *calibrating* or *fishing* is the more accurate verb for characterizing psychiatric biological research.

Buckley, P., Stack, J. P., Madigan, C., O'Callaghan, E., Larkin, C., Redmond, O., Ennis, J. T., & Waddington, J. L. (1993). Magnetic resonance imaging of schizophrenia-like psychoses associated with cerebral trauma: Clinicopathological correlates. 150, 146–148.

This study has five subjects and eight authors. The authors state:

> Four of our patients had no family history of schizophrenia, but an uncle of patient 1 had himself experienced a head injury prior to the onset of psychosis. The modest number of patients studied precludes definitive inferences as to genetic risk, but our findings are consistent with the idea that the risk for schizophrenia among relatives of patients with a schizophrenia-like psychosis is considerably lower than the risk in relatives of patients with schizophrenia.

The phraseology partially disguises the preposterous nature of the authors' comments.

Quitkin, F. M., Stewart, J. W., McGrath, P. J., Nunes, E., Ocepek-Welikson, K., Tricamo, E., Rabkin, J. G., & Klein, D. F. (1993). Further evidence that a placebo response to antidepressants can be identified. 150, 566–570.

The authors studied response to placebo and active medication in depression and concluded that rapid responses are placebo responses, and do not last as long as slower-onset true medication responses. They view more gradual-onset responses to placebo as true spontaneous remissions. This is a biased viewpoint because rapid onset of anxiety to benzodiazepines and of psychotic agitation to neuroleptics is commonplace, and both are regarded as true medication responses.

The most interesting implication of the paper, which the authors do not discuss, is the unavoidable conclusion, following from their line of logic, that the placebo plus spontaneous remission response rate must be subtracted from the apparent medication response rate in drug trials, in order to yield the true medication response rate, which will be much closer to the sum of placebo plus spontaneous remission. This is the argument I made in the preceding chapter.

Miller, L. J., O'Connor, E., & DiPasquale, T. (1993). Patients' attitudes towards hallucinations. 150, 584–588.

The ideological bias that extrasensory experiences are a symptom of mental illness is enshrined in the DSM-IV criteria for schizotypal personality disorder, and this false assumption confounds all studies of schizophrenia spectrum disorders. The idea that hallucinations are always pathological, and presumably due to organic brain dysfunction, also pervades psychiatry and confounds research. The authors of this paper demonstrate these biases, and remark: "In medical practice, symptoms of an illness are usually assumed to be undesirable. It is notable, therefore, that more than one-half of the subjects in this study reported that their hallucinations served adaptive functions, and a sizable minority wished to continue experiencing the hallucinations."

The final sentence of the paper is: "The findings also suggest, but do not prove, that psychological factors contribute toward the expression of hallucinations in patients with psychotic illnesses." The possibility that hallucinations can be normal psychic phenomena, and not always pathological, is inconceivable to bioreductionist psychiatry, even when psychological factors are accepted. The paper illustrates pathologizing of normal human experience—a characteristic of contemporary psychiatry.

Faraone, S. V., Biederman, J., Lehman, B. K., Keenan, K., Norman, D., Seidman, L. J., Kolodny, R., Kraus, I., Perrin, J., & Chen, W. J. (1993). Evidence for the independent transmission of attention deficit hyperactivity disorder and learning disabilities: Results from a family genetic study. 150, 891–895.

This study could have been titled a family environmental study just as easily, because the methodology cannot differentiate genetic from environmental causes. The only reason to call it genetic is ideological bias, fueled by cognitive errors.

Cloninger, C. R. (1993). Unraveling the causal pathway to major depression. 150, 1137–1138.

Kendler, K. S., Kessler, R. C., Neale, M. C., Heath, A. C., & Eaves, L. J. (1993). The prediction of major depression in women: Toward an integrated etiological model. 150, 1139–1148.

In an editorial that precedes the Kendler et al. (1993) paper, Cloninger (1993) states of the study: "It was possible to draw etiologic conclusions about both genetic and environmental influences because the sample included both monozygotic and dizygotic twins." The Kendler study was a major project, and worth doing; however, the genetic factors included in the study are entirely artifactual.

Kendler et al. explain:

> The genetic liability to major depression was assessed by a dummy variable given the value of 0 if the co-twin had no history of major depression

and 1 if the co-twin had had one or more lifetime episodes. This dummy variable was multiplied by 1.0 if the twin pair was monozygotic and 0.5 if the twin pair was dizygotic. This method of modeling genetic effects in a regression analysis assumes that the familial transmission of the liability to major depression is largely due to additive genetic effects (which are correlated perfectly in monozygotic twins but only 0.5 in dizygotic twins).

If monozygotic twins have environments that are purely equal, while those of dizygotic twins are only half equal, and if the causes of depression are purely environmental, a similar dummy variable could be constructed to yield an environmental contribution to depression. The "genetic factor" in this study is a pure artifact that confirms its own assumptions through a tautology. The analysis should be redone with the dummy variable removed. This study should never be cited as providing any evidence of any kind on the genetics of depression. It is a worthwhile study of environmental factors, but nothing more.

Oliver, J. E. (1993). Intergenerational transmission of child abuse: Rates, research, and clinical implications. 150, 1315–1324.

This is a good paper. I include it here because the findings and the literature review could have been used to support the idea that there is a gene for child abuse, given that child abuse is clearly familial. This would be the usual bioreductionist inference from such data. This inference is never encountered in the child abuse literature because that literature is not driven by reductionist ideology. The putative gene for child abuse could be used as a defense in a court of law.

Walker, E. F., Grimes, K. E., Davis, D., & Smith, A. J. (1993). Childhood precursors of schizophrenia: Facial expressions of emotion. 150, 1654–1660.

The authors studied the facial expressions of adult schizophrenics in home movies taken during their childhoods, and compared them to childhood home movies of their healthy siblings. The authors viewed the reduced frequency of expressions of joy in the children who would later develop schizophrenia as early signs of the illness: "[T]he fact that these occur in the domain of emotion suggests that constitutional vulnerability to schizophrenia has implications for affective functioning long before the onset of clinical symptoms."

One could just as logically conclude that the subjects had a constitutional predisposition to joylessness, and that the schizophrenia was a secondary psychosocial consequence of being born with this constitution, in this culture, in these families. Alternatively, one could simply conclude that the schizophrenics received less love than their siblings, which caused both their joylessness and their schizophrenia. The data cannot differentiate between these two hypotheses versus the one the authors chose on ideological grounds.

> *Stoll, A. L., Tohen, M., Baldessarini, R. J., Goodwin, D. C., Stein, S., Katz, S., Geenens, D., Swinson, R. P., Goethe, J. W., & McGlashan, T. (1993). Shifts in diagnostic frequencies of schizophrenia and major affective disorder at six North American psychiatric hospitals. 150, 1972–1988.*

In this study, the authors found that diagnoses of schizophrenia declined from a peak of 27% of all diagnoses in 1976 to 9% in 1989, while major affective disorders rose from 10% in 1972 to 44% in 1990. The authors concluded: "Although a real decrease in new cases of schizophrenia may have occurred, this effect was probably minor and dominated by a larger shift of such diagnoses to affective categories." They also remarked: "The changes in the reported frequency of the disorders and their diagnostic criteria underscore the limited accuracy and usefulness of psychiatric diagnosis due to lack of knowledge of the etiological basis of major mental disorders."

The authors are saying that this major shift in diagnostic patterns was based predominantly on bias and ideology, not on science.

> *Goldman, S. J., D'Angelo, E. J., & DeMaso, D. R. (1993). Psychopathology in the families of children and adolescents with borderline personality disorder. 150, 1832–1835.*

The authors measured psychopathology in the relatives of 44 child and adolescent patients with borderline personality disorder and the relatives of 100 comparison subjects without that diagnosis. They found more depression, substance abuse, and antisocial behavior in the borderline relatives. Then, making a characteristic bioreductionist assumption, they reach a conclusion that is not supported by their data to the least degree:

> The impact of finding greater rates of family psychopathology associated with the diagnosis of borderline personality disorder in children is twofold. First, it suggests an associated biological diathesis. Numerous studies have shown that the rates of depression, substance abuse, and antisocial disorder are higher in the offspring of parents with those same disorders. We have demonstrated, for the first time, that children with borderline personality disorder appear to be at significant biological risk for the development of certain types of psychopathology.

> Second, and harder to evaluate, is the impact of familial psychopathology on the developmental experiences of these children. (p. 1834)

In fact, the environmental influences on these children are much easier to study than the biological ones, and the authors present data on environmental factors but none on biology. However, the authors have developed a rationale for reducing even demonstrated environmental factors to a genetic basis. They postulate that abusive behavior by parents is genetically driven:

> What appears to shine as a beacon through the foggy nature of this disorder is its association with abuse and parental psychopathology. This makes the next logical step the development of an etiologic hypothesis that is grounded in these factors. This hypothesis would initially build on the role of abuse and parental psychopathology in the development of the disorder in a biologically vulnerable population. It might then be refined to a more genetic type of critical environmental failure that, when combined with biological vulnerability, would be an etiologic factor across a wide range of developmental circumstances. (p. 1835)

By this logic, parents abuse their children because they are genetically driven to do so, and children develop psychiatric disorders in response to their childhood trauma because of biological vulnerability. The environment is reduced to a mere vector of biological determinism, and biology has become destiny. Eugenics follows logically as a "treatment intervention" from this biogenetic model, although, in the twenty-first century, the genetic interventions are expected to be "refined," involving genetic engineering rather than sterilization or execution.

THE STRONGEST BIOLOGICAL FINDINGS CORRELATE WITH SYMPTOMS, NOT DIAGNOSES

The ideology of bioreductionist psychiatry is that depression, schizophrenia, and other illnesses are biomedically distinct and genetically driven. Decades of fishing for supporting data have yielded nothing of substance, however. The meaningful biological findings in psychiatry and general medicine demonstrate correlations between biological variables and psychiatric symptoms—not illnesses—and these symptoms can occur in many different disorders. This means that even the findings of biological psychiatry are destroying the ideology that dominates the field.

| *Marin, R. S. (1990). Differential diagnosis and classification of apathy. 147, 22–30.*

In this review paper, the author notes that there is solid evidence for apathy occurring as a symptom of numerous biomedical illnesses, including Parkinson's disease, Korsakoff's syndrome, Huntington's chorea, progressive supranuclear palsy, akinetic mutism, delirium, dementia, Kluver–Bucy syndrome, hypoparathyroidism, the amotivational syndrome associated with chronic marijuana abuse, and a wide variety of drug toxicities. In psychiatry, apathy, when it occurs in schizophrenia, is considered to be a "negative symptom" of schizophrenia, and to have a specific genetic cause.

| *Jones, J. S., Stanley, B., Mann, J. J., Frances, A., Guido, J. R., Traksman-Bendz, L., Winchel, R., Brown, R. P., & Stanley, M. (1990). CSF 5-HIAA and HVA concentrations in elderly depressed patients who attempted suicide. 147, 1225–1227.*

This study compared the levels of metabolites of serotonin and dopamine in the cerebrospinal fluid of 12 depressed elderly people who had attempted suicide, 9 depressed elderly people who had not attempted suicide, and 7 controls. The study involves 28 subjects and 9 authors. The Bonferroni correction would eliminate all significant findings. There were no significant differences between the two clinical groups on any measures of psychopathology, including level of depression, but the suicidal group had lower levels of both metabolites. The implication drawn is that suicide is directly caused by a depletion of dopamine and serotonin, rather than by environmental stressors.

The biological finding therefore correlates with a *behavior* but not with diagnosis or level of symptomatology. One might object that this is not a strong finding, and argue that the paper should be included in the fishing expedition section.

| *Barta, P. E., Pearlson, G. D., Powers, R. E., Richards, S. S., & Tune, L. E. (1990). Auditory hallucinations and smaller superior temporal gyral volume in schizophrenia. 147, 1457–1462.*

The authors used MRI scans to measure different areas of the brain in 15 schizophrenics and 15 controls. They found a robust significant correlation ($r = 0.71$) between degree of difference in superior temporal gyrus volume (subjects versus controls) and degree of auditory hallucinations, but no significant correlation for somatic/tactile, visual, or olfactory hallucinations, a finding consistent with what is known about the brain and language. The diagnostic specificity of this finding requires replication in other diagnostic groups—most interestingly, dissociative identity disorder. As they stand, the data support a relationship between a symptom and a biological finding, but not a relationship with a diagnosis.

> *Darko, D. F., Risch, S. C., Gillin, J. C., & Golshan, S. (1992). Association of beta-endorphin with specific clinical symptoms of depression. 149, 1162–1167.*

Plasma endorphin levels were measured in 20 depressed patients and 23 controls, with no difference between groups. Within the pooled group of 43 subjects there were significant correlations between two clinical measures (psychic anxiety and phobia) and endorphin levels, out of five variables measured; out of the 20 depressed patients alone, there were significant correlations for three out of four (psychic anxiety, phobia, and obsessions/compulsions). The authors state in their discussion: "There were no significant correlations between beta-endorphin and the SADS interview items in the comparison group." One wonders whether the authors added the secondary analyses after getting a negative finding concerning their original hypothesis.

> *Goldman, M. B., Blake, L., Marks, R. C., Hedecker, D., & Luchins, D. J. (1993). Association of nonsuppression of cortisol on the DST with primary polydipsia in chronic schizophrenia. 150, 653–655.*

The authors found that the DST was positive in 38% of 13 polydipsic and 5% of 40 nonpolydipsic schizophrenics ($X2 = 6.9$, df $= 1$, $p < .01$ with Yates's correction). The same phenomenon might occur among nonschizophrenic subjects, if controls were included, confirming that the biological finding is diagnostically nonspecific.

BIOLOGICAL FISHING EXPEDITIONS WITH NO SIGNIFICANT FINDINGS

In a serious, developed scientific field, the pressure on journals to publish new findings leaves little or no room for studies with negative results. These either should not be published or should be included as letters to the editor, except for the occasional major failure to replicate an important previous piece of research. This is not the situation in psychiatry.

The American Journal of Psychiatry publishes numerous biological studies in which there are no significant results. This occurs because of ideological enthusiasm for reductionism, lack of critical thinking, an insufficient quantity of meaningful studies, and the mistaken idea that negative fishing expeditions are scientifically exciting. The gestalt of the published studies as a whole is a blunderbuss approach with everything possible (usually a neurotransmitter or hormone) being tested in every possible disorder.

It would be impossible to publish similar papers on topics to which mainstream psychiatry is ideologically hostile. Reviewers would simply dismiss such papers as meaningless because they contained no significant findings. In fact, significant findings that are ideologically offensive are more difficult to publish than insignificant results on favored and acceptable topics. The negative studies often have lengthy author lists.

> *Martinot, J-L., Pernon-Magnan, P., Huret, J-D., Mazoyer, B., Baron, J-C., Boulenger, J-P., Loch, C., Maziere, B., Caillard, V., Loo, H., & Syrota, A. (1990). Striatal D2 dopaminergic receptors assessed with positron emission tomography and 76Br bromospiperone in untreated schizophrenic patients. 147, 44–50.*

The authors did PET scans on 12 schizophrenics and 12 controls and found no differences in an indirect measure of striatal dopamine receptor density in the two groups. The discussion section of the paper occupies 216 lines.

> *Kaye, W. H., Ballenger, J. C., Lydiard, B., Stuart, G. W., Laraia, M. T., O'Neil, P., Fossey, M. D., Stevens, V., Lesser, S., & Hsu, G. (1990). CSF monoamine oxidase levels in normal-weight bulimia: Evidence for abnormal noradrenergic activity. 147, 225–229.*

The authors measured cerebrospinal fluid levels of HVA (a metabolite or breakdown product of dopamine), 5-HIAA (a metabolite of serotonin), and norepinephrine (also called noradrenalin) in 27 bulimics and 14 controls. These are currently fashionable neurotransmitters in psychiatry. They did 14 t tests and 14 Pearson correlations on their data, two of each kind of test being significant at $p < .05$. If they had applied the Bonferroni correction for multiple comparisons, there would have been no significant results, meaning that this paper belongs in the category of biological fishing.

The authors state in their introduction: "Theoretically, greater than normal noradrenergic activity or low serotonergic or dopaminergic activity could contribute to binge-eating." Without the Bonferroni correction applied, their findings were that there were no differences between bulimics and controls on dopaminergic and serotonergic activity, and that bulimics had lower noradrenergic activity than controls ($t = 2.24$, df $= 38$, $p < .03$)!

These negative findings did not constrain the authors from concluding: "We theorize that normal-weight bulimia is not a subtype of depressive disorder and should be considered an illness with a unique and characteristic neurobiological profile."

> *Pelonero, A. L., Pandurangi, A. K., & Calabrese, V. P. (1990).*
> *Autoantibodies to brain lipids in schizophrenia. 147, 661–662.*

In this study, levels of autoantibodies to brain lipids in 38 schizophrenics were compared to those in 22 controls, with no significant findings.

> *Lopez, O. L., Boller, F., Becker, J. T., Miller, M., & Reynolds,*
> *C. F. (1990). Alzheimer's disease and depression:*
> *Neuropsychological impairment and progression of the illness.*
> *147, 855–860.*

As stated in the abstract, "The authors longitudinally evaluated the cognitive functions of patients with probable Alzheimer's disease who also met criteria for major depression and compared them with matched patients with Alzheimer's disease who were not depressed." They found "no significant difference in the pattern of neuropsychological deficits between the two groups." This study involved 10 subjects and 10 controls, and would have never been published in *The American Journal of Psychiatry* if the subjects had a disorder presumed to be nonbiological in nature.

> *Jenike, M. A., Baer, L., Summergrad, P., Minichiello, W. E.,*
> *Holland, A., & Seymour, R. (1990). Sertraline in*
> *obsessive-compulsive disorder: A double-blind comparison*
> *with placebo. 147, 923–928.*

This drug study involved 10 subjects on sertraline and 9 on placebo. Findings were negative. The discussion is 196 lines long. Although this is a drug study, not a biological fishing expedition, I include it here because of the negative findings.

> *Tancer, M. E., Stein, M. B., Gelernter, C. S., & Uhde, T. W.*
> *(1990). The hypothalamic-pituitary axis in social phobia. 147,*
> *929–933.*

The authors compared 26 patients with social phobia and 26 controls and found: "There were no significant differences in measurements of T3, T4, free T4, or TSH between patients with social phobia and normal control subjects."

> *Andreasen, N. C., Swayze, V., Flaum, M., Alliger, R., & Cohen, G. (1990). Ventricular abnormalities in affective disorder: Clinical and demographic correlates. 147, 893–900.*

This study occupies 7 pages and has 73 references, yet the findings are negative. As stated in the abstract:

> Ventricular-brain ratio was measured by CT scan in 24 bipolar patients, 27 unipolar patients with major depression, 108 schizophrenic patients, and 75 normal control subjects. The male bipolar patients had significantly larger ventricles, but the depressive patients did not. The findings suggest the possibility that ventricular enlargement in bipolar patients is independent of age, as it appears to be in schizophrenia, whereas in depressed patients it may be related to the aging process. Ventricular enlargement in bipolar patients was not related to relevant clinical correlates, such as response to treatment, history of substance abuse, history of ECT, or cognitive impairment.

There were no significant findings between diagnostic groups, which shows that, in this sample, there is no biological specificity to ventricular-brain ratios with respect to psychiatric diagnosis. The groups were therefore divided into male and female subjects and 8 comparisons were done (4 diagnoses $\times$ 2 genders). Of these, only one was significant at $p < .01$, but this would not survive the Bonferroni correction for multiple comparisons. Subsequent to this, another analysis with age as a covariate was done. The amount of speculation in the paper can be inferred from the abstract.

> *Mayerhoff, D. I., Lieberman, J. A., Lemus, C. Z., Pollack, S., & Schneider, B. S. (1990). Growth hormone response to growth hormone-releasing hormone in schizophrenic patients. 147, 1072–1074.*

The authors compared growth hormone function in 10 schizophrenics and 5 controls: "No significant differences between the schizophrenic and control groups were found on any of the variables." The discussion section is quoted here in full because of its surrealistic quality:

> The GH responses to GH-RH elicited in the control subjects and schizophrenic patients appear to be consistent with those reported in

normal subjects in the endocrinologic literature. The data suggest that the pituitary somatotrophic cells in patients with schizophrenia are capable of normal GH responses when stimulated directly. The results of this pilot study are consistent with the hypothesis that pathology at a level above the pituitary affects GH responses to dopamine agonists in schizophrenia. However, these findings must be viewed as preliminary because of the low statistical power resulting from the small number of subjects. The importance of applying the method used in this study to a larger sample is that any abnormalities found in GH responses of schizophrenic patients can be better localized in the brain.

Besides confirming these results by the study of larger numbers of subjects, future research in this area should also use selective pharmacologic probes for possible neurotransmitters that regulate GH-RH secretion from the hypothalamus. These measurements of GH should be coupled with GH-RH stimulations of GH in the same subjects in order to obtain a more complete characterization of neuroendocrine function in schizophrenia.

For those who have only time to read the abstract, the authors' key conclusion is: "The results suggest suprapituitary dysfunction in schizophrenia, but replication in a larger study is required."

The authors are emphasizing the importance of the replication of their negative findings in one area of the brain based on the assumption that this means positive findings will later be confirmed elsewhere in the brain—in this instance, at a level above the pituitary gland. Logically, this is equivalent to stating that analysis of one quadrant of the haystack suggests that the needle must be in another quadrant, although replication is required. Positive morale and continued funding for such research depend absolutely on the conviction that there is a needle to find, which is a matter of faith, not empirical science.

Roy, A., DeJong, J., Ferraro, T., Adinoff, B., Ravitz, B., & Linnoila, M. (1990). CSF gamma-aminobutyric acid in alcoholics and control subjects. 147, 1294–1296.

Cerebrospinal fluid levels of GABA were measured in 53 dry alcoholics and 22 controls and did not differ.

Sharma, R. P., Janicak, P. G., Javaid, J. I., Pandey, G. N., Gierl, B., & Davis, J. M. (1990). Platelet MAO inhibition, urinary MHPG, and leukocyte beta-adrenergic receptors in depressed patients treated with phenelzine. 147, 1318–1321.

Various biochemical variables were measured in 36 depressed inpatients treated with phenelzine. Except for confirmation of the known fact that phenelzine reduces levels of monoamine oxidase, which is not a publishable result, there were no significant findings.

> *Flaum, M., Arndt, S., & Andreasen, N. C. (1990). The role of gender in studies of ventricle enlargement in schizophrenia: A predominantly male effect. 147, 1327–1332.*

Brain ventricle size was measured by MRI or CT scan in four different studies with a total of more than 200 subjects and 200 controls. There were no significant findings.

> *Mutchler, K., Crowe, R. R., Noyes, R., & Wesner, R. W. (1990). Exclusion of the tyrosine hydroxylase gene in 14 panic disorder pedigrees. 147, 1367–1369.*

This genetic study yielded no significant findings in 145 individuals in 14 pedigrees, and this was conceptualized as an important exclusion.

> *Nelson, J. C., Mazure, C. M., & Jatlow, P. I. (1990). Value of the DST for predicting response of patients with major depression to hospitalization and desipramine. 147, 1488–1492.*

The authors did dexamethasone suppression tests on 51 depressed patients treated with desipramine, and found no differences between DST-positive and DST-negative subjects in response to hospitalization or medication.

> *Bowers, M. B. (1991). Characteristics of psychotic inpatients with high or low HVA levels at admission. 148, 240–243.*

The author measured pretreatment homovanillic acid levels in 85 psychotic inpatients and found only one significant result out of 25 different dependent variables measured separately in high and low HVA groups, with these two groups subdivided into male and female for all comparisons. This one significant finding, at $p < .05$ out of 100 analyses, is a chance finding.

> *Darko, D. F., Wilson, N. W., Gillin, J. C., & Golshan, S. (1991). A critical appraisal of mitogen-induced lymphocyte proliferation in depressed patients. 148, 337–344.*

The authors measured in vitro proliferation of lymphocytes in reaction to stimulants called mitogens, using blood from 23 depressed patients and 23 controls. There were no significant differences between the two groups. They conducted numerous nonsignificant secondary analyses on various subgroups of subjects, and got one spurious statistically significant finding on a subgroup of 10 patients.

| *Garver, D. L., Bissette, G., Yao, J. K., & Nemeroff, C. B. (1991). Relation of CSF neurotensin concentrations to symptoms and drug response of psychotic patients. 148, 484–488.*

Twenty patients with mood-incongruent psychoses and 6 controls were compared on cerebrospinal fluid neurotensin levels, with no significant findings. Significant subsidiary analyses would not survive the Bonferroni correction for multiple comparisons. This is a repeated pattern in fishing expeditions with negative findings in the primary analysis: the authors then conduct numerous subanalyses and discuss a handful of statistically significant findings at length without correcting for chance.

| *Christenson, G. A., MacKenzie, T. B., Mitchell, J. E., & Callies, A. L. (1991). A placebo-controlled double-blind crossover study of fluoxetine in trichotillomania. 148, 1566–1571.*

Fluoxetine (Prozac) was found to be no more effective than placebo in treatment of chronic hair pulling. The discussion section is 215 lines long.

| *McNeil, T. F., Blennow, G., & Lundberg, L. (1992). Congenital malformations and structural developmental anomalies in groups at high risk for psychosis. 149, 57–61.*

The authors compared the rates of congenital malformations in the offspring of 84 women with histories of nonorganic psychosis, and those of 100 control women, and found no significant differences between groups. Yet, in their abstract, the authors state: "The inferred genetic risk for psychosis does not appear to be associated with greater rates of early somatic developmental anomalies, suggesting that early developmental anomalies do not represent an expression of genetic influence toward psychosis." This is a good example of how negative findings do not inhibit reductionist editorializing or the faith in a genetic predisposition to psychosis.

In their final paragraph, the authors reiterate their belief in an established genetic risk for psychosis: "[T]he findings appear more to suggest that there is no relation between greater genetic risk and the occurrence of congenital malformations." A parsimonious explanation of the negative finding is that the study has no bearing on whether there is a genetic factor in schizophrenia.

Nothen, M. M., Erdman, J., Korner, J., Lanczik, M., Fritze, J., Fimmers, R., Grandy, D. K., O'Dowd, B., & Propping, P. (1992). Lack of association between dopamine D1 and D2 receptor genes and bipolar affective disorder. 149, 199–201.

This paper is one of five biological fishing expeditions (out of 16 papers in the issue) with no significant findings, in the February 1992 issue of the *Journal*. The authors tested 56 bipolar patients and 69 controls for restriction fragment length polymorphism alleles at the D1 and D2 receptor loci, and found no differences between the two groups.

Simeon, D., Stanley, B., Frances, A., Mann, J. J., Winchel, R., & Stanley, M. (1992). Self-mutilation in personality disorders: Psychological and biological correlates. 149, 221–226.

This is a negative fishing expedition disguised with spurious statistically significant findings. The authors measured cerebrospinal fluid 5-HIAA levels and platelet imipramine binding and affinity sites in 26 self-mutilators and 26 controls. The two groups did not differ on CSF 5-HIAA, number of platelet imipramine binding sites, or imipramine affinity. The positive finding was two significant correlations, between number of platelet imipramine receptor sites and self-mutilation and impulsivity, in the self-mutilator group but not the controls, at $p < .05$, out of 15 correlations reported. 5-HIAA levels did not correlate significantly with any clinical variable in either group, yet the authors concluded in their abstract that their results "provide preliminary support for the hypothesis of underlying serotonergic dysfunction facilitating self-mutilation."

Garber, H. J., & Rivto, E. R. (1992). Magnetic resonance imaging of the posterior fossa in autistic adults. 149, 245–247.

Twelve autistic adults and 12 controls were compared on MRI scans of a number of different brain regions, with no differences between groups.

Kumar, A., Yousem, D., Souder, E., Miller, D., Gotlieb, G., Gur, R., & Alavi, A. (1992). High-intensity signals in Alzheimer's disease without cerebrovascular risk factors: A magnetic resonance imaging evaluation. 149, 248–250.

There were no differences between 16 Alzheimer's patients and 23 controls on MRI brain scan.

Pomara, N., Singh, R., Deptula, D., Chu, J. C.-Y., Schwartz, M. B., & LeWitt, P. A. (1992). Glutamate and other CSF amino acids in Alzheimer's disease. 149, 251–254.

The authors measured the levels of 20 amino acids in the cerebrospinal fluid of 10 Alzheimer's patients and 10 controls. There were five significant differences out of 20 comparisons at $p < .05$, but two showed higher levels in the Alzheimer's group, and three showed lower. None of these findings was significant with the Bonferroni correction applied, which the authors failed to do. They ignored the three amino acids that were lower in the Alzheimer's group, and stated in their abstract: "The authors speculate that the excitotoxic effects of glutamate may contribute to progressive neuronal loss in Alzheimer's disease."

Gorman, J. M., Warne, P. A., Begg, M. D., Cooper, T. B., Novacenko, H., Williams, J. B., Rabkin, J., Stern, Y., & Ehrhardt, A. A. (1992). Serum prolactin levels in homosexual and bisexual men with HIV infection. 149, 367–370.

The authors compared 121 HIV-positive and 79 HIV-negative men on serum prolactin levels with no significant findings.

Wang, Z. W., Crowe, R. R., & Noyes, R. (1992). Adrenergic receptor genes as candidate genes for panic disorder: A linkage study. 149, 470–474.

Various adrenergic receptor loci were studied in 14 panic disorder pedigrees with no significant results. Because this was a genetic linkage study, the authors could conceptualize it as an important exclusion study: this conceptualization, of course, requires the prior assumption that panic disorder is inherited.

Brown, F. W., Lewine, R. J., Hudgins, P. A., & Risch, S. C. (1992). White matter hyperintensity signals in psychiatric and nonpsychiatric subjects. 149, 620–625.

Brain MRI scans of 229 psychiatric patients and 154 controls yielded no significant findings.

Zilbovicius, M., Garreau, B., Tzourio, N., Mazoyer, B., Bruck, B., Martinot, J.-L., Raynaud, C., Samson, Y., Syrota, A., & Lelord, G. (1992). Regional cerebral blood flow in childhood autism: A SPECT study. 149, 924–930.

Brain scans of 21 autistic children and 14 controls showed no significant findings. The study had 10 authors and 35 subjects.

Geracioti, T. D., Liddle, R. A., Altemus, M., Demitrack, M. A., & Gold, P. W. (1992). Regulation of appetite and cholecystokinin secretion in anorexia nervosa. 149, 958–961.

Six patients and 6 controls showed no significant differences on plasma cholecystokinin levels.

Birmaher, B., Dahl, R. E., Ryan, N. D., Rabinovich, H., Ambrosini, P., Al-Shabbout, M., Novacenko, H., Nelson, B., & Puig-Antich, J. (1992). The dexamethasone suppression test in adolescent outpatients with major depressive disorder. 149, 1040–1045.

The DST was given to 44 depressed and 38 control adolescents with no significant differences between groups.

Gelertner, J., Kennedy, J. L., Grandy, D. K., Zhou, Q.-Y., Civelli, O., Pauls, D. L., Pakstis, A., Kurlan, R., Sunahara, R. K., Niznik, H. B., O'Dowd, B., Seeman, P., & Kidd, K. K. (1993). Exclusion of close linkage of Tourette's syndrome to D1 dopamine receptor. 150, 449–453.

The authors established that Tourette's syndrome is not linked to the D1 receptor gene. In the abstract the authors stated: "This exclusion extends the authors' earlier work with the dopamine system in Tourette's syndrome to exclude the two best characterized dopamine receptors from linkage with Tourette's syndrome."

Gorman, J. M., Papp, L. A., Coplan, J., Martinez, J., Liebowitz, M. R., & Klein, D. F. (1993). The effect of acetazolamide on ventilation in panic disorder patients. 150, 1480–1484.

The authors replicated a previous finding that acetazolamide has no effect on panic patients.

Kertzner, R. M., Goetz, R., Todak, G., Cooper, T., Lin, S.-H., Reddy, M. M., Novacenko, H., Williams, J. B., Ehrhardt, A. A., & Gorman, J. M. (1993). Cortisol levels, immune status, and mood in homosexual men with and without HIV infection. 150, 1674–1678.

The authors found no differences between HIV-positive and HIV-negative subjects.

STATISTICALLY SIGNIFICANT FINDINGS OF DOUBTFUL CLINICAL SIGNIFICANCE

In many biological papers, there are statistically significant findings, but the magnitude of the differences is of doubtful clinical or biological meaning. Irrelevant statistically significant results are often reported when they do not support the study hypothesis, and when there were no significant findings concerning the key study variables. Considerable effort is often expended to disguise the fact that the results have no real meaning by hiding things in sections on methods or results, not mentioning them in the discussion, creating statistical artifacts, or glossing over the negative findings.

All of this is evidence of ideology driving the field, rather than disinterested curiosity. The effort is to support the cognitive errors analyzed in the previous chapter, not to understand nature. Many of these papers could be characterized as biological fishing expeditions with significant findings.

> *Denicoff, K. D., Joffe, R., Lakshmanan, M. C., Robbins, J., & Rubinow, D. R. (1990). Neuropsychiatric manifestations of altered thyroid state. 147, 94–99.*

As stated in the abstract: "The authors assessed the mood and cognitive effects of sequential T4, T3, and withdrawal of thyroid replacement on 25 patients who had had thyroidectomies for cancer." T3 and T4 are two different forms of thyroid hormone. The problem with the study is imbedded in the tables but not discussed. The main measure of depressed mood used was the Beck Depression Inventory (BDI). To be clinically depressed and enrolled in a drug study, one should usually score above 20 on the BDI, and one will be counted as a drug responder if the score drops to 10 by study end.

The Beck scores of the 25 subjects when not on thyroid replacement averaged 10.14 (S.D. 8.78), compared to 5.50 (S.D. 6.40) on T4 and 5.42 (S.D. 5.53) on T3. An ANOVA on these figures was significant ($F = 12.14$; $df = 2.36$; $p < .01$). The problem is that scores of 5 and 10 are not meaningfully different clinically. Out of 25 patients, only 2 had BDI scores above 20 when not on thyroid replacement, and only 2 experienced BDI score increases of greater than 10 when taken off one of the two forms of thyroid hormone.

It is doubtful that blind independent clinicians could correctly assign these subjects to on-thyroid or not-on-thyroid replacement groups at a level above chance, based on assessment of depression symptoms alone. The depressive response to low thyroid hormone levels should be one of the most robust and clinically meaningful findings in all of biological psychiatry, but it is in fact very weak.

Another problem with this study is that BDI scores reported to *one* decimal place, let alone two, are meaningless, because the precision of the BDI does not permit such fine discrimination.

Gillin, J. C., Smith, T. L., Irwin, M., Kripke, D. F., Brown, S., & Shuckit, M. (1990). Short REM latency in primary alcoholic patients with secondary depression. 147, 106–109.

This study looks good on first glance, but closer inspection reveals a serious problem. The study was done in a sleep laboratory with sleep EEGs performed on alcoholics with secondary depressions (N = 12), alcoholics without secondary depressions (N = 21), and controls (N = 31). The Bonferroni correction for multiple comparisons was used, but it was applied in a fashion that made insignificant results appear significant. Significance was set at $p < .05$ and Newman–Keuls tests were done on the dependent variables for the three groups. In the table, 34 variables were presented, which means that the corrected significance level should be $p < .0015$. There would then be only one significant difference between groups, which is in the total amount of non-REM sleep.

Instead, the authors applied the Bonferroni correction "on 23 sleep measures on which analyses of variance were performed," which could be regarded as reasonable, given that the other variables in the table are demographic or clinical. This would yield a corrected significance level of $p < .0022$. Using this significance level, the total amount of sleep time (REM plus non-REM) also becomes significant at $p < .002$). However, these results are meaningless, so the authors salvaged significance for the variables they wanted to differ between groups by limiting the Bonferroni correction to only "the five sleep measures of particular interest." Now significance was set at $p < .01$, and the key variable of short REM latency, which ties into sleep findings in the depression literature, became significant.

However, REM latency itself was still not significant ($p < .02$), so the authors constructed a variable they called corrected REM latency, which just made significance at $p < .01$. Corrected REM latency is calculated by subtracting the intervening awake time from the REM latency. For those unfamiliar with sleep physiology, REM latency is the period of time between falling asleep and the onset of the first period of REM sleep, and is shorter than normal in clinically depressed patients.

To get statistical significance, the authors of this study had to pull a statistical sleight of hand with the Bonferroni correction and then create a dummy variable. Yet they titled their paper *Short REM Latency in Primary Alcoholic Patients with Secondary Depression* and opened their discussion with these sentences: "These results are consistent with the concept that short REM latency is a biological state marker associated with formally diagnosed (i.e., by DSM-III criteria) depression, secondary as well as primary or endogenous. It should be noted that REM latency was not correlated with scores on the Hamilton depression scale."

Coffey, C. E., Figiel, G. S., Djang, W. T., & Weiner, R. D. (1990). Subcortical hyperintensity on magnetic resonance imaging: A comparison of normal and depressed elderly subjects. 147, 187–189.

In this study, MRI scans were done on 35 depressed elderly patients referred for ECT with no neurological history, 16 depressed elderly patients referred for ECT who had histories of neurological problems, and 22 controls. The authors did this study because "the significance of subcortical hyperintensity in patients with depression remains unclear." They wanted to control for the effect of neurological problems, which was a good idea. They found significant differences between the group of depressed with no neurological history and the controls, on number of subjects with grade 2 or grade 3 MRI changes (chi square = 4.9, df = 1, p < .03). However, they excluded subjects with grade 1 changes from the analysis, although these are reported in the table. Of the controls, 77% showed grade 1 periventricular hyperintensity, compared to 43% of the nonneurological subjects and 25% of the neurological subjects; 64% of controls showed grade 1 deep white matter hyperintensity, compared to 37% of the nonneurological subjects and 19% of the neurological subjects. This is the reverse of the pattern for grade 2 and grade 3 changes.

The explanation for exclusion of grade 1 subjects was: "On the basis of the reported occurrence and severity of subcortical hyperintensity in normal elderly subjects, we hypothesized that grade 2 and grade 3 periventricular and deep white matter hyperintensity would be more common in our depressed inpatients than in the control group." Did they really mean that failure to exclude grade 1 changes would introduce too much noise and threaten significance? The decision to exclude grade 1 subjects makes both the findings and the methodology questionable.

Karasjgi, B., Rifkin, A., Doddi, S., & Kolli, R. (1990). The prevalence of anxiety disorders in patients with chronic obstructive pulmonary disease. 147, 200–201.

The authors interviewed 50 subjects with chronic obstructive pulmonary disease and found a lifetime prevalence of anxiety disorders of 16%, compared to 15% in the general population. They observed that 8% of their subjects had panic disorder, however, compared to 1.5% of the general population, which they considered to be significant, although they did not do a statistical test such as a z score to determine whether this was actually significant. They also noted a lifetime prevalence of mood disorders of 18% in their sample, but did not return to this at all in the discussion section. Nor did they point out the reciprocal of their finding concerning panic disorder—namely, that 7% of their sample had nonpanic anxiety disorders compared to 13.5% of the general population. Finally, they did not say anything about the age at onset of the panic disorder in their subjects which, given the natural history of panic disorder and obstructive lung disease, was probably 20 to 30 years before the onset of pulmonary symptoms (the mean age of their subjects was 64.96 years, S.D. 9.70).

If age-at-onset data were included, the findings would be that obstructive lung disease has an onset decades later than mood and anxiety disorders; that the rate of mood and anxiety disorders is equal in their sample and no different from the general population; and that a future history of lung disease protects against the onset of nonpanic anxiety disorders occurring decades earlier. These are meaningless findings. The authors, as could be predicted from the title of their paper, discuss bioreductionist theories of panic focused on the locus ceruleus, and try to connect the physiology of chronic obstructive pulmonary disease to that of panic disorder.

Siever, L. J., Keefe, R., Bernstein, D. P., Coccaro, E. F., Klar, H. M., Zemishlany, Z., Peterson, A. E., Davidson, M., Mahon, T., & Mohs, R. (1990). Eye tracking impairment in clinically identified patients with schizotypal personality disorder. 147, 740–745.

The authors of this paper concluded from their data: "[O]ur results are the first to demonstrate impaired tracking in clinically identified schizotypal patients and thus support the hypothesis that schizotypal personality disorder, as diagnosed in clinical settings, may be considered a schizophrenia-related disorder." Abnormalities of eye tracking have been shown to correlate with schizophrenia in previous research, which I am not disputing. The problem here is with differential reporting of statistical analyses to support the bioreductionist concept of the schizophrenia spectrum.

The authors measured smooth eye pursuit movement in 26 subjects with clinically diagnosed schizotypal personality disorder, 17 with other personality disorders, 44 with schizophrenia, and 29 controls. They did not address the problem of the low interrater reliability of even the most rigorous structured-interview Axis II diagnoses, which is crucial for their research. They did report the rates of other personality disorders in their two key groups, however, which were as follows:

	Schizotypal Group: Percent Positive	Other Personality Disorder Group: Percent Positive
Paranoid	53.8%	—
Borderline	38.5	52.9%
Histrionic	23.1	41.2
Avoidant	23.1	11.8
Antisocial	19.2	5.9
Compulsive	19.2	47.1
Schizoid	7.7	—
Dependent	3.8	11.8
Mixed	—	17.7
Narcissistic	—	17.7
Passive-Aggressive	—	5.9

The authors did not report whether there were any significant differences between the two groups on the rates of any of these other personality disorders; to do so would have called their conclusions into question. It is obvious by visual inspection that chi-square analyses would reveal no significant difference in the frequency of many of the personality disorders in the two groups. Like the extensive overall Axis II comorbidity of both groups, this is a crucial limitation of their study.

In their analyses of the eye-tracking findings, the authors pointed out that the schizotypal and schizophrenia groups both differed from normal controls, but the other personality disorder group did not. However, they strategically failed to report the result of comparing the schizotypal and schizophrenic groups to the other personality disorder group, which is nonsignificant, saying only that "mean qualitative ratings for the patients with other personality disorders were intermediate between those of the schizotypal and normal control cohorts." The data are as follows:

	Eye Tracking Value	
	Mean	S.D.
Schizotypal	2.9	0.8
Other personality	2.6	0.7
Schizophrenia	3.0	0.9
Control	2.1	0.6

The data show that there is no significant difference among the three clinical groups; therefore one could as easily conclude, logically, that schizophrenia is a personality disorder. Instead, the authors reach a reductionist conclusion:

> The finding of impaired tracking in schizotypal patients is consistent with evidence from other studies suggesting that schizotypal personality disorder may be related to schizophrenia with respect to its genetics, biology, treatment response, and outcome. The refinement of biological measures with a substantial genetic basis such as eye tracking in schizotypal patients and control subjects thus may enhance resolution of selection of affected phenotypes in molecular genetic linkage studies of schizophrenia, as well as advance our knowledge of the pathophysiology of the schizophrenia-related disorders.

It is remarkable how many of the cognitive errors analyzed in the previous chapter are packed into these two sentences.

Southwick, S. M., Yehuda, R., Giller, E. L., & Perry, B. D. (1990). Altered platelet alpha-2-adrenergic receptor binding sites in borderline personality disorder. 147, 1014–1017.

In this study, 13 nonmedicated borderlines, 11 borderlines medicated with benzodiazepines, and 18 controls were assayed for platelet alpha-2-adrenergic binding sites. The anxiety subscale scores on the Hamilton Depression Scale (HAM-D) of the two borderline groups did not differ. The finding was that the nonmedicated borderlines had fewer receptors than the other two groups, which the authors speculated might be due to down-regulation of receptors by the greater catecholamine release occurring in the nonmedicated borderlines. This doesn't make any sense. The effect should occur only if the nonmedicated group is more anxious and therefore releasing more catecholamines. The data are in the opposite direction of the conclusion.

To support their conclusion, the authors did correlational analyses separately in the two borderline groups, and found that there was a significant correlation between HAM-D anxiety subscore and receptor density at one of 2 sites where assays were done, but no significant correlation at either site in the medicated group. This is an artifact that is overridden by the lack of difference in anxiety between the two groups.

Walker, E., & Lewine, R. J. (1990). Prediction of adult-onset schizophrenia from childhood home movies of the patients. 147, 1052–1056.

This is an interesting study in which blind raters tried to predict adult schizophrenia from watching home movies from childhood of schizophrenic patients and their siblings. In the analysis used by the authors, they obtained significant diagnostic hit rates for 1 sibship on 2 out of 4 film segments, and on 1 sibship on 1 out of 2 segments. There were 4 patients and 5 unaffected siblings; films of 2 siblings were reviewed for 1 patient. Four different segments at different ages were reviewed for each of 3 patients, and 2 segments for the patient with 2 siblings. Altogether, 302 judgments of schizophrenic versus non-schizophrenic were made by the varying numbers of independent raters for each sibship.

Out of these 302 judgments, there were 84 true positive, 45 false positive, 111 true negative, and 58 false negative diagnoses made (I had to calculate these figures from the table; they were not given). This means that the overall rate of agreement between adult clinical diagnosis and diagnosis by childhood home movies was 195/302 = 65%. Applying Cohen's kappa to this result yields an interrater reliability of kappa = 0.30, which is not clinically significant. This paper is included in this section because the findings are of doubtful clinical significance using the authors' analyses, and of no significance when overall hit rate corrected for chance is calculated.

Breier, A., Wolkowitz, O. M., Roy, A., Potter, W., & Pickar, D. (1990). Plasma norepinephrine in chronic schizophrenia. 147, 1467–1470.

This study involves measurement of plasma and cerebrospinal fluid (CSF) norepinephrine levels resting and standing in 14 schizophrenics and 33 controls. A variety of positive results are presented but they obscure the core finding, which is no difference between the two groups on CSF levels. The significant findings were limited to plasma and correlations between CSF and plasma levels. The plasma levels have nothing to do with the brain or any possible brain pathology in schizophrenia.

Yet, undaunted, the authors concluded: "Thus, it is possible that the above-normal peripheral sympathetic nervous system activity found in this and other studies of schizophrenia reflects altered central processes involving dopaminergic and noradrenergic function."

Spivak, B., Radwan, M., Brandon, J., Molcho, A., Ohring, R., Tyano, S., & Weizman, A. (1991). Cold agglutinin autoantibodies in psychiatric patients: Their relation to diagnosis and pharmacological treatment. 148, 244–247.

The authors measured cold agglutinin titers, which are indirect indicators of infection and autoimmune activity, in 90 schizophrenics, 54 bipolar patients, and 22 subjects with depression. They found positive titers in 42.4% of the schizophrenics, 11.1% of the bipolars, and 8.1% of the depressives, which was statistically significant. They noted, however, that, "titers up to 1:4, such as were found in our patients, are not considered to be evidence of pathology, and can be found in healthy populations too." Their finding had no biological meaning.

Yehuda, R., Lowy, M. T., Southwick, S. M., Shaffer, D., & Giller, E. L. (1991). Lymphocyte glucocorticoid receptor number in posttraumatic stress disorder. 148, 499–504.

In this study, 15 Vietnam vets with posttraumatic stress disorder were compared to 11 controls on serum cortisol levels alone, correlation of cortisol levels with glucocorticoid receptor densities, and receptor densities alone. The only significant finding was in number of receptors, but given the lack of differences on the other two measures, this finding is of dubious biological significance.

Volkow, N. D., Fowler, J. S., Wolf, A. P., Hitzemann, R., Dewey, S., Bendriem, B., Alpert, R., & Hoff, A. (1991). Changes in brain glucose metabolism in cocaine dependence and withdrawal. 148, 621–626.

The authors measured brain metabolism in cocaine addicts at 1 week and again at 2 to 4 weeks postwithdrawal using PET scans. There were 17 addicts and 15 controls. The two groups differed significantly only at week one. Although this is interesting, it must be attributed to biologically nonspecific characteristics of the withdrawal state pending further research, which must include withdrawal from various substances. Additionally, the finding of increased activity in the orbitofrontal cortex and basal ganglia, noted during week one of cocaine withdrawal, has also been observed in obsessive-compulsive disorder, according to the authors. This fact completely erodes any biological specificity to the finding in the cocaine addicts.

Lewine, R. J., Risch, S. C., Risby, E., Stipetic, M., Jewart, D., Eccard, M., Caudle, J., & Pollard, W. (1991). Lateral ventricle–brain ratio and balance between CSF HVA and 5-HIAA in schizophrenia. 148, 1189–1194.

The authors compared 45 patients with schizophrenia, 28 with mood disorders, and 91 controls on ventricle–brain ratio (VBR), HVA, and 5-HIAA, with no significant findings. In a subsidiary analysis, they found that the ratio of HVA to 5-HIAA was significantly correlated with VBR, however, and they were able to construct reasons for this being a publishable finding, despite its questionable biological meaning.

Siever, L. J., Amin, F., Coccaro, E. F., Bernstein, D., Kavoussi, R. J., Kalus, O., Horvath, T. B., Warne, P., Davidson, M., & Davis, K. L. (1991). Plasma homovanillic acid in schizotypal personality disorder. 148, 1246–1248.

The authors measured plasma HVA, which has no consistent relationship with psychiatrically significant levels of HVA in the brain, in 11 subjects with schizotypal personality disorder, 7 with other personality disorders, and 6 controls. They found that the schizotypal group differed from the controls, and concluded: "These findings suggest dopaminergic mechanisms underlying the psychotic-like symptoms of schizotypal personality disorder and support the concept that the psychotic-like symptoms of schizotypal personality disorder and psychotic symptoms of schizophrenia are not only phenomenologically similar but are biologically related as well."

The problem with the study is that the other personality disorder group did not differ from either the schizotypal group or the controls. HVA levels were: schizotypal 12.9 (S.D., 4.60); other personality disorders 9.1 (S.D., 2.53); and controls 7.8 (S.D., 1.30). This pattern was observed in other studies published over the four-year period. One could as well conclude that symptoms of other personality disorders are biologically normal, or alternatively, that they are related to the biology of schizophrenia. For the authors' conclusions to make sense, the other personality disorder group *must* be no different from controls and significantly different from schizotypals.

Those not familiar with DSM-IV criteria might be alarmed to know that the symptoms of biologically driven schizophrenia-spectrum brain illness listed in DSM-IV under criteria for schizotypal personality disorder include "odd beliefs or magical thinking that influence behavior and are inconsistent with subcultural norms (e.g., superstitiousness, belief in clairvoyance, telepathy, or "sixth sense . . . ."

This study had 24 subjects and 10 authors.

Cartwright, R. D., Kravitz, H. M., Eastman, C. I., & Wood, E. (1991). REM latency and the recovery from depression: Getting over divorce. 148, 1530–1535.

The authors measured REM latency in 100 subjects who were undergoing marital separation; of these, 70 were clinically depressed. The study was interesting and well done, but the finding directly contradicts all previous biological thinking about the significance of shortened REM latency in depression, a replicated and consistent finding. Shortened REM latency is supposed to tap into the diagnostically specific biology of depression. The problem is that, in this study, shortened REM latency predicted a better outcome at one-year followup. This author concluded: "Depressed individuals with normal REM latencies may need more aggressive treatment interventions." According to this logic, being biologically normal is a sign of being psychiatrically sicker.

Bajwa, W. K., Asnis, G. M., Sanderson, W. C., Irfan, A., & van Praag, H. M. (1992). High cholesterol levels in patients with panic disorder. 149, 376–378.

The authors compared cholesterol levels in 30 patients with panic disorder, 30 with depression, and 30 controls. The cholesterol levels of the panic patients were significantly higher: mean of 224.7 (S.D., 43.5) compared to 189.8 (S.D., 32.8) for depression and 183.6 (S.D., 37.7) for controls (F = 10.10; df = 2, 87; p < .001), but "the cholesterol levels of the patients with panic disorder as a group remained within the normal range (150–250 mg/dl). In addition, we did not measure high-density lipoprotein (HDL) or low-density lipoprotein (LDL) cholesterol levels, which are considered to be more specifically correlated with risk of coronary artery disease."

Wu, J. C., Gillin, J. C., Buchsbaum, M. S., Hershey, T., Johnson, J. C., & Bunney, W. E. (1992). Effect of sleep deprivation on brain metabolism of depressed patients. 149, 538–543.

The authors did PET scans on 15 depressed patients and 15 controls. There were 18 comparisons, and no findings would survive the Bonferroni correction. This paper is noteworthy because in the main table the authors reported that, for some brain regions, the sleep-deprivation responders had a higher baseline metabolic rate than the nonresponders; of these comparisons, they noted that the finding was not significant after application of the Bonferroni correction for only one comparison, when that was true for all data in the study. This is an example of selective application of the Bonferroni correction within a single table, which violates the most elementary rules of scientific research. The Bonferroni correction was perhaps not applied to the cingulate findings in this study because: "In a previous study [by the same group], the cingulate gyrus was the only cortical structure with a significantly higher glucose metabolic rate during REM sleep than during the normal waking state."

Williamson, P., Pelz, D., Merskey, H., Morrison, S., Karlik, S., Drost, D., Carr, T., & Conlon, P. (1992). Frontal, temporal, and striatal proton relaxation times in schizophrenic patients and normal comparison subjects. 149, 549–551.

This is a good study with no methodological problems or reductionist editorializing. MRI values in a specific brain region were significantly different, in a comparison of 10 schizophrenics and 10 controls. I include it because, in the footnotes to the table, each of 5 statistical footnotes states that the findings were significant after correction for multiple comparisons. This paper appeared in the same issue as the previous paper, therefore this quality of methodology should have been demanded of the Wu et al. (1992) paper as well.

> Lydiard, R. B., Ballenger, J. C., Laraia, M. T., Fossey, M. D., & Beinfeld, M. C. (1992). CSF cholecystokinin concentrations in patients with panic disorder and in normal comparison subjects. 149, 691–693.

CSF cholecystokinin levels were compared in 25 panic patients and 16 controls. The findings were statistically significant but the difference in absolute values and the size of the *t* statistic make the findings of doubtful biological significance. The patients had a mean value of 20.6 (S.D., 7.7) and the controls 16.2 (S.D., 5.9) (t = 2.05, df = 39, p < .05).

> Petitto, J. M., Folds, J. D., Ozer, H., Quade, D., & Evans, D. L. (1992). Abnormal diurnal variation in circulating natural killer cell phenotypes and cytotoxic activity in major depression. 149, 694–696.

The authors measured immunological variables in 24 depressed patients and 24 controls. They studied two immunological cell markers, Leu-7 and Leu-11, and found more diurnal variation in cell activity in normals than in patients for one type of cell, but not for the other. They could not account for the difference between cell types and did not comment on the biological meaning of their finding.

> Luchins, D. J., Cohen, D., Hanrahan, P., Eisdorfer, C., Pavexa, G., Ashford, J. W., Gorelick, P., Hirschman, R., Freels, S., Levy, P., Semla, T., & Shaw, H. (1992). Are there clinical differences between familial and nonfamilial Alzheimer's disease? 149, 1023–1027.

This study is of doubtful clinical significance because of the poor performance of clinicians in predicting Alzheimer's, as discussed below, and because the Alzheimer's disease of the relatives was "reported" in an unspecified fashion. The two groups, supposed familial and nonfamilial Alzheimer's, did not differ on numerous variables.

> Coryell, W., & Tsuang, D. (1992). Hypothalamic-pituitary-adrenal axis hyperactivity and psychosis: Recovery during an 8-year followup. 149, 1033–1039.

This study is remarkable because of its finding that biologically normal patients have a poorer clinical outcome than those with an abnormal dexamethasone suppression test. This finding is the exact opposite of that predicted by bioreductionist psychiatry.

> Cleghorn, J. M., Franco, S., Szechtman, B., Kaplan, R. D., Szechtman, H., Brown, G., Nahmias, C., & Garnett, E. S. (1992). Toward a brain map of auditory hallucinations. 149, 1062–1069.

There were many comparisons and many significant findings in this PET scan study, but none would survive the Bonferroni correction for multiple comparisons.

> Schwartz, J. M., Aylward, E., Barta, P. E., Tune, L. E., & Pearlson, G. D. (1992). Sylvian fissure size in schizophrenia measured with the magnetic resonance imaging rating protocol of the consortium to establish a registry for Alzheimer's disease. 149, 1195–1198.

Various brain areas were measured using MRI scans in 48 schizophrenics and 51 controls, with a specific finding that the only difference was that the schizophrenics had wider sylvian fissures. This finding is of potential interest because it implies tissue loss in the temporal lobes, which could be related to the cause of schizophrenia. However, the sylvian fissure was measured on a scale that goes from zero, for no atrophy, to 3.0 for severe atrophy, and no schizophrenics scored above 1.0, meaning that the range of variation may have been biologically trivial. The table in the paper looks like this:

Rating of Sylvian Fissure Atrophy	Number of Subjects	
	Schizophrenic (N = 48)	Normal (N = 51)
Right		
0.0	19	38
0.5	25	13
1.0	4	0
Left		
0.0	30	46
0.5	18	5

This does not present a robust, meaningful biological finding. The kappa for interrater reliability on reading the scans was modest (only

"0.60 or greater"), making the biological significance of these fine differences even more doubtful.

> *Peselow, E. D., Sanfilipo, M. P., Difiglia, C., & Fieve, R. R. (1992). Melancholic/endogenous depression and response to somatic treatment and placebo. 149, 1324–1334.*

A total of 231 patients entered into drug trials for depression were analyzed for response to placebo and medication. The data showed: "Moderately depressed patients with DSM-III melancholia had a significantly better response to active medication than did severely depressed patients with melancholia and showed the greatest difference between active medication and response to placebo." Yet, given that this finding contradicts the reductionist assumption that more severe illness means more severe biological abnormalities and greater need for medication, the authors concluded: "This finding suggests that patients who have DSM-III melancholia may be unresponsive to nonsomatic treatments." One could just as easily conclude that the more severe the depression, the less biological it is, and therefore the less responsive to medication.

The data are twisted in their interpretation, because the moderately depressed patients with melancholia had a complete response rate to medication of 38.2% and to placebo of 5.0%; the severely depressed patients with melancholia had a complete response rate to medication of 14.3% and to placebo of 4.2%. The greater gap between medication and placebo is an artifact of the result that the severe patients had a lower response rate to medication while placebo response rates were equal, which supports a conclusion that more severe illness does not affect the placebo response rate but reduces the efficacy of medication.

In examining the rates of partial response of the two groups, one finds that the moderate group had a medication response rate of 35.3% and placebo response rate of 25.0%; the severe group had a medication response rate of 23.8% and placebo response rate of 12.5%. If one were to base conclusions on rates of partial response, the gap between drug and placebo response rates would be equal for the two groups, which is not consistent with the authors' conclusions. Close examination of the table in which these data appear shows an erratic, inconsistent pattern when placebo and drug responses are rated as complete or partial and when severe and moderate patients with and without melancholia are compared. For instance, moderately depressed patients without melancholia have the same gap between drug and placebo responses as severely depressed patients with melancholia (11.0 and 10.1, respectively).

The data do not support any consistent conclusions, and there are no significant findings when the Bonferroni correction is applied.

Andreason, P. J., Altemus, M., Zametkin, King, A. C., Lucinio, J., & Cohen, R. M. (1992). Regional cerebral glucose metabolism in bulimia nervosa. 149, 1506–1513.

PET scans were done in 11 bulimics and 11 controls. The main table in the paper gives 51 comparisons of the two groups, of which 5 are significant at p < .05, but none of which would survive the Bonferroni correction. In Table 2, there are 9 comparisons, of which none is significant at p < .05; in Table 3, all 8 comparisons are significant at p < .05. Table 3 also deals with degree of asymmetry between hemispheres, which was greater in 5 brain regions for bulimics and 3 for controls. These simply are not robust findings.

Buchanan, R. W., Breir, A., Kirkpatrick, B., Elkashef, A., Munson, R. C., Gellad, F., & Carpenter, W. T. (1993). Structural abnormalities in deficit and nondeficit schizophrenia. 150, 59–65.

The authors did MRI scans on 17 deficit-symptom schizophrenics, 24 nondeficit schizophrenics, and 30 normal controls. Total brain volume did not differ among the three groups; there were scattered, inconsistent differences among the groups on degree of volume asymmetry between hemispheres for certain brain regions. None of these would survive correction for multiple comparisons.

Yehuda, R., Southwick, S. M., Krystal, J. H., Bremner, D., Charney, D. S., & Mason, J. W. (1993). Enhanced suppression of cortisol following dexamethasone administration in posttraumatic stress disorder. 150, 83–86.

In this study, 21 subjects with posttraumatic stress disorder and 12 controls were given the DST. The paradoxical finding was that the PTSD patients were more biologically normal than the controls. Using a cutoff of 5 ug/dl, 5 out of 12 controls were DST nonsuppressors at both 8:00 A.M. and 4 P.M., a very unusual finding of high significance. The rate of nonsuppression in controls should be 5%. The so-called positive finding about PTSD is an artifact of using a highly abnormal control group.

Andreasen, N. C., Flaum, M., Swayze, V., O'Leary, D. S., Alliger, R., Cohen, G., Ehrhardt, J., & Yuh, W. T. C. (1993). Intelligence and brain structure in normal individuals. 150, 130–134.

The authors did MRI scans and IQ tests in 67 normal volunteers. Table 3 includes 72 correlation coefficients, none of which would be significant with the Bonferroni correction. The authors could not advance any specific hypotheses as to why males and females differed on many values.

> *Volkow, N. D., Wang, G.-J., Hitzemann, R., Fowler, J. S., Wolf, A. P., Pappas, N., Bigon, A., & Dewey, S. L. (1993). Decreased cerebral response to inhibitory neurotransmission in alcoholics. 150, 417–422.*

This study compared PET scans in 10 alcoholics and 12 controls, after they had been given lorazepam. There was no difference between the groups in whole brain metabolic rates, and there would have been no significant differences between the groups in any brain regions if the Bonferroni correction had been applied. The greater reduction in brain metabolism in three brain regions in response to lorazepam among the controls, the key observation of the paper, was an artifact of the lower resting metabolic rate of the alcoholics on placebo.

> *Altemus, M., Pigott, T., L'Heureux, F., Davis, C. L., Rubinow, D. R., Murphy, D. L., & Gold, P. W. (1993). CSF somatostatin in obsessive-compulsive disorder. 150, 460–464.*

The authors found higher CSF somatostatin levels in 15 obsessive-compulsive patients than in 27 controls. Values were 58.3 pmol/liter (S.D. 13.8) for patients and 45.8 (S.D. 9.0) for controls (t = 3.6, df = 40, p < .001). However, the authors stated: "The functional importance of the high CSF levels of somatostatin and the positive correlations between CSF somatostatin and CSF, CRH, and CSF arginine vasopression in patients with obsessive-compulsive disorder remains to be determined."

> *Haggery, J. J., Stern, R. A., Mason, G. A., Beckwith, J., Morey, C. E., & Prange, A. J. (1993). Subclinical hypothyroidism: A modifiable risk factor or depression? 150, 508–510.*

The authors found a lifetime history of depression in 56% of 16 subjects with subclinical hypothyroidism and 20% of 15 controls, a difference significant at p < .04. The two groups did not differ on levels of thyroid hormone, but the subclinical hypothyroid group had higher thyroid-stimulating hormone levels. The authors had no data as to whether the depressions occurred prior to or after the onset of the subclinical hypothyroidism, and commented: "It is also conceivable, however, that the association we observed was not due to the effects of subclinical hypothyroidism but rather to the influence of depression on the development of hypothyroidism, mediated perhaps by altered autoimmune processes."

That depression could cause hypothyroidism is highly unlikely, although it is conceivable that a cause of depression could also be a cause of hypothyroidism.

DeBellis, M. D., Gold, P. W., Geracioti, T. C., Listwak, S. J., & Kling, M. A. (1993). Association of fluoxetine treatment with reductions of CSF concentrations of corticotropin-releasing hormone and arginine vasopressin in patients with major depression. 150, 656–657.

There was no correlation between the magnitude of reduction in Hamilton Depression Scale scores and the magnitude of changes in CSF, CRH, or CSF arginine vasopressin in 9 depressed patients, when measurements were taken before and after treatment with fluoxetine. The observed reduction in the biological variables is therefore clinically spurious.

Nunes, E. V., McGrath, P. J., Quitkin, F. M., Stewart, J. P., Harrison, W., Tricamo, E., & Ocepek-Welikson, K. (1993). Imipramine treatment of alcoholism with comorbid depression. 150, 963–965.

In this study, 45% of depressed alcoholics responded to an open trial of imipramine, but this does not differ from the placebo response rate recognized in the literature on depression.

Lydiard, R. B., Brewerton, T. D., Fossey, M. D., Laraia, M. T., Stuart, G., Beinfeld, M. C., & Ballenger, J. C. (1993). CSF cholecystokinin octapeptide in patients with bulimia nervosa and in normal comparison subjects. 150, 1099–1101.

Brambila, F., Bellodi, L., Perna, G., Barberi, A., Panerai, A., & Sacerdote, P. (1993). Lymphocyte cholecystokinin concentrations in panic disorder. 150, 1111–1113.

I am discussing these two papers together because they appear a few pages apart in the same issue of the *Journal*, and both deal with cholecystokinin octapeptide (CCK-8), although the measurements are done differently. The findings from the two studies concerning CCK levels are:

Bulimia	13.5	S.D.	6.5
Bulimia controls	20.5	S.D.	7.5
Panic disorder	35	S.D.	21
Panic controls	58	S.D.	32

The same finding in two unrelated disorders means that the results are of doubtful clinical and biological importance or specificity. One might want to postulate a CCK-spectrum disorder, however, including panic disorder and bulimia, given the logic of biological psychiatry.

> *Maddock, R. J., Cater, C. S., Magliozzi, J. R., & Gietzen, D. W. E. (1993). Evidence that decreased function of lymphocyte beta adrenoreceptors reflects regulatory and adaptive processes in panic disorder with agoraphobia. 150, 1219–1225.*

The basic finding in this study is that increased anxiety leads to down-regulation of beta adrenoreceptors, and treatment with benzodiazepines reduces anxiety and results in up-regulation of receptors. Although this is an acceptable study methodologically, the findings are scientifically banal.

> *Siegel, B. V., Buchsbaum, M. S., Bunney, W. E., Gottschalk, L. A., Haier, R. J., Lohr, J. B., Lottenberg, S., Najafi, A., Nuechterlein, K. H., Potkin, S. G., & Wu, J. C. (1993). Cortical-striatal-thalamic circuits and brain glucose metabolic activity in 70 unmedicated male schizophrenic patients. 150, 1325–1336.*

The tables in this paper present 101 rows of PET scan data on 70 schizophrenics and 30 controls. Each row has 4 to 6 data points in it. The authors stated:

> For exploratory analyses, because of the large number of correlations and t tests calculated, significance levels of $p < .05$ were considered a trend, and $p < .001$ was considered significant. Bonferroni corrections were not reported; we believe that using less stringent corrections in a large exploratory study such as this one is useful for comparison to findings of other investigators. Thus, we attempted to reduce the possibilities of Type I errors in three ways: by using repeated measures ANOVA, by labeling some analyses as exploratory and correcting them for multiple comparisons, and by attempting to match already published findings.

In this literature, the Bonferroni correction can be used only some of the time in a dataset to avoid the result of no significant findings, a softened informal Bonferroni correction can be used to preserve significance, and insignificant data can be reported so that they can be validated by similar insignificant data from other investigators.

> *Morgan, M. J., Cascella, N. G., Stapleton, J. M., Phillips, R. L., Yung, B. C. K., Wong, D. F., Shya, E. K., & London, E. D. (1993). Sensitivity to subjective effects of cocaine in drug abusers: Relationship to cerebral ventricle size. 150, 1712–1717.*

In this study, the authors correlated ventricle–brain ratios with subjective response to intravenous cocaine in 20 male polydrug users. They stated, in a footnote to Table 1, that the findings are "significant at $p < .05$ without correction for multiple comparisons." One assumes that, with correction, none would be significant. They also noted that "none of these subjects was considered to show pathological ventriculomegaly when the CT scans were inspected by a radiologist." The study, then, involves nonsignificant findings within the normal range. The nature of the demand characteristics in the study and the ethics of giving drug addicts I.V. cocaine to study a scientifically weak hypothesis are not discussed.

TWIN, FAMILY, AND GENETIC STUDIES

Twin and genetic studies strike to the heart of our thesis in this book, so I paid special attention to any such research, looking for conceptual and methodological flaws. I have included here several examples of studies that are well conducted and free of ideological distortion, to demonstrate that my analysis is not based on hostility to this category of research.

Segal, N. L., Dysken, M. W., Bouchard, T. J., Pedersen, N. L., Eckert, E. D., & Heston, L. L. (1990). Tourette's disorder in a set of reared-apart triplets: Genetic and environmental variables.

This is a good study and worth publishing, but the question is: What do the findings mean? The methodology is flawless, and the twins actually were reared apart. The pattern in the pedigree is incomprehensible genetically, however. The pedigree chart consists of four generations: in the oldest, two brothers had Tourette's. One of these brothers had no children, and the other married twice. By one wife he had no Tourette's progeny out of 9 relatives (2 children, 4 grandchildren, 3 great-grandchildren). By the other, he had 5 Tourette's progeny out of 10 relatives, including a set of triplets—2 monozygotic girls and a boy—all of whom had Tourette's. One of the girls and the boy each had three unaffected children and no grandchildren. One of the MZ girls had two affected children, a boy and a girl, one unaffected son, and an unaffected grandson by her affected daughter.

The authors concluded: "The presence of Tourette's disorder in an adult monozygotic/dyzygotic set of triplets raised apart from early infancy provides unique evidence that genetic factors are important in the development of this disorder. The presence of this disorder among the first-degree relatives of the triplets, both those living together and those living apart, also underlines the importance of genetic effects."

In fact, the data do not differentiate genetic factors from intrauterine trauma. An alternative hypothesis is that there is no genetic component to Tourette's and that two mothers in this pedigree had infections or were exposed to other toxins during pregnancy. The girl with Tourette's in the third generation, whose mother and brother had Tourette's, also had myasthenia gravis, which suggests some diagnostically nonspecific factor at work.

> *Pearlson, G. D., Ross, C. A., Lohr, W. D., Rovner, B. W., Chase, G. A., & Folstein, M. F. (1990). Association between family history of affective disorder and the depressive syndrome of Alzheimer's disease. 147, 452–456.*

This paper is useful because it contains a direct statement of the fallacy that if a disorder runs in families, that is evidence of a genetic cause or contribution. It is a study comparing the rate of depression in relatives of 41 depressed Alzheimer's patients to the rate in relatives of 71 non-depressed Alzheimer's patients. The authors state in their abstract: "The depressed patients had significantly more first- and second-degree relatives with depression than did control subjects. The lifetime risk for major depression, adjusted for differences in age distribution, was significantly greater in first-degree relatives of index patients, suggesting that depression in Alzheimer's disease is genetically related to primary affective disorder."

> *Klein, D. N. (1990). Symptom criteria and family history in major depression. 147, 850–854.*

The author interviewed 82 outpatients with a current major depressive episode but no bipolar history, and 27 outpatients with no affective diagnoses, most of whom had anxiety and personality disorders. All subjects reported on lifetime history of depression in their first-degree relatives via Family History Research Diagnostic Criteria, but no first-degree relatives were interviewed directly.

The study yielded a negative finding: "The rates [of depression] in relatives of neither group differed significantly from the rates in relatives of patients with nonaffective disorders. Finally, the rates of bipolar disorder in the relatives of all three groups of probands did not differ significantly." Why is the author talking about three groups when the study contained only two groups in its original design? This is because of the negative findings. The author divided the depressed group (N = 82) into two subgroups in order to generate significant data: (a) depressed subjects positive for 4 or 5 symptoms, and (b) those positive for 6, 7, or 8 symptoms. Using these subgroups, he was able to generate sufficient findings to produce a publication. This is analogous to creating an affective spectrum or schizophrenia spectrum to create significant findings in genetic studies, when there are negative findings with respect to schizophrenia alone, as analyzed by Dr. Pam in Chapter 1.

> *Torgersen, S. (1990). Comorbidity of major depression and anxiety disorders in twin pairs. 147, 1199–1202.*

This is a study of three diagnostic subgroups in a sample of 177 twin pairs: major depression only, major depression with anxiety disorders, and anxiety disorders only. It contains all the flaws of logic analyzed by Dr. Pam in Chapter 1. The author mentions the equal environments problem, but then ignores it in the rest of the paper: "The difference between concordance rates among monozygotic and dyzygotic twins might also be due to chance. Furthermore, a higher concordance among monozygotic than dyzygotic twins might be a consequence of a more similar environment for monozygotic twin partners than for dyzygotic twin partners."

What do the data look like? The author presents two tables, one with anxiety disorders in general, one limited to panic attacks alone. This results in 18 cells in the two tables combined, with a concordance rate for monozygotic and another for dyzygotic twins in each cell. Each table lists three proband diagnoses in the vertical column versus three co-twin diagnoses in the horizontal row.

Out of the 18 cells, the frequency of a positive co-twin diagnosis in the monozygotic pairs exceeds that in the dyzygotic pairs by 10% only 4 times. Only two of these show what could be called a *breeding true* pattern: anxiety disorder only is more common in co-twins of anxiety disorder only monozygotic probands than in co-twins of dyzygotic probands in both tables. In none of the 6 comparisons involving probands with major depression only was there a difference in frequency of depression of 10% between co-twin rates in monozygotic and dyzygotic pairs. The data therefore rule out a genetic component to pure depression in this sample and are consistent with, but do not rule in or out, a genetic component to pure anxiety disorder. With application of the Bonferroni correction, there would be no significant findings.

The significant findings in the study are typified by an odds ratio of 9.6 for monozygotic co-twins versus dyzygotic co-twins of affected probands; however, the 95% confidence interval for this value is 1.1–115.5.

This finding applies to the higher frequency of major depression with anxiety in monozygotic co-twins of probands with major depression only, compared to that in dyzygotic twin pairs. The absolute values are an 18.8% frequency in monozygotes and 8.0% in dyzygotes, neither of which is notably different from the range of norms in the general population.

Winokur, G., & Coryell, W. (1991). Familial alcoholism in primary major depressive episode. 148, 184–188.

This is a good study without intrusion of reductionism.

Biederman, J., Faraone, S. V., Keenan, K., Steingard, R., & Tsuang, M. T. (1991). Familial association between attention deficit disorder and anxiety disorders. 148, 251–256.

This is a good paper, except for the cognitive error that *if it runs in families it must be genetic,* which the authors make in their introduction: "Converging evidence implicates a genetic component in anxiety disorders and ADD. In a study of children with anxiety disorders, Last et al. reported that mothers of anxious children had a significantly higher risk for adult and childhood anxiety disorders than mothers of normal children."

Reiss, D., Plomin, R., & Hetherington, E. M. (1991). Genetics and psychiatry: An unheralded window on the environment. 148, 283–291.

This paper would make an excellent chapter in the present book, except that the authors have not grasped the seriousness of the methodological limitations to the biogenetic literature on psychiatric disorders. These limitations, once analyzed and understood, lead to the irrefutable conclusion that no genetic component to schizophrenia or bipolar mood disorder has yet been demonstrated. The authors write:

> As the research in molecular genetics has gathered momentum, it has partially broken loose from its original moorings. The search for specific genes in unipolar, bipolar, and schizophrenic illness began with the demonstration of significant genetic effects, but not exclusive genetic effects, for both disorders. That is, bipolar and related illnesses occurred among family members of probands with these illnesses more frequently than in the general population, concordances were generally higher in monozygotic twins than in dyzygotic twins, and, in studies with the most rigorous designs, the frequency of the illness was higher in biological than in adopted relatives.

The same patterns hold for schizophrenia. What is often forgotten is that although the evidence for a genetic contribution to the etiology of these disorders is beyond dispute, no studies indicate that the genetic effects account for all the variation between ill and not ill individuals.

The authors of this paper do not recognize the pseudoscientific nature of biological psychiatry, although, judging from the following statement, they might appreciate the chapter by Kemker and Khadivi in the present book: "Psychiatry derives a remarkable portion of its self-image from pictures of its future. For example, images of a psychiatry based on molecular biology, of the kind rendered by Mullan and Murray and Pardes et al., have had an enormous impact on the types of research that currently receive public funding."

O'Callaghan, E., Larkin, C., Kinsella, A., & Waddington, J. L. (1991). Familial, obstetric, and other clinical correlates of minor physical anomalies in schizophrenia. 148, 479–483.

In this study, 41 schizophrenics were divided into two groups based on histories of obstetrical complications while they were in utero. A disorder running in families is taken, pure and simple, as evidence of genetic influence. The thinking, therefore, is flawed in the extreme.

> The principal finding was both a greater number of body regions affected by minor physical anomalies and a higher prevalence of mouth abnormalities in the subgroup of patients who had family histories of schizophrenia but whose mothers had not had any obstetric complications. This relationship suggests that familial/genetic factors may determine not only the development of minor physical anomalies but also a particular topography of developmental abnormality. More speculatively, it might suggest that genetic factors relevant to schizophrenia are related in some way to those which determine oral morphogenesis.

The authors are suggesting that the gene for mouth shape and the gene for schizophrenia might be linked. Familial and genetic are treated as synonyms in this intellectual universe.

Maj, J., Starace, F., & Pirozi, R. (1991). A family study of DSM-III-R schizoaffective disorder, depressive type, compared with schizophrenia and psychotic and nonpsychotic major depression. 148, 612–616.

This is a well done study with no ideological biases.

Silverman, J. M., Pinkham, L., Horvath, T. B., Coccaro, E. F., Klar, H., Schear, S., Apter, S., Davidson, M., Mohs, R. C., & Siever, L. J. (1991). Affective and impulsive personality disorder traits in relatives of patients with borderline personality disorder. 148, 1378–1385.

The authors emphasize genetic factors in a study whose methodology cannot differentiate environmental from genetic influences: "Although environmental influences may play a role in accounting for these familial factors and, as noted, cannot be excluded on the basis of family diagnostic data, the results raise the possibility of a role for genetically heritable personality traits." The phrase *genetic/familial factors* is used by the authors in a fashion that makes the two words seem like synonyms, when actually genetic is a subset of familial from a logical classification point of view, and environmental factors may be intra- or extrafamilial.

Kendler, K. S., Silberg, J. L., Neale, M. C., Kessler, R. C., Heath, A. C., & Eaves, L. J. (1991). The family history method: Whose psychiatric history is measured? 148, 1501–1504.

Very interesting data show that an affected twin reports a higher incidence of her disorder among first-degree relatives than the discordant, nonaffected twin. This is a major confound not addressed in any other family studies during the four years.

Weinberger, D. R., Berman, K. F., Suddath, R., & Torrey, E. F. (1992). Evidence of dysfunction of a prefrontal-limbic network in schizophrenia: A magnetic resonance imaging and regional cerebral blood flow study of discordant monozygotic twins. 149, 890–897.

I include this paper to emphasize that any studies finding biological differences between twins discordant for psychiatric illness point completely and exclusively to environmental etiology. This is one of the best possible research strategies for proving environmental etiology in psychiatric disorders. Concerning the specific findings, the authors say, ". . . the correlation reported here between a small reduction in size of the anterior hippocampus measured on an MRI scan and a slight diminution in rCBF related to a specific cognitive task may not be found in other groups unless very large numbers of subjects are studied. If this prediction is correct, it raises the question of whether the correlation itself is so rarefied as to be neurobiologically trivial."

*Bracha, H. S., Torrey, E. F., Gottesman, I. I., Bigelow, L. B., &
Cunnif, C. (1992). Second-trimester markers of fetal size in
schizophrenia: A study of monozygotic twins. 149, 1355–1361.*

The authors studied fingertip dermal ridges in 23 twin pairs discordant
for schizophrenia, because fingertip dermal ridge counts are regarded
as a marker of toxic effects on the fetus during the second trimester.
The findings were that discordant twins had greater intrapair differences than 7 control sets of twins without schizophrenia. However, of
the 23 affected twinships, the affected twin had a higher score in 13,
and a lower score in 10. The authors state that ridge count is increased
in Turner's syndrome (45XO) and decreased in Klinefelter's syndrome
(47XXY).

This means that biological insults with opposite effects occur in different syndromes with different known genetic abnormalities, and in a
syndrome with a presumed but unproven genetic basis (schizophrenia,
which is variably either 46XX or 46XY). The authors conclude: "The
study suggests that various second-trimester prenatal disturbances in
the epigenesis of one twin pair discordant for schizophrenia may be related to the fact that only one of the twins expresses his or her genetic
predisposition toward schizophrenia. This is consistent with a 'two-
strike' etiology of schizophrenia: a genetic diathesis plus a second-
trimester environmental stressor."

The authors have not explained why one second trimester twin is not
affected by the environmental stressor. A more parsimonious explanation for the data is a "one-strike" etiology that is purely environmental,
because there is no scientific reason to postulate a genetic diathesis in
order to account for the data.

*Grove, W. M., Clementz, B. A., Iacono, W. G., & Katsanis, J.
(1992). Smooth pursuit ocular motor dysfunction in
schizophrenia: Evidence for a major gene. 149, 1362–1368.*

The authors studied eye tracking abnormalities in first-degree relatives
of 92 schizophrenics and 171 controls. This was a total of 146 proband
relatives and 171 control relatives. The study assumed the existence of a
gene for schizophrenia and proposed that a gene for eye tracking abnormalities could be used to study and locate it. However, the authors
stated that "eye tracking accounts for approximately 25% of the variance in risk for a spectrum diagnosis (schizophrenia in addition to
schizotypal personality) in schizophrenic patients' families." This is a
modest amount of variance, and the prior research should be examined

for spectrum-type cognitive errors and for failure to show a finding when schizophrenia alone is considered.

| **Simpson, S. G., Folstein, S. E., Meyers, D. A., & DePaulo, J. R. (1992). Assessment of lineality in bipolar I linkage studies. 149, 1660–1665.**

Unilineal families are ones in which only one parent has a given disorder; in bilineal families, both parents are affected. The mating patterns of the unilineal family parents are far from genetically random, as noted in another study: "Eighty-five percent of their bipolar inpatients had spouses with histories of some psychiatric disorder, compared to 45% of the unipolar patients." This raises a question as to how unilineal most bipolar families are: many parents rated as unaffected in inadequately designed studies must have "affective spectrum disorders." In a study of children, such cases would be rated as affected in order to support the affective spectrum hypothesis; in a study of parents, they would be rated as unaffected in order to generate a sample of unilineal families. Such methodology destroys the studies.

The only way to avoid this problem is to scrupulously screen potentially unilineal bipolar families for affected coparents. The problem then becomes the massive logistical effort required to locate enough families, given the number of loci to be screened in genetic marker studies. At best, one could detect a minute number of apparently mendelian pedigrees through such research, but these would be an infinitesimal subsample from a public health point of view, and the number of families required to correct for chance findings would be astronomical.

The authors screened 1,800 bipolar pedigrees and entered 34 families into their study, which involved 96 siblings. Out of five comparisons of rates of different mood disorder categories (bipolar I, bipolar II, unipolar, uncertain, and unaffected) in unilineal and probably bilineal sibs, they found a higher rate of unipolar depression in the bilineal sibs (29% versus 6%), which was the only significant finding (chi square = 5.60, df = 1, p < .02). This would not survive the Bonferroni correction.

The authors also assumed that recurrent depressions are genetic and sporadic ones are not, an assumption for which there is no logical or scientific basis. They stated: "The issue of whether even recurrent cases of depression should be considered genetic cases of depression will be reviewed before linkage analysis." Fortunately, they understood, as stated in their conclusions, that "[t]he mode of inheritance of bipolar I disorder is unknown." However, in the succeeding sentences they propose future projects that would cost tens of millions of dollars: "While there may be mendelian dominant forms of the disorder, they may be uncommon. If the current searches for mendelian forms of the disorder are to have the best chance of success, an adequate resource of unilineal families must be studied with DNA markers spanning the entire genome."

A methodological question is whether there are enough unilineal bipolar families in North America to support such a project.

Maier, W., Lichterman, D., Minges, J., Heun, R., Halmayer, J., & Benkert, O. (1992). Schizoaffective disorder and affective disorders with mood-incongruent psychotic features: Keep separate or combine? Evidence from a family study. 149, 1666–1673.

Rates of affective disorders and psychoses in relatives of 118 patients with schizoaffective disorder or mood disorder with incongruent psychotic features were compared to those in relatives of 109 controls. This involved 475 proband relatives and 432 control relatives. All disorders under consideration (schizophrenia, schizophreniform, schizoaffective, bipolar and unipolar with and without incongruent psychotic features, cyclothymia, and dysthmia) were more common in both sets of proband relatives than in the normal comparison group. The families of the two types of probands did not differ in rates of affective disorder. The data can best be understood in terms of severe mental illness running in families with little or no diagnostic specificity and with no conclusions as to genetic versus environmental causes being possible.

Maziade, M., Roy, M.-A., Fournier, J.-P., Cliche, D., Merette, C., Caron, C., Garneau, Y., Montgrain, N., Shriqui, C., Dion, C., Nicole, L., Potvin, A., Lavallee, J.-C., Piers, A., & Raymond, V. (1992). Reliability of best-estimate diagnosis in genetic linkage studies of major psychoses: Results from the Quebec pedigree studies. 149, 1674–1686.

The authors reviewed 38 "major linkage studies and workshop reports." They found that in 21 studies it was not reported whether the same diagnostic procedures were used for all subjects, and could confirm that they were in only 8 studies; blindness of interviewers was not reported in 16 studies and could be confirmed in only 2; independence of diagnosticians reviewing study diagnoses could be confirmed in only 7 studies. The literature contains major methodological flaws that prevent replication or meaningful conclusions being drawn from meta-analyses, and many individual studies.

The authors stated that "unblind diagnosticians tended, for instance, to diagnose more affective disorders in bipolar pedigrees than the blind psychiatric board did." They also commented:

Most of all, our review again indicates that it is imperative that researchers enter only the most severe or definite diagnosis in the first hierarchical level for linkage analysis and that publications provide a minimal description of the diagnostic procedure according to current standards in order to permit replication. Several of the most recent reports do not even provide this information. Finally, our results call for further studies of the impact and origin of this field on diagnosis in pedigree studies.

The authors are setting a low and minimal standard for genetic research, which has not been met by psychiatry.

Thaker, G., Adami, H., Moran, M., Lahti, A., & Cassady, S. (1993). Psychiatric illnesses in families of subjects with schizophrenia-spectrum personality disorders: High morbidity risk for unspecified functional psychoses and schizophrenia. 150, 66–71.

The authors studied 259 first- and second-degree relatives of 30 probands with Cluster A personality disorders (schizoid, schizotypal, and paranoid), and 225 first- and second-degree relatives of 8 controls and 12 subjects with other personality disorders. The pattern of findings was different in first- and second-degree relatives, and there were no significant findings when first-degree relatives only were considered: rates of schizophrenia, unspecified functional psychoses, schizophrenia spectrum personality disorders, depression, bipolar disorder, alcoholism, anxiety disorder and antisocial personality disorder were no more frequent in the first-degree relatives of schizophrenia spectrum probands than in control first-degree relatives. Significance was obtained when second-degree relatives were added, but would have been lost if the Bonferroni correction for multiple comparisons had been done. Adding second-degree relatives to obtain significance violates the genetic principle of higher prevalence in first- than in second-degree relatives. Adding second-degree relatives should *reduce* the degree of difference between groups in a genetic disorder.

This study is close to being a fishing expedition with negative findings.

Bailey, M. J., & Bemishay, D. S. (1993). *Familial aggregation of female sexual orientation. 150*, 272–277.

This study does not suffer from major methodological flaws; however, the authors make an interesting statement about the observed low rate of homosexuality in sisters of index homosexual females:

> Because the 12.1% rate implies that the large majority of sisters of female homosexuals are heterosexual, one might be tempted to conclude that familial factors are of minor etiological importance. However, a multifactorial model of transmission, in which one's sexual orientation depends on a continuous underlying etiological dimension that is influenced by many genetic or environmental factors each of small effect, can reconcile powerful familial factors with rates such as ours.

The authors are saying that familial factors with weak effects can still be regarded as powerful if analyzed within a "model" that could be used to "explain" everything about human behavior. The model amounts to no more than a statement that human behavior is influenced by many genetic and environmental factors in a complicated fashion. Such statements can be published only in a field with low scientific standards.

Taylor, M. A., Berenbaum, S. A., Jampala, V. C., & Cloninger, C. R. (1993). *Are schizophrenia and affective disorder related? Preliminary data from a family study. 150*, 278–285.

In this study, 1,895 first-degree relatives of 166 probands with schizophrenia, 949 first-degree relatives of 71 probands with affective disorders, and 85 controls were studied for their rates of schizophrenia and affective disorder. The risk of both forms of illness was equal in the two clinical pedigrees, and higher in both clinical pedigrees than in control relatives. The findings indicate that there is no familial, and therefore no genetic, specificity to the two forms of major mental illness.

Silverman, J. M., Siever, L. J., Horvath, T. B., Coccaro, E. F., Klar, H., Davidson, M., Pinkham, L., Apter, S. H., Mohs, R. C., & Davis, K. L. (1993). *Schizophrenia-related and affective personality disorder traits in relatives of probands with schizophrenia and personality disorders. 150*, 435–442.

The rates of schizophrenia-related and affective personality disorder traits were measured in 588 nonpsychotic first-degree relatives of 55 schizophrenics, and 67 probands with personality disorders. Affective personality disorder traits were defined as "one of the hallmark trait of borderline personality disorder, chronic affective instability not attributable to a concurrent major affective disorder." Schizophrenia-related personality disorder traits were defined as "a condensation of DSM-III criteria for schizotypal and paranoid personality disorders."

In the relatives of pure schizophrenic probands, the rate of pure schizophrenia-related personality disorder traits was 12.3%; in the relatives of pure borderline probands, it was 3.9%. Inversely, in the relatives of pure schizophrenic probands, the rate of affective personality traits was 1.7%, compared to 6.7% in relatives of pure borderline probands.

The authors concluded: "[T]he features associated with schizotypal personality disorder, while familially related to schizophrenia, lack specificity for this disorder and may also be found in relatives of probands with prominent affective-related symptoms such as borderline personality disorder." The finding of lack of specificity echoes the previous study.

An assumption of the study is that borderline personality disorder is in the affective spectrum and schizotypal personality disorder is in the schizophrenia spectrum. However, it is well known that borderline and schizotypal personality disorders overlap extensively in clinical samples, so there is no reason to predict specific findings in family studies. This makes the expenditure of effort required for such family studies questionable, from the point of view of budgeting psychiatric research resources.

Allen, J. M., Lam, R. W., Remick, R. A., & Sadovnick, A. D. (1993). Depressive symptoms and family history in seasonal and nonseasonal mood disorders. 150, 443–448.

The authors stated in their abstract: "[T]he genetic loading for mood disorders (of unspecified seasonality), as determined by the family history method, is similar for seasonal and nonseasonal mood disorders." In the last paragraph of their discussion, they stated: "The demonstration of a genetic contribution to seasonality in mood disorders will require rigorous methods for identifying patterns of mood disorders in family history data collection." Two pages earlier in the same issue of the *Journal*, Silverman et al. (1993) made this statement: "Family data cannot distinguish between genetic and environmental factors and hence preclude a determination of a *genetic* relationship between nonaffective symptoms of schizotypal personality disorder and schizophrenia."

One wonders how such discrepant statements survive the peer review process. Allen et al. (1993) committed the cognitive error that *it if runs in families it must be genetic.*

Mathew, R. J., Wilson, W. H., Blazer, D. G., & George, L. K.
(1993). Psychiatric disorders in adult children of alcoholics:
Data from the epidemiological catchment area project. 150,
793–800.

The pattern of data in this study is entirely explicable by environmental factors. In Table 2, the authors present 14 comparisons of the rates of various psychiatric disorders in 408 children of alcoholics and 1,477 matched comparison subjects. The significant findings do not involve an odds ratio above 2.02 for any of these disorders except panic disorder, which has an odds ratio of 4.06 for the children of alcoholics. These are very modest increases in risk. If a Bonferroni correction had been applied, given that the entire Diagnostic Interview Schedule was administered, there would have been only two significant chi-square values: (a) for panic disorder, and (b) for generalized anxiety disorder. However, the prevalence of panic disorder (2.7%) in the children of alcoholics is not much different from general population norms and yields an odds ratio of 4.06 only because the controls have a low prevalence of 0.7%.

Fulton, M., & Winokur, G. (1993). A comparative study of
paranoid and schizoid personality disorders. 150, 1363–1367.

The authors "found no statistically significant differences in the prevalence of either paranoid traits or schizoid traits among family members of probands with paranoid or schizoid personality disorder."

Torgersen, S., Onstad, S., Skre, I., Edvardsen, J., & Kringlen,
E. (1993). "True" schizotypal personality disorder: A study of
co-twins and relatives of schizophrenic probands. 150,
1661–1667.

The authors compared 176 nonschizophrenic co-twins and first-degree relatives of schizophrenic probands to 101 co-twins and first-degree relatives of depressed probands on the frequency of 12 different personality disorders. Table 3 contains 48 comparisons, none of which would survive correction for multiple comparisons. Paranoid and schizoid personality disorders were more common among dizygotic co-twins than monozygotic co-twins of schizophrenic probands; the reverse was true for schizotypal personality disorder. This finding contradicts the schizophrenia spectrum hypothesis and the idea that these three personality disorders belong to a single cluster (Cluster A in DSM-IV). In addition, antisocial, borderline, narcissistic, and passive-aggressive personality disorders were more common in dizygotic co-twins of schizophrenic probands than in monozygotic ones.

Among the twins of depressed probands, paranoid personality disorder was more common among dizygotes, and schizoid and schizotypal disorders were more common among monozygotes. The frequency of a given personality disorder was greater among dizygotic co-twins of schizophrenic probands than among monozygotic co-twins for 2/3 Cluster A, 3/4 Cluster B, and 1/5 Cluster C personality disorders. For co-twins of depressed probands, the frequency was greater in dizygotes for 1/3 Cluster A, 0/4 Cluster B, and 1/5 Cluster C personality disorders. These data are very difficult to fit into any model of true schizotypal personality disorder.

The authors concluded: "[T]he genetic link even between true schizotypal features and schizophrenia is a modest one." In terms of absolute values, schizotypal personality disorder was found in 3/15 monozygotic co-twins of schizophrenic probands, 1/13 monozygotic co-twins of depressed probands, 4/27 dizygotic co-twins of schizophrenic probands, and 0/23 dizygotic co-twins of depressed probands. "Modest" would appear to be the correct term in this context, given the magnitude of the findings and the fact that the problem of equal environments is ignored.

Livesley, W. J., Jang, K. L., Jackson, D. N., & Vernon, P. A. (1993). Genetic and environmental contributions to dimensions of personality disorder. 150, 1826–1831.

Subjects in this study were 90 monozygotic and 85 dizygotic twin pairs from the general population who were reared in the same homes. They completed the Dimensional Assessment of Personality Pathology— Basic Questionnaire. The authors claimed to have controlled for the assumption of equal environments, but their attempt to do so was methodologically crude. The most interesting aspect of the authors' thinking is the following:

> The estimates of genetic contributions to some dimensions warrant further comment. Statistically significant genetic differences were not observed for several dimensions, including insecure attachment, intimacy problems, and submissiveness. These dimensions describe interpersonal problems relating to close interpersonal relationships. This is a novel finding that requires replication. One might speculate that these scales refer to problems in the way the attachment behavioral system develops and that, although the system is genetically controlled, differential experiences within the family are primarily responsible for its expression and development. (p. 1829)

The authors were saying that when they find a genetic effect, it is truly present, given that they have demonstrated the validity of the equal environments assumption in their population. However, when they do not find a genetic effect, it is still truly present, but masked by the effect of unequal environments. In reality, the authors have not demonstrated either equal or unequal environments, and the genetic effect they claimed to have demonstrated is a statistical artifact. Their language and tone are those of reductionist biology: they might as well have been talking about ducklings or earthworms.

INABILITY OF CLINICIANS TO PREDICT BIOLOGICAL FINDINGS

If the ideological system of bioreductionist psychiatry is sound, clinicians should be able to match clinical diagnosis to hard physical findings, when these are available. Yet they can't, as demonstrated by the following study.

> *Risse, S. C., Raskind, M. A., Nochlin, D., Sumi, S. M., Lampe, T. H., Bird, T. D., Cubberley, L., & Peskind, E. R. (1990). Neuropathological findings in patients with clinical diagnoses of probable Alzheimer's disease. 147, 168–172.*

In this study, autopsies were done on 25 demented patients who had received diagnoses of Alzheimer's disease on an Alzheimer's Disease Research Unit, and 68% actually had Alzheimer's on postmortem. This would seem reasonably good, but the authors failed to correct for chance using Cohen's kappa, a procedure that is part of the basic methodology of any study in which there are two possible categories for subjects' assignment by clinicians (Alzheimer's or non-Alzheimer's, in this study). Using Cohen's kappa, the chance-corrected level of agreement between clinician and autopsy is 0.36, which is far below the level required to be clinically meaningful.

FAILURE TO CONSIDER SEVERE CHILDHOOD TRAUMA

The failure to consider the biopsychosocial consequences of severe, chronic childhood trauma is a flaw in the methodology of every biological paper reviewed in this chapter. I will discuss only a few papers illustrative of this category of error.

| *Teicher, M. H., Glod, C., & Cole, J. (1990). Emergence of intense suicidal preoccupation during fluoxetine treatment. 147, 207–210.*

This was the most influential paper published in *The American Journal of Psychiatry* from 1990 to 1993. It gave rise to a tremendous amount of discussion in psychiatry, in the pharmaceutical industry, on TV talk shows, and in the general media, and it generated many lawsuits and court actions. The paper consisted of six brief case histories of patients who became acutely suicidal while taking fluoxetine (Prozac). Among them were:

> Case 3, Ms. C., a 19-year-old college freshman hospitalized "with symptoms of depression, paranoia, bulimia, agoraphobia, and dissociation." While on fluoxetine, she superficially scratched herself, banged her head, and had to be physically restrained. This profile is not uncommon in individuals with a childhood sexual trauma history and a dissociative disorder.
>
> Case 4, Ms. D., a 39-year-old former executive who "had a history of recurrent major depression, episodic alcohol abuse (in remission), and borderline personality disorder." Her symptoms included "severe suicidal ruminations, dissociative feelings, and the belief that she could not fight or control her suicidal impulses." This is also a trauma-dissociative profile.
>
> Case 5, Ms. E., "a 39-year-old woman with major depression, borderline personality disorder, and temporal lobe epilepsy" who also had "prominent dissociative symptoms." There is no comment on whether she had an abnormal EEG, but a false-positive diagnosis of temporal lobe epilepsy is common in people with undiagnosed dissociative identity disorder.
>
> Case 6, Ms. F., had "multiple personality disorder," according to the authors.

It looks to me like these reactions of Prozac had more to do with the psychobiology of trauma than with anything studied by bioreductionist psychiatry. If this is correct, psychiatry has created a major amount of adverse publicity for itself by failing to consider trauma and dissociation systematically in these six cases.

| *Signer, S., & Benson, D. F. (1990). Three cases of anorexia nervosa associated with temporal lobe epilepsy. 147, 235–238.*

This paper is interesting because these authors reported cases of dual personality associated with temporal lobe epilepsy, but the cases did not come close to meeting criteria for a dissociative disorder, and are the best examples of false-positive diagnoses of multiple personality disorder in the entire psychiatric literature (Benson, Miller, & Signer, 1986).

In this study, the authors presented three cases of coexisting temporal lobe epilepsy and anorexia nervosa, and they indulged in lengthy bioreductionist speculations about the etiology of anorexia nervosa.

> Case 1, Ms. A., "justified not eating on the basis of examples of Biblical figures, starvation in the world, and God's command." As well, "Her affect was flattened, and hyposexuality, hyperreligiousness, and philosophical concerns were noted." This is far from a typical case of anorexia nervosa, and the woman appears to be chronically psychotic. The authors stated that for 7 months following a right frontotemporal lobectomy she displayed "agitation, overactivity, extroverted behavior, thought disorder, and refusal to eat; she had lost 77 lb. She responded partially to neuroleptics."
>
> This woman has an organic brain syndrome and a psychosis: no conclusions about anorexia nervosa of any kind can be reached from her case.
>
> Case 2, Ms. B., "had occasional ideas of reference and auditory hallucinations (not directed at her), but hyperreligiousness and hypergraphia were not present." The woman's father was an alcoholic, her mother had been treated with antidepressants, and one sister and two brothers had unknown psychiatric disorders. This is again an atypical profile for anorexia nervosa.
>
> Case 3, Ms. C., "reported frequent episodes of depression with suicidal ideation, including six suicide attempts. Her mood was labile, with almost continuous ruminations over how she would feel or react. She was hypergraphic, maintaining copious diaries over many years. Libido was absent. There was no nascent philosophical or religious concern, but she was unable to distinguish important from trivial events. It was uncertain which neurovegetative symptoms had appeared during past episodes, but neither these nor signs of mania were present on examination; many of these episodes had been associated with amnesia."

For those unfamiliar with the literature, the authors are preoccupied with religiosity, philosophical concerns, and hypergraphia (writing a lot) because these are supposed to be signs of a personality syndrome caused by epilepsy. I suspect that case three had an undiagnosed chronic, complex dissociative disorder and kept journals like many sexual abuse survivors do.

This paper represents biomedical reductionism extended to its extreme.

> *Rotheram-Borus, M. J. (1993). Suicidal behavior and risk factors among runaway youths. 150, 103–107.*

The author studied risk factors for running away from home and attempting suicide in 260 male and 316 female adolescents. Childhood physical and sexual abuse were not mentioned or referenced at any point in the paper, except that sexual abuse was noted to be an immediate precipitant of attempting suicide in 4% of cases: this figure was buried in a list of other precipitants in the results section, and not discussed. I expect that the rate of childhood physical and/or sexual abuse in this sample, if measured, would have been higher than the most prevalent risk factor identified, which was depression (54% of children). This was not a biological research study, but I include it to illustrate the extreme nature of contemporary psychiatry's refusal to consider severe childhood trauma, even in populations in which it is likely to be a key factor.

PSEUDOSCIENCE CONCERNING THE AFFECTIVE SPECTRUM DISORDERS

The idea that many different psychiatric disorders are variants of depression is one of the fixed ideas of bioreductionist psychiatry. Pervasive cognitive errors are to be found in this sector of the literature.

> *Hudson, J. I., & Pope, H. G. (1990). Affective spectrum disorder: Does antidepressant response identify a family of disorders with a common pathophysiology? 147, 552–564.*

The authors postulated that bulimia, panic disorder, obsessive-compulsive disorder, and attention deficit disorder with hyperactivity belong to a physiologically caused affective spectrum disorder. They tried to get cataplexy, migraine, and irritable bowel syndrome to fit in the spectrum as well, but classified these as possible forms of affective spectrum disorder, as opposed to the probable ranking given the first four disorders. Their rationale for creation of the spectrum was that these disorders all respond to antidepressant medications, a core cognitive error of bioreductionist psychiatry analyzed in the previous chapter. I also refer the reader to Dr. Pam's discussion of the schizophrenia spectrum in Chapter 1.

The authors mentioned: "It should also be noted that the choice of the word 'affective' is arbitrary, reflecting simply the historical fact that antidepressants were generally first used to treat depression and only later found to be effective in other disorders." If the choice of terminology is scientifically arbitrary, on what was it based? I venture to guess that it was politically strategic in the climate of bioreductionism to call the spectrum affective because this would harness the maximum amount of biomedical prestige, yet clarify that the turf was owned by psychiatrists rather than gastroenterologists (specialists in irritable bowel spectrum disorders) or neurologists (specialists in migraine spectrum disorders).

The findings of subsequently published papers reviewed in this section illustrate the chaotic, contradictory state of findings in biological psychiatry.

Wu, J. C., Hagman, J., Buchsbaum, M. S., Blinder, B., Derrfler, M., Tai, W. Y., Hazlett, E., & Sicotte, N. (1990). Greater left cerebral hemispheric metabolism in bulimia assessed by positron emission tomography. 147, 309–312.

This paper could be used as an example of a statement of ideological bias. The authors concluded: "In summary, our findings suggest that women with bulimia nervosa have some specific metabolic brain abnormalities when compared with normal women, anorexic patients, and depressed patients. This suggests that bulimia nervosa represents a distinctive psychiatric illness."

The study involved doing PET scans on 8 bulimics and 8 controls. There would have been no significant findings with application of the Bonferroni correction for multiple comparisons; there were 13 comparisons in the table, and all significance levels were p > .03. The basic finding was that the women with bulimia, when compared to the controls, had lost the normal hemispheric asymmetry in the cerebral cortex.

Martinot, J. L., Hardy, P., Feline, A., Huret, J-D., Mazxoyer, B., Attar-Levy, D., Pappata, S., & Syrota, A. (1990). Left prefrontal glucaose hypometabolism in the depressed state: A confirmation. 147, 1313–1317.

The authors did PET scans on 10 severely depressed patients before and after treatment with antidepressants, and 10 controls. They observed that the abnormal brain asymmetry found in the depressed state normalizes after successful treatment with antidepressants—the opposite finding from the bulimia study just reviewed. In the depression study, asymmetry is viewed as abnormal; in the bulimia study, lack of asymmetry is abnormal. It is hard to see how opposite findings can occur in related conditions.

Jeike, M. A., Hyman, S., Baer, L., Holland, A., Minichiello, W. E., Buttolph, L., Summergrad, P., Seymour, R., & Ricciardi, J. (1990). A controlled trial of fluvoxamine in obsessive compulsive disorder: Implications for a serotonergic theory. 147, 1209–1215.

In this nicely done paper, the authors found that the less relatively potent and the less relatively selective for serotonin receptors four antidepressants were, the more effective they were for obsessive-compulsive disorder. In decreasing order of clinical efficacy, the medications are: chlomipramine, fluoxetine, fluvoxamine, and sertraline. This finding is inconsistent with the affective spectrum hypothesis, but is consistent with the view that there is no biological specificity to any of the disorders on the spectrum.

Goff, D. C., Brotman, A. W., Waites, M., & McCormick, S. (1990). Trial of fluoxetine added to neuroleptics for treatment-resistant schizophrenic patients. 147, 492–494.

In this paper, the authors found that, in 9 schizophrenics, fluoxetine reduced both positive and negative symptoms of schizophrenia over a 6-week period at p < .05. This finding, if replicated, would mean that neuroleptic-resistant schizophrenia would also have to be placed on the affective spectrum, but this would violate the central dogma of bioreductionist psychiatry, which states that affective disorders and schizophrenia are biologically distinct, genetically driven diseases.

McDougle, C. J., Goodman, W. K., Price, L. H., Delgado, P. L., Krystal, J. H., Charney, D. S., & Heninger, G. R. (1990). Neuroleptic addition in fluvoxamine-refractory obsessive-compulsive disorder. 147, 652–654.

In this study, the reverse strategy of the previous study was tried. One of three neuroleptics was added to fluoxetine in 17 patients who had what was supposed to be an affective spectrum disorder, and statistically significant improvement in the obsessive-compulsive symptoms was observed.

Kagan, B. L., Sultzer, D. L., Rosenlicht, N., & Gerner, R. H. (1990). Oral S-adenosylmethionine in depression: A randomized, double-blind, placebo-controlled trial. 147, 591–595.

In this small-N study, 9 subjects received active drug and 6 received placebo, with significant differences in antidepressant effect favoring the active drug. The authors stated: "The biological effects of S-adenosylmethionine are myriad, and it is difficult to determine which effects contribute to its therapeutic action." The study is interesting because it reviews the history of methylation hypotheses of mental illness, and concludes that the current fishing expedition is on the right track (if this is correct, the affective spectrum hypothesis will receive another blow if it is based on serotonergic dysfunction):

> Perhaps the most exciting implications of the effectiveness of S-adenosylmethionine are those regarding the role of methylation in psychiatric illness. The original transmethylation hypothesis of schizophrenia postulated that schizophrenic patients have an overactive methylation system, which puts too many methyl groups on neurotransmitters during their metabolism, thus creating endogenous "psychotoxins." While the search for these compounds was ultimately fruitless, this hypothesis inspired nearly a dozen studies of methionine loading, which all achieved the same finding: an oral challenge of 10 g of methionine (the immediate precursor of S-adenosylmethionine) causes 40%–50% of patients diagnosed as "chronic schizophrenic" to have acute, transient, reversible psychotic reactions even without overt signs of organic delirium. This highly reproducible finding remains unexplained to this day. Our present results suggest an explanation. It seems possible that many of the patients then diagnosed as "chronic schizophrenic" might today be diagnosed as bipolar or schizoaffective. Thus, the 40%–50% psychosis rate found might represent a consistent rate of misdiagnosed bipolar and/or schizoaffective patients who experienced an acute manic psychosis in response to challenge with methionine. It will be interesting to test this hypothesis with today's more stringent diagnostic criteria. A more modern version of the transmethylation hypothesis postulates an under-active methylation system in depression and an over-active system in mania.

This is an example of the lurching from enthusiasm to enthusiasm, always with a pretense of progress, that Dr. Pam discussed in Chapter 1.

Wender, P. H., & Reimherr, F. W. (1990). Bupropion treatment of attention-deficit hyperactivity disorder in adults. 147, 1018–1020.

This was an open trial of bupropion in treatment of attention deficit in adults, with positive results. The authors stated: "There is a theoretical basis for a therapeutic effect of bupropion in attention-deficit hyperactivity disorder. The drug has dopaminergic activity and attention-deficit hyperactivity is proposed to be the result of a deficiency in dopaminergic function."

There is a "theoretical" basis for an excess or deficit of every transmitter in every disorder, at this level of usage of the term theoretical, which is its standard usage in biological psychiatry. By theoretical, bioreductionist psychiatrists mean a level of intellectual function that falls far below any serious scientific threshold for the theoretical.

According to this author's reasoning, attention deficit disorder should be placed on a spectrum with schizophrenia and should occur when the dopamine hyperactivity of schizophrenia is overcorrected with neuroleptics, which never occurs. Similarly, attention deficit should be treatable with L-Dopa according to this model, but this has never been reported.

> *McCann, U. D., & Agras, W. S. (1990). Successful treatment of nonpurging bulimia nervosa with desipramine: A double-blind, placebo-controlled study. 147, 1509–1513.*

In this standard drug study, the authors treated 10 bulimics with desipramine and 13 with placebo, with significant results. However, based on a variety of measures administered, they concluded that the desipramine worked by suppressing appetite, a mechanism that is biologically nonspecific and unrelated to the affective spectrum hypothesis.

> *McElroy, S. L., Hudson, J. I., Pope, H. G., Keck, P. E., & Aizley, H. G. The DSM-III-R impulse control disorders not elsewhere classified: Clinical characteristics and relationship to other psychiatric disorders. 149, 318–327.*

The authors added intermittent explosive disorder, kleptomania, pathological gambling, pyromania, and trichotillomania to the affective spectrum, using the same logic as in the Hudson and Pope (1990) paper described above.

> *Wolkowitz, O. M., Reus, V. I., Manfredi, F., Ingbar, J., Brizendine, L., & Weingartner, H. (1993). Ketoconazole administration in hypercortisolemic depression. 150, 810–812.*

The authors showed that depression can be treated with ketoconazole, a "commonly used imidazole antifungal drug, [which] has prominent cortisol biosynthesis inhibition and glucocorticoid receptor antagonist properties." According to the logic of the affective spectrum hypothesis, we must now consider classifying depression as a fungal infection.

> *Kahn, R. S., Davidson, M., Siever, L., Gabriel, S., Apter, S., & Davis, K. L. (1993). Serotonin function and treatment response to clozapine in schizophrenic patients. 150, 1337–1342.*

Although serotonin is supposed to be the biological foundation of the affective spectrum, these authors showed that the serotonin system is implicated in the response of schizophrenia to clozapine.

O'Flynn, K., & Dinan, T. G. (1993). Baclofen-induced growth hormone release in major depression: Relationship to dexamethasone suppression test result. 150, 1728–1730.

This study demonstrates an abnormality in GABA in depression, yet another brain chemical that must be accounted for in the affective spectrum hypothesis. The benzodiazepine receptor is close to the GABA receptor on the neuron cell wall, and activation of the benzodiazepine receptor–chloride ion channel–GABA receptor complex is widely presumed to be the basis of the anxiolytic efficacy of benzodiazepines in biological psychiatry. This study raises yet another problem for those who believe in the diagnostic specificity of neurotransmitters.

Altamura, C. A., Mauri, M. C., Ferrara, A., Moro, A. R., D'Andrea, G., & Zamberlan, F. (1993). Plasma and platelet excitatory amino acids in psychiatric disorders. 150, 1731–1733.

The authors measured plasma and platelet levels of 8 amino acids in 38 psychiatric patients and 19 controls. The patients included 3 with organic mental disorders, 15 with mood disorders, 13 with schizophrenia, and 7 with anxiety disorders. High levels of plasma glutamate were found in the depressed subjects, coupled with low levels of platelets. This led them to suggest that reduced uptake of amino acids may play a role in depression, yet another complication that must be resolved by any adequate affective spectrum hypothesis.

CONCLUSION

This completes a detailed analysis of pseudoscience in *The American Journal of Psychiatry* from 1990 to 1993. The January 1994 issue of the *Journal* indicates that logical errors and bioreductionist ideology will continue to dominate psychiatry for some time. A similar analysis could not be made of a leading journal in a truly scientific field.

REFERENCES

Benson, D. F., Miller, B. L., & Signer, S. F. (1986). Dual personality associated with epilepsy. *Archives of Neurology, 43*, 471–474.

Carlson, E. B., Putnam, F. W., Ross, C. A., Torem, M., Coons, P., Diil, D. L., Loewenstein, R. J., & Braun, B. G. (1993). Validity of the Dissociative Experiences Scale in screening for multiple personality disorder: A multicenter study. *American Journal of Psychiatry, 150*, 1030–1036.

Ross, C. A., Anderson, G., Fleisher, W. P., & Norton, G. R. (1991). The frequency of multiple personality disorder among psychiatric inpatients. *American Journal of Psychiatry, 148,* 1717–1720.

Ross, C. A., Joshi, S., & Currie, R. (1990). Dissociative experiences in the general population. *American Journal of Psychiatry, 147,* 1547–1552.

Ross, C. A., Miller, S. D., Reagor, P., Bjornson, L., Fraser, G. A., & Anderson, G. (1990). Structured interview data on 102 cases of multiple personality disorder from four centers. *American Journal of Psychiatry, 147,* 596–601.

4

THE GENETICS OF PREPOSTEROUS CONDITIONS

Harry Wiener

Four years ago, Alvin Pam (1990) published a detailed and thorough "critique of the scientific status of biological psychiatry." I enjoyed his convincing exposure of flaws, errors, spurious assumptions, discredited citations, and work below scientific standard in what I think is now the dominant orthodoxy in psychiatry—the geneticist, organic, blame-the-patient's-body ideology as opposed to the previously regnant environmentalist, interpersonal, blame-the patient's-family ideology.

At one point, however, I felt Pam went too far. Discussing a notion of Goodwin (see, e.g., Goodwin, Schulsinger, Hermansen, Guze, & Winokur, 1973) that divorce and alcoholism may perhaps be covariants of a single or related genetic predisposition, Pam commented: "Talk about neo-Lamarckism: it seems even acquired legal status can be inherited these days!"

This type of criticism has been made by many others, particularly in connection with the genetics of schizophrenia. The belief that schizophrenia is a specific organic disease or a group of organic brain diseases has never been confirmed. We have been on the verge of confirming it

193

since the dawn of modern psychiatry, and we are still on the verge. The recent discoveries of ventricular and electroencephalographic changes are irrelevant to this question. There is no hint as to the direction of the cause-effect arrow: Do the brain changes lead to an organically caused schizophrenia, or do the social dysfunctions of schizophrenia lead to a disuse-type brain atrophy?

Many observers, including Pam, remain unconvinced. If, as they believe, schizophrenia involves unusual ways of living, toxic family environments, labeling, and scapegoating, is it not preposterous to suggest that these kaleidoscopic and unpredictable events might be subject to the rigid rules of genetic predestination? This indeed is what I suggest, and so I call this approach "preposterous genetics" or "the genetics of preposterous conditions."

To be specific: unlike my fellow devotees of behavioral genetics, I accept the evidence that schizophrenia and its congeners are not well-defined brain diseases, inexorably unrolling according to a pattern laid down in the central nervous system; that they are, instead, ill-defined personal problems as much under the sway of the human environment as of the bodily milieu-interieur. But still, my aim is to show that, in theory, *it is possible* for genetic predisposition to affect the relative vulnerability of different population groups to unpleasant events that are clearly determined by fate's roll of dice.

THE MOST PREPOSTEROUS GENETIC SCHEME: INHERITANCE OF IMPOLITENESS

To get a lead on specific applications of the approach I have just mentioned, let me start with the notion that impoliteness might be inherited. Alvin Pam and Harry Wiener agree that this is not just preposterous, but positively side-splitting. But when we stop laughing, I begin to suspect that the clownish garb of this notion veils a sad problem of human relations.

In an abstract of a Danish study of behavioral precursors of the schizophrenia spectrum, Parnas, Schulsinger, Schulsinger, Mednick, and Teasdale (1982a, 1982b) stated: "S-subjects were described as impolite children." S-subjects were children averaging 15 years of age who had been considered at high risk of schizophrenia, and who 10 years later were in fact diagnosed as having schizophrenia. In the full report of this study (Parnas, et al., 1982a), such a finding was shown to be based on a forced-choice report from the parents of these children: "Schizophrenics were described as being impolite children, corresponding to their disturbing school behavior." Why was this forced choice included? I assume that the researchers concluded that there was a genetically shared predisposition to schizophrenia and to impoliteness, or that impoliteness was a premorbid social marker for schizophrenia. But they might have felt that it would be more diplomatic to let so unusual an observation come from the parents rather than from themselves.

The notion that the predisposition to schizophrenia is also a predisposition to impoliteness is somewhat strange, yet I can show how it is at least *possible.* Imagine that you were a fly on the wall in Copenhagen, and that in fact you saw this impoliteness. Did you see the children being impolite to *everyone?* The report fails to answer this question, but from the general tenor of the article we may surmise: no, they were just being impolite to the researchers and their parental allies. They were not necessarily impolite to each other, nor were they necessarily impolite to people in general. So, we may have one specified group of people being impolite to another. We know something about one group: at the time of the study, they were believed predisposed to schizophrenia— a belief supported by the 10-year follow-up. What do we know about the other group? Parnas et al. are part of the United States–Danish adoptee study group that was set up to settle, once and for all, the question of whether the contribution of genetics to schizophrenia is clearcut, while the contribution of environment is vague.

The children and the researchers therefore might be considered to represent two population groups. I suspect that these are not some obscure groupings, but the two most commonly recognized polarities of personality. There are hundreds of terms for these pairs of trait groups, many of which are judgmental, prescriptive, or polarized; they express a positive judgment about one side and a negative one about the other. Reviews of the literature have shown (Adams, 1954; MacKinnon, 1954) that these many names can be easily grouped in two columns, left and right. The choice of name then depends only on your personal preference; the two groupings remain the same.

I use the nonjudgmental and non-Manichean abbreviations D and C, short for Liam Hudson's (1966) personality types: "diverger" and "converger." In Hudson's research on British schoolboys, convergers had a commitment to practical action and did well on tests requiring right-or-wrong answers; divergers avoided practical action and did well on open-ended tests, where their imagination could roam freely. Hudson also has two neutral types: (a) "none-of-the-above," which I call O, and (b) "all-rounder," which I call CD. Some fairly well known approximate synonyms are:

Theorist	Practical (Type C)	Imaginative (Type D)
F. Dostoievski	Man of action	Man of consciousness
L. Hudson	Converger	Diverger
C. Jung (original usage)	Extravert	Introvert
F. Nietzsche	Apollonian	Dionysian
G. B. Shaw	Philistine	Idealist
W. James	Tough-minded	Tender-minded

In this case, we could guess that the children might seem somewhat more flaky, and the researchers somewhat more rigid, than your average Joe Citizen. We also note that the children belong to a population group said to be predisposed to schizophrenia, and that the researchers belong to a population group predisposed to viewing schizophrenia as an organic/genetic disease! I therefore think of the children as D (divergers) and the researchers as C (convergers). These groups, by themselves, are not pathologic (although a person in group C is likely to think someone in group D is sick or needs help, and vice versa). For argument's sake, these two groups can be considered *normal personality types,* perhaps the two "practical" and "imaginative" columns tabulated above.

To discuss impoliteness, we can ignore everything we know about the personality characteristics these two groups represent, except that they dislike and irritate each other. Each wishes the other would go away. This is of personal interest to me. Twenty-five years ago, when I started out on the road that led me to my present conclusions, I wrote a short programmatic note (Wiener, 1966) that included the following, copied from "Familiar Medical Quotations" (Strauss, 1968):

> Schizophrenia . . . splits psychiatrists into two cultures, the psychologic (psychodynamic) and the organic (somatic). Each group ignores the other and wishes it would go away.

If two types of people (convergers vs. divergers; psychologic psychiatrists vs. organic psychiatrists; researchers vs. children) were in a symmetrical situation, equally valued and empowered, then we could say nothing more about impoliteness. But the situation described here is highly asymmetrical and unequal.

Where one type is up and one is down, or where one type has the power to force itself into the presence of the other, the mutual hostility between the two will charge the atmosphere. The preposterous genetics of impoliteness depends in part on context: if, as in this case, respected and powerful C authority figures come to inspect disrespected and powerless D child specimens, the latter will have much incentive to resist, to dissimulate, to be resentful, uncooperative, or impolite. Interestingly, this sounds like *oppositional defiant disorder*, an allegedly common psychiatric disorder in children characterized in DSM-III as "disobedient, negativistic, and provocative opposition to authority figures" (Loeber, 1991). But if the situation were reversed, I fear, the genetic predisposition to impoliteness would appear to reside in personality type C.

It also depends on who tells the tale. If the children were doing the evaluating and reporting, we might come to suspect that a genetic predisposition to blaming the body of the schizophrenic victim is also a genetic predisposition to impoliteness. But what actually happened is that the researchers told the story. Under these limited circumstances, preposterous as it may seem, I do believe that it is *possible* for impoliteness to be genetically determined.

GENETICS-BETWEEN VERSUS GENETICS-WITHIN

If there is any semblance of reality in the story I have just told, its importance lies entirely in the notion that the impact of genetics on any one behavioral or social trait (impoliteness, in this case) sometimes resides not in single persons, but in pairs: dyads composed of one person predisposed (among other things) to schizophrenia and another person predisposed (among other things) to genetic explanations of psychiatric problems. I do agree with Pam that *genetics-within* (intrapersonal) interpretations of impoliteness, divorce, criminality, schizophrenia, and the like are truly preposterous. But *genetics-between* (interpersonal) interpretations deserve a closer look.

This reframing affects the notion of typology as well as of genetics. I have long considered the ancient science of typology as my hobby, in spite of the fact that some experts, when typology was more in vogue than it is now, viewed it as a reprehensible field of study, linked to racists and Nazis. There is some merit to this view as far as *typology-within* is concerned. Because each typologist has his or her own firm values and pet hates, typology-within has struck me as a riotous celebration of bias and prejudice. It has given moral support to murderous regimes of the hyperfascist (Hitler) as well of the hypersocialist (Pol Pot) persuasion, each of which postulates a fundamental distinction between "good" and "bad" types of people.

Typology-between, on the other hand, requires that opposing types or contrasting trait-groups be viewed as symmetrical, with dysfunction and pathology located not in any one personality type, but in negative interactions between different cognitive organizations. It also requires that the terms used for different genetic structures be neutral, neither triumphalist nor condemnatory, and that they be based on observable descriptions rather than on theoretical mechanisms. Ornstein (1973), a theorist, has related the polarities tabulated above to brain function, arguing that left-brain operations tend to control imaginative and verbal functions (the "night" side of consciousness), as opposed to practical and mechanical functions (the "day" side of consciousness) for the right brain. I find this terminology useful, but observable evidence for the relation between left-brain predominance and converger function is unavailable. In Rusu's (1939) typology-within, the C-side is termed sympathetic and the other "demoniac [sic]," which tells us only that Rusu was, in Ornstein's terms, an extreme left-brain personality, and that he viewed the disapproved trait-group as spawn of the devil. In the model of typology-between, which I prefer, the two sides are called convergers/divergers or Cs/Ds, respectively. These are neutral terms, and they inhibit the expression of personal prejudice.

The between-rather-than-within concept (interactional psychology) has a long history and has recently gained considerable attention and recognition, as in the work of Thomas and Chess (1980) on goodness and poorness of temperamental fit between organism and environment; Hampson's (1982) integration of internal processes and social environment; the work of Lerner, Lerner, and Zabski (1985) on the relation between temperament and context ("contextualism") in psychosocial adaptation; and the conclusion by Sameroff and Emde (1989) that early childhood psychological disorders are best understood as a dysfunction of the infant-caretaker dyad. As far as I know, however, this concept has been applied to genetics only in my own work (Wiener, 1977, 1979).

BAD MARRIAGES, AND OTHER POSSIBLE APPLICATIONS OF TYPOLOGY-BETWEEN

Concerning marital dysfunction and divorce, when blood from persons of type A and of type B is brought together, a severe reaction ensues. Pretransfusion blood-type testing is intended to avoid these dysfunctions. But there is no premarriage personality type testing! Thus, it often happens that persons of antithetical personality structures enter into the intimate social contact and contract of marriage. These are people predisposed to repel each other once the masks of the courting dance are dropped. Some dysfunctional marriages involve other causes, but some are a result of C-vs.-D (converger-vs.-diverger) mismatch.

Even in these cases, however, cover stories will usually be invented to avoid facing the taboo notion of instinctive antipathy.

What does this have to do with the preposterous genetics of divorce? Let us assume 15 percent divergers, 30 percent convergers, and random mating. Let us assume further that divergers and convergers are equally predisposed to good or bad marriages. Unfortunately, they are not equally predisposed to run into marriage partners who are good for them or bad for them. You can see that the random chance of a diverger to form a hostile dyad is 30 percent (the proportion of convergers), while the chance of a converger to enter into a hostile dyad is only 15 percent. The rarer diverger personality type is twice as likely to be exposed to marital dysharmony—only because it is rarer, not because it is more dysfunctional. Assortative mating could reduce, but would not eliminate, this differential risk. And genetic studies are likely to show, preposterous as it may seem, that certain population groups are twice as likely as others to be involved in divorce, an acquired legal status. To conclude from such findings that divorce and alcoholism may be covariants of a single or related genetic predisposition (Goodwin et al., 1973) is to stretch the notion of "genetics-within" to the breaking point. The alternative "genetics-between" explanation may sound preposterous, but it does not require suspension of disbelief in the possibility that acquired legal status can be inherited.

The same sort of reasoning can be used to suggest a "preposterous" genetic linkage to dyadic (environment-responsive) conditions or events such as alcoholism, child abuse, criminality, schizophrenia, stress, and suicide. I will go into some detail on schizophrenia.

WHAT IS THE NATURE OF THE PREDISPOSITION TO SCHIZOPHRENIA?

Looking over the first attempts by geneticists, in the early 1900s, to prove genetic causation in schizophrenia, I find that three unstated assumptions were common to all of them:

1. Heritability—schizophrenia is inherited. An understandable assumption because, by definition, a geneticist is biased to find genetic solutions to clinical problems. However, in practice, psychiatrists found this assumption to be false, and it had to be modified into: "The" *predisposition* to schizophrenia is inherited.

2. Mendelian genes—there are simple mendelizing *genes*, perhaps one, perhaps many, that produce schizophrenia. The role of nongenetic factors may be ignored.

3. Gene-types come in twos—there are two forms *(two alleles or gene-types)* of each gene involved in the inheritance of schizophrenia, like Gregor Mendel's wrinkled and smooth peas. I shall here refer to these gene-types as *a gene-type that codes for proneness to schizophrenia* and *a gene-type that codes for proneness to normality*. Traditionally, these two are abbreviated as *s* (schizophrenic) and *n* (normal).

The results of these 80 years' research are clear and indisputable: nothing has come of it to date except utter confusion. I know of three reactions to this failure: the environmentalist response, the geneticist response, and my own.

The environmentalist response is to conclude that enough rope has been given to the geneticists/organicists, and that assumption 1 is simply untrue. Clinical evidence for environmental, particularly familial, impact on the etiology of schizophrenia seems to point in this direction (Lidz, Blatt, & Cook, 1981).

The geneticist response is to conclude that assumption 2 has been shown to be false: that the role of environmental factors cannot be ignored, and that no simple Mendelian system can explain the genetics of schizophrenia; instead, that the predisposition to schizophrenia is a complex concatenation of genetic elements with also some role for environmental triggers. For example, McGuffin (1989) stated at an international symposium that although schizophrenia is substantially genetic in origin, its inheritance does not follow a regular Mendelian pattern.

My own response is to cast an evil eye on assumption 3, which, so far as I know, has never been questioned. No matter what mechanism is assumed by geneticists working on schizophrenia, the contrast has always been between one normal and one pathological gene-type. I suspect, instead, that two gene-types have gotten us into deep quicksand, and that, paradoxically, three gene-types may get us out, back onto the Mendelian highway.

MULTIPLE GENE-TYPES

Current work on the genetics of schizophrenia directly descends from the studies first done around the turn of the century, when a simple legume-type 1900s Mendelian model was the only one available: two forms of a gene, one dominant, one recessive. But what if this research had arisen *de novo* in the 1980s, without historical antecedents? Then, I believe, researchers would automatically have used the 1980s human-type Mendelian model: in the study of the inheritance of human variants ("polymorphisms"), it has become apparent that two-only gene-types are quite rare (please note that I use the phrase *gene-type* for the sake of the reader who has no experience in Mendelian terminology; to a professional geneticist, *allele* is the only correct term).

Multiple gene-types are far more common, from 3 to 10 to 50 gene-types for each gene. Often, some of these gene-types are codominant, rather than recessive-vs.-dominant as in the pea-scheme. And sometimes (as I think is the case for schizophrenia), traits originally thought to be controlled by two gene-types have later been found to have more than two. Some illustrative applications follow:

> Major histocompatibility complex: *more than 50 gene-types* at some loci encoding transplantation antigens (Steinmetz & Hood, 1983).
>
> Anodal tear protein: five *codominant gene-types* (Azen, 1976).
>
> Phenylketonuria: twenty years ago, suggestion of a third gene-type at the phenylketonuria locus, rather than just the 2 previously thought to control predisposition to this disease (Woolf et al., 1968); by now we are up to *10 or more* gene-types (Okano et al., 1991).

I shall ignore my belief that there are dozens or scores of gene-types on each gene coding for the predisposition of schizophrenia, and that there are many such separate multi-gene-type genes. I cannot handle the arithmetic for 12, nor for 4. I only know how to deal with 3 gene-types. Just that alone can be surprisingly illuminating.

WHAT IS THE THIRD GENE-TYPE?

So far, we have described 2 of the 3 gene-types: *(1/3)* —a gene-type that codes for proneness to schizophrenia—and *(2/3)* a gene-type that codes for proneness to nonschizophrenia (or what the classifiers themselves call "normality").

Now we look for *(3/3)* —a gene-type that codes for some as-yet-unspecified predisposition. I think we have three points of information—enough to make a viable guess as to what the predisposition is.

1. The two common personality types have been viewed from many angles. One view was that of Ernst Kretschmer (1931), dominant in German psychiatry between the world wars. To him, one type was schizothymic (normal, but predisposed to schizophrenia), the other cyclothymic (normal, but predisposed to affective disorder).

The personality that we, now as then, perceive as flaky, cogitative, right-brained, people-minded, tender-minded, antiauthoritarian ("liberal") and divergent, he observed to be predisposed to schizophrenia. The personality that we, now as then, perceive as stolid, jovial, left-brained, thing-minded, tough-minded, authoritarian ("conservative"), and convergent, he observed to be predisposed to "MDD" (an abbreviation for what was then called manic-depressive disease and is now termed "the major affective disorders," including depression and manic-depressive illness).

According to Kretschmer, we can then hypothesize that gene-type ($\frac{1}{3}$) corresponds to the normal personality predisposed to schizophrenia, and that its counterpart, gene-type ($\frac{3}{3}$) corresponds to the normal personality predisposed to "MDD." The three gene-types, according to this hypothesis, now can be called: ($\frac{1}{3}$)—a gene-type that codes for predisposition to schizophrenia, corresponding to Liam Hudson's diverger, which I abbreviate as type D; ($\frac{2}{3}$)—a gene-type that codes for predisposition to neither schizophrenia nor "MDD," corresponding to Hudson's none-of-the-above, which I abbreviate as type O (we can no longer say that this gene-type codes for normality; types C, D, and O are *all* normal personality types); and ($\frac{3}{3}$)—a gene-type that codes for predisposition to "MDD," corresponding to Hudson's converger, which I abbreviate as type C.

2. From the example of impoliteness above, we might suspect that the gene-types ($\frac{1}{3}$) and ($\frac{3}{3}$) are in some sort of antagonistic, hostile, push-pull relation to each other.

3. The examples of multiple gene-types above are all taken from the laboratory and not from the doctor's office. But in clinical practice, there is only one set of human polymorphisms for which we have a working genetic model: the blood groups and their interactions. The first system to be examined was the clearest and simplest: the ABO blood group system. And, ideally for what we are discussing, in its simplified version it has three gene-types, two dominant (A, B) and one recessive (O).

Perish the thought that the ABO types have anything to tell us about predisposition to psychiatric illness. Instead, the ABO system is useful as a *structural* example, a show-and-tell, of three gene-types in humans. And so we have O clearly as analog to blood type O, and D as analog to, say, A. Type C (converger) thus becomes the analog to blood type B. That fits nicely, for B ("anti-A") reacts unfavorably with A in the blood stream—it triggers transfusion reactions—and I have already mentioned a possible antagonistic reaction between the converger and the diverger types. I am therefore led to propose that the gene-type ($^3/_3$) also codes for another aspect of type C, "predisposition to anti-schizophrenia"—predisposition to trigger schizophrenic reactions in other persons predisposed to them.

Yes, yes; I know that you never heard of genetic predisposition to hostility to the schizophrenic patient and others of his genotype, and that it sounds strange if not sick. And I can't even claim that I thought of the notion that the high-EE parent, the schizogenic mother and the like, might carry a genetic predisposition, just as the schizophrenic patient presumably does. The originator is Martti Siirala, the most extreme environmentalist I know (which is by no means a recommendation). Siirala (1961) pointed out that, for 100 years, psychiatrists have been preoccupied with the question:

> Is there a special hereditary predisposition toward a later schizophrenic illness? And if so, what does it look like?

But there is, he cautioned, a reverse side to this question:

> Is there amongst us a special predisposition to view unusual tendencies in our fellow humans as undesirable blots on an otherwise perfect humanity, as disturbances of an otherwise ideal reality? Is it perhaps just this, our predisposition, that blocks the growth of human beings so much that we end up labeling them schizophrenic?

Commenting on this idea, Rümke (1964) said: "I reject this notion, but I cannot help thinking: this is something that can be thought of only in the case of schizophrenia. In any other case the thought would be ridiculous. This confronts us once more with the mystery of the disease." Arieti (1974) stated: "For several years I have been quite intolerant of Siirala's views, but recently I believe I understand him better and some of his ideas seem to me partially acceptable."

If, like me, you do not believe that schizophrenia "is" a genetic disease, then the term "predisposition to schizophrenia" can be a source of discomfort. Technically, all it means is that some persons are more likely than others to develop schizophrenia. But in common parlance—lay and psychiatric—it implies things like "doomed to deviance" or "intended for illness." I therefore would prefer to use the term "conditional predisposition." Conditional predisposition to develop schizophrenia (type D) means that in the presence of an unfavorable (type C) environment, illnesses of the schizophrenic-spectrum type are indeed more likely to occur. But in the presence of a favorable (type D) human environment, type D is also a conditional predisposition to creativity. Heston (1966) has shown that about half of a group of adopted-away children of schizophrenic mothers developed various behavior problems, including schizophrenia; but the other half "were notably successful adults. They possessed artistic talents and demonstrated imaginative adaptations to life which were uncommon in the control group. . . . They held the more creative jobs: musician, teacher, home-designer; and followed the more imaginative hobbies: oil painting, music, antique aircraft."

Summing all this up, I think that the following oversimplified description of the 3 gene-types (alleles) involved in schizophrenia—all on the same gene—could be helpful: ($\frac{1}{3}$)—a gene-type that codes for type D, that is, among other things, predisposition to creativity or, depending on human context, predisposition to schizophrenia; ($\frac{3}{3}$)—a gene-type that codes for type C, that is, among other things, predisposition to affective disorder or, depending on human context, predisposition to antischizophrenia; and ($\frac{2}{3}$)—a gene-type that codes for type O, that is, none of the above. Or, more briefly:

($\frac{1}{3}$) A schizophrenic gene-type
($\frac{2}{3}$) A neutral gene-type
($\frac{3}{3}$) An antischizophrenic gene-type

Summarizing further, it would seem that predisposition to schizophrenia-or-creativity is genetically determined. Schizophrenia is not genetically determined; it is one possibility resulting from a series of chance encounters. In line with the widely accepted diathesis–stress theory of schizophrenia, each encounter is between diathesis (type D in one individual) and stress (type C in another significant individual or individuals nearby). If someone must be blamed, I am blaming the dyad: not the schizophrenic patient nor the schizogenic significant other, but the fall of the dice that made each the victim of the other.

SUGGESTED GENETIC INFLUENCE ON POLITICAL ALLEGIANCE AND OTHER SOCIAL ATTITUDES

I have now managed to draw a tenuous connection from *genetics-between* to social dysfunction (impoliteness), to marital dysfunction (divorce), and to psychotic dysfunction (schizophrenia); I might as well take a step into seemingly even more absurd territory: the genetics of political dysfunction, of being out of step with the politics of those around you. My knowledge of the subject of the *inheritance* of political allegiance is largely limited to the fundamental finding of Sir William Schwenck Gilbert, that "every boy and every gal, that's born into the world alive, is either a little Liberal, or else a little Conservative!"

Let me explore this idea further. Political allegiance is not, I suspect, likely to be an independent variable. Genetic conditional predisposition is not likely to affect *how you vote*, but it may well help determine *who you are*. A human being born as a little Liberal is a potential liberal thinker (type D), not necessarily a liberal voter. "Every boy and every gal," in this view develops into either a little diverger/D-type (Democrat), or a little converger/C-type (Conservative), or a little Middle-of-the Roader (type O or type CD). The human personality types differ in all aspects of human relations, including politics.

The two basic political styles have in fact been shown to be linked to many other interesting and surprising interactional traits. Take, as one example, tolerance of ambiguity: the diverger/liberal tends to see shades of gray, the converger/conservative tends to see black and white. This manifests itself in philosophy (Occam's sharp C-razor vs. D shades-of-gray), in religion (the C-fundamentalist vs. the D-unitarian), in art (the sharp contours and primary colors of "socialist" realism vs. the deeper sensitivity of the creative D-artist), and in personal habits (neat/rigid-C vs. messy/free-D).

Another example deals with traits concerning one's relationship to others. Divergers ("communitarians") tend to be more empathic, more likely to weep, verbally more explicit about their feelings, more altruistic, more prosocial, more intellectually gifted, less bellicose, more affiliative, more advanced on measures of moral judgment, and more apt to volunteer than convergers ("solitarians").

The two main political-and-personality types (Conservative/C-type/Converger and Democratic/D-type/Diverger) may be almost as important a division among humans as are the two main sexual types (male and female). That is because "politics" involves much more than voting or preaching or conniving or electioneering. It is, as the word originally indicated, the way of humans in society, the style in which human-among-others relates to these others. Some alternative terms for political-psychological attitudes are: Liberalism (solidarism, progressivism, socialism); Conservatism (capitalism, traditionalism, authoritarianism).

Inevitably, the holders of each of these two attitudes will view their own as morally more advanced and the other as morally less developed. Typology-between, however, suggests that we could view both the political types (C—conservative, bourgeois, authoritarian; D—democratic, liberal, socialist) as normal variants of the human race, symbiotically interacting with each other for some common, extrapersonal, societal good.

Inevitably also, the more active Cs and Ds will view *each other* as abnormal, bad, strange, out of touch, deviant, psychotic, or dysfunctional. But these knee-jerk eye-of-the-beholder reactions cannot be accepted as valid descriptions. True political dysfunction comes from one individual's being in the position of an outsider among others of the opposite type.

The preposterous models I have used in other areas can therefore be usefully applied here too, with one important exception. In all the examples mentioned so far—impoliteness, divorce, crime, schizophrenia—there is face-to-face contact between the opposing human types. When political or social polarities involve close contact (microculture: families, at work, town meetings), the rule remains as before: the majority (more common) polymorph has the advantage. But in the macroculture, in politics as we generally understand it, contact is mainly by printed or broadcast words rather than by face-to-face social signals (the Germans say: paper does not blush). Here, the opposite is true: the minority (rarer) polymorphic form has the advantage.

In the macroculture, therefore, Socratic doctrine applies today as it did 2,500 years ago: the few (*hoi oligoi*), those *who know,* should rule; the others, the many (*hoi polloi*) should obey. In our day, public opinion largely accepts the doctrine that "the best and the brightest" (Ds favorably described by Ds) should conduct public affairs for the benefit of the others, who are only implicitly thought of as "the worst and the dumbest" (Cs unfavorably described by Ds) when they vote against their own best interests, as defined by the rarer polymorphic form.

As to the microculture, statistical studies of political dysfunction have usually been based on samples of American college students, often at universities reputed to be liberal in climate. For this reason, the majority of published studies show a link between right-wing attitude and personal pathology. McClosky (1958), for example, found conservative students to be submissive and alienated, as well as poorly integrated psychologically. However, replicating this study in the conservative climate of apartheid/white South Africa, Orpen (1972) found significant correlations among conservatism, prejudice, and higher levels of mental health.

This contextual effect on political dysfunction (the association between political attitude and social dysfunction) can even be found in a single locality. At Harvard, the authoritarian (C-type) student was likely to come across as more disturbed, confused, and alienated. He was the outsider there. But at the nearby University of Massachusetts, students who rated low on the F-scale (antiauthoritarians, D-types) were in a distinct minority. When the dean there saw a list of the low-F students, he commented, without knowing what it was: "Why, you have the names of almost all of my problem children!" (Marquis, 1973).

This is the perspective of the authoritarian. Just the opposite could be expected from the antiauthoritarian. For example, the relation between political dysfunction and lack of fit was emphasized by Keniston (1967) who, unlike the University dean cited above, saw himself as deeply in tune with these young people:

The "fit" between individuals and society, culture and history is never a perfect fit and is not always even a good fit. In this book, for example, I have been chiefly concerned with those who do not fit, who reject what their society demands of them.

Though their goals are often confused and inarticulate, they converge on a passionate yearning for openness and immediacy of experience, on an intense desire to create, on a longing to express their perception of the world, and above all, on a quest for values and commitments that will give their lives coherence.

Political dysfunction (failure to fit in) can be minimized by escape hatches. One is *mobility:* activist individuals who feel temporarily out of place where they live or where they work can find a location where their political and personal values are ascendant, where they feel more at home. Another is Montesquieu's *separation of powers,* a device that permits outsiders (Xs-among-Ys: conservatives-among liberals, liberals-among-conservatives) to opt out into an insider (Xs-among-Xs: conservatives-among-conservatives, liberals-among-liberals) area. It seems messy, illogical, and gridlocked—if your entering assumption is that we are all more or less alike and that we all seek similar goals, such as neatness and logic in political governance. But the bloody history of the world shows that we are *not* all alike. More centralized governments tend to be controlled by one side, the in-group. The out-group is thus condemned to political impotency and dysfunction, with resulting growth in extremist sentiment and social instability. On the other hand, Montesquieu's system is embedded in the U.S. Constitution: Congress, Executive, and Judiciary all oscillate between the Liberal and the Conservative visions, often each with a different frequency of the pendulum. This offers something for everybody. In other words, a healthy political body need not vilify its opponents, but it makes space for them in the community.

SUMMARY

It is suggested that genetic influences on social dysfunction and pathology can act not on single individuals, but on pairs of individuals. This approach may help explain how genetics might affect even such preposterous conditions as impoliteness, and how schizophrenia may be viewed with equanimity as either a genetic or an environmental condition. Accordingly, there is no warrant for blaming the body of the victim, *for genetics is not fate.* Instead, I argue, fate is the combination of genetics and environment, that is, the result of the interaction of the individual's genes with the genes of his or her counterparts in the human environment.

REFERENCES

Adams, D. K. (1954). *The anatomy of personality.* New York: Random House.

Arieti, S. (1974). An overview of schizophrenia from a predominately psychological approach. *American Journal of Psychiatry, 131,* 241–249.

Azen, E. A. (1976). Genetic polymorphism of human anodal tear protein. *Biochemical Genetics, 14,* 225–235.

Goodwin, D. W., Schulsinger, F., Hermansen, L., Guze, S. B., & Winokur, G. (1973). Alcohol problems in adoptees raised apart from alcoholic biological parents. *Archives of General Psychiatry, 28,* 238–243.

Hampson, S. E. (1982). *The construction of personality.* Boston: Routledge.

Heston, L. L. (1966). Psychiatric disorders in foster home reared children of schizophrenic mothers. *British Journal of Psychiatry, 112,* 819–825.

Hudson, L. (1966). *Contrary imaginations: A psychological study of the young student.* New York: Schocken.

Keniston, K. (1967). *The uncommitted—alienated youth in American society.* New York: Dell.

Kretschmer, E. (1931). *Körperbau and charakter.* Berlin: Springer.

Lerner, J. V., Lerner, R. M., & Zabski, S. (1985). Temperament and elementary school children's actual and rated academic performance—a test of a "goodness of fit" model. *Journal of Child Psychology and Psychiatry, 26,* 125–136.

Lidz, T., Blatt, S., & Cook, B. (1981). Critique of the Danish–American studies of the adopted-away offspring of schizophrenia parents. *American Journal of Psychiatry, 138,* 1063–1068.

Loeber, R. (1991). Oppositional defiant disorder and conduct disorder. *Hospital and Community Psychiatry, 42,* 1099–1102.

MacKinnon, D. W. (1954). The structure of personality. In J. M. Hunt (Ed), *Personality and the behavior disorders,* Vol. 1 (pp. 3–48). New York: Ronald Press.

Marquis, P. C. (1973). Experimenter-subject interactions as a function of authoritarianism and response set. *Journal of Personality and Social Psychology, 25,* 289–296.

McClosky, H. (1958). Conservatism and personality. *American Political Review, 42,* 27–45.

McGuffin, P. (1989). Cited in note "Genes aren't everything." *Lancet, 1,* 1402.

Okano, Y., Eisensmith, R. C., Güttler, F., Lichter-Konecki, U., Konecki, D. S., Trefz, F. K., Dasovich, M., Wang, T., Henriksen, K., Lou, H., & Woo, S. L. C. (1991). Molecular basis of phenotypic heterogeneity in phenylketonuria. *New England Journal of Medicine, 324,* 1232–1238.

Ornstein, R. E. (1973). *The psychology of consciousness.* New York: Viking.

Orpen, C. (1972). A cross-cultural investigation of the relationship between conservatism and prejudice. *Journal of Psychology, 81,* 297–300.

Pam, A. (1990). A critique of the scientific status of biological psychiatry. *Acta Psychiatrica Scandinavica, 82* (Suppl. 362), 1–35.

Parnas, J., Schulsinger, F., Schulsinger, H., Mednick, S. A., & Teasdale, T. W. (1982a). Behavioral precursors of schizophrenia spectrum. A prospective study. *Archives of General Psychiatry, 39,* 658–664.

Parnas, J., Schulsinger, F., Schulsinger, H., Mednick, S. A., & Teasdale, T. W. (1982b). Behavioral precursors of schizophrenia spectrum (abstract). *Digests of Neurology and Psychiatry, 50,* 362.

Rümke, H. C. (1964). Aspects of the schizophrenia problem. *Psychiatric and Neurological Neurochemistry, 67,* 79–94.

Rusu, L. (1939). Contributions to typology. *Reviews of Physiology, 2,* 35–43.

Sameroff, A. J., & Emde, R. N. (1989). *Relationship disturbances in early childhood— a developmental approach.* New York: Basic Books.

Siirala, M. (1961). *Die schizophrenie des einzelnen und der allgemeinheit.* Gottingen: Vandenhoek.

Steinmetz, M., & Hood, L. (1983). Genes of the major histocompatibility complex in mouse and man. *Science, 222,* 727–733.

Strauss, M. B. (1968). *Familiar medical quotations.* Boston: Little, Brown.

Thomas, A., & Chess, S. (1980). *The dynamics of psychological development.* New York: Brunner/Mazel.

Wiener, H. (1966). External chemical messengers. *Journal of the American Medical Association, 197,* 216–217.

Wiener, H. (1977). *Schizophrenia and anti-schizophrenia. The symmetrical theory of mental illness.* New York: Arrow House.

Wiener, H. (1979). Environment and inheritance—opposing forces? *Schizophrenia Bulletin, 5,* 218–219.

Woolf, L. I., Goodwin, B. L., Cranston, W. I., Wade, D. N., Woolf, F., Hudson, F. P., & McBean, M. S. (1968). A third allele at the phenylalanine-hydroxylase locus in mild phenylketonuria (hyperphenylalaninaemia). *Lancet, 1,* 114–117.

5

A SOCIAL CRITIQUE OF BIOLOGICAL PSYCHIATRY

Ellen M. Borges

The dream of reason did not take power into account.
—Paul Starr, 1982:3

In this chapter, I explore the social construction of the dominant paradigm in American psychiatry today, biological psychiatry, and examine some of the consequences that follow from "blaming the body." Determinism excludes all other views. Biological psychiatry, a form of determinism, effectively excludes consideration of social and psychodynamic factors when it constructs the "truth" about normality and abnormality.

Despite research that discredits genetic bases for human behavior, bioreductionist views of mental illness have become solidly entrenched over the past several decades, not just within psychiatry and the medical profession, but within the general public as well. In this chapter, I apply a sociological perspective to gain an understanding of contemporary biological psychiatry. Because of the recent emergence of many sources of competition for the care of people's minds, psychiatry has needed to ensure its dominant position, which it has attempted to do by adhering to a bioreductionist model of mental illness.

I believe in the reality and the pain of mental illness, but I have difficulty with theories, ideologies, and practices that define normality and set standards for behavior without awareness of how these theories, ideologies, and practices originate and persist, or to whom benefits accrue. Biological psychiatry does not consider a full range of possible explanations for human behavior and human misery. Kleinman (1988) argued that up to two-thirds of medical practice deals with life problems that are socially constructed. But social dimensions, too little considered in psychiatry, vanish altogether with an excessive focus on biological factors.

As a field, psychiatry developed without a great deal of attention to social diversity. Diversity, in biological psychiatry, means a range of pathological conditions, all of which exist within the category of *sick*. The underlying assumption is that sickness is a response to a physical defect; there is a shared belief in the presence of a physical defect; and a belief that a mechanism exists to "fix" the defect and to restore "normalcy." Sickness and medical conditions are viewed as objective biomedical entities. But why accept this particular viewpoint, given scientific evidence that refutes biological determinism in many psychiatric conditions (Ingleby, 1980)? Why, as psychiatry transformed itself from a local, custodial occupation into an internationally recognized and influential medical field, has there been so much concern with biology and so little with social diversity?

Intellectual processes are constrained by social context, one's sociocultural position influences one's perspective, and ideology biases thinking in a way that can distort reality (Mannheim, 1936). All human knowledge is socially constructed (Berger & Luckmann, 1967). The knowledge created depends on the social characteristics of its creators and on political processes. What people choose to study, how information is filtered and censored, the stance a researcher takes, and what gets published and accepted as knowledge are all the results of social process. There may be an objective reality, but social processes bias perceptions and create ideologies.

Our perspectives and our political processes determine what we view as "truth." Using the framework of the sociology of knowledge, it becomes easier to understand why biological psychiatrists increasingly view life through electron microscopes in order to find causes for different behavior patterns, rather than studying the rich, social diversity of human culture.

THE SOCIAL CONSTRUCTION OF MEDICAL DEVIANCE

At least three things occur when biological psychiatry performs its tripartite mission of healing individuals, protecting the social order, and protecting its own interests. Biological psychiatry redefines social deviance as a medical problem. By doing so, it transforms social norms, which are subjective and political, into medical norms, presumed to be objective and scientific. Deviation from these norms becomes defined as medical deviance, as sickness, not as social deviance. This transformation has been called the medicalization of deviance (Conrad & Schneider, 1985). Because of this transformation, the boundaries that separate true deviance, sickness, and social difference become blurred, with corresponding lack of clarity about how to react to each category.

Belief in the superordinacy of biology is not new in psychiatry, nor should it be unexpected. This ideology exists because of psychiatry's historical foundation, itself a product of social forces. Historically, American psychiatry developed in response to two separate but related concerns. During the early nineteenth century in this country, humanitarian concerns about poor treatment of the "mad" marked the point at which society redefined bizarre, or "evil" behaviors as illness (Jiminez, 1987; Sullivan, 1964). The separate but related public health concern was how to contain these behaviors in order to protect the larger society. Psychiatry began with a dual mandate: (a) to focus concern on the plight of afflicted individuals, and (b) at the same time, contain and isolate potentially harmful social conditions. Physicians assumed agency on behalf of individuals and on behalf of society. They assumed a protector role both for helpless victims of madness and for the larger society. In both cases, concerns for physical safety were primary. In its early stages, psychiatry aligned with a fledgling neuroscience (Sullivan, 1964). Psychiatry, as a subfield of medicine, emerged as a source of social control that focused on human emotions but based its practice on natural science models. Physicians now took the role of administrators in asylums that confined society's misfits, and the number of asylums grew to meet the needs of the larger society. A dual asylum system, public and private, emerged to keep the poor isolated from the less poor (Starr, 1982).

No significant change came until after World War I, during which psychiatrists tested men for military suitability and treated "shell shock" (Showalter, 1987). Not until after the 1930s, with the influx of European refugee psychiatrists, was there a shift from administrative, custodial psychiatry to a psychoanalytic model, and from asylum to private practice (Starr, 1982). Further change occurred after World War II, during which social scientists collaborated with psychiatrists to develop field treatments for service personnel. In spite of this collaboration, successful both in terms of treatment outcome and the development of insights into the role of social factors in psychiatric conditions (Janowitz, 1960), many psychiatrists held tenaciously to a biomedical ideology.

During the 1960s and 1970s, society was ripe for change. There was widespread cynicism, questioning of legitimacy, and mistrust of established institutions and social patterns. Psychiatry did not escape criticism during this period. The radical British psychiatrist, R. D. Laing, attempted to upturn psychiatry from within with his argument that those who are labeled mentally ill are, in fact, reacting to a loss of authenticity and the construction of a false self demanded by modern society (Laing, 1960; Laing & Esterson, 1964). He argued that schizophrenia is a defensive and "healthy" response to an existential crisis created by a "crazy" family. Reality is so bizarre and untenable for a "healthy" individual within this family constellation that psychosis is a "sane" alternative to participating in a shared "craziness."

Laing developed a substantial following, but partly because of a lack of supporting research, partly because of patient mismanagement, and partly because of his personal characteristics and behaviors, Laing lost what following he had. He was never viewed as credible by the majority of psychiatrists. Still, he raised questions within psychiatry and directed attention away from biological explanations for schizophrenia and toward the relevance of social systems and psychodynamics. He focused attention, too, on the potential for psychiatry's misconstruing and mislabeling behaviors of its clientele. Family systems theory carried on Laing's social orientation toward psychopathology and succeeded in gaining a measure of respectability within the psychiatric establishment (Pam, personal communication, 1993).

There were other critics. Sociologist Erving Goffman studied the effects of institutions on the labeling and perpetuation of mental illness and the changes in identity that emerge from internalizing labels, particularly negative ones (Goffman, 1961, 1963). Goffman's perspective, a dramaturgical one, deals with the impact of structure and others' expectations on how we play our social roles, as well as how we incorporate others' opinions of us. Relevant for biological psychiatry, Goffman's research showed that, given the powerlessness associated with institutionalization, people will exhibit symptoms authorities expect of them, and they deteriorate further in situations of structural powerlessness. Similarly, the conferring of a negative label by someone in a position of authority creates social stigma.

Scheff (1966) focused on the process by which diagnostic labeling directs people toward careers of deviant behavior. He argued that, regarding mental illness, symptoms are violations of social norms that occur in a social context. Those behaviors that are labeled "symptoms" are behaviors that somehow offend or puzzle those around them. The biomedical diagnostic process created expectations about patients' future behaviors. In social situations, people respond to the stigmatizing label rather than to the person. Worse, the stigmatized person will try to hide the stigma by behaving "as if normal," or may come to believe the label and act accordingly. The relevant point for biological psychiatry is that behavior is often a product of social situations and conferred identity, regardless of the individual's biological condition.

This perspective originally developed to explain the persistence of many forms of deviant behavior (Lemert, 1951). Initially, it evolved from the study of criminal behavior and recidivism. Researchers using this perspective argue that sometimes the behavior labeled as deviant is less offensive to society than the label itself. For example, the term "ex-convict," which carries highly negative expectations about behaviors, may be out of proportion to the actual criminal activity. Partly because of stereotyped ideas, people who become labeled negatively (and it is people, not behaviors that carry the label) are denied access to opportunities for leading ordinary lives—for example, obtaining jobs or mortgages. Because of the way society responds to and blocks opportunities for people with negative labels, ex-convicts may have fewer options open to them and therefore be more likely to return to crime. This perspective is constructivist: what constitutes deviance in any society depends on what offends those who have the power to define behaviors as criminally deviant rather than simply annoying. For example, calling someone "vagrant" has significantly different connotations than calling the person "homeless."

The other pertinent observation is that negative labels accrue more frequently to the socially disadvantaged, regardless of behavior, because less advantaged people are more likely to be arrested. As an example, common wisdom once assumed that child abuse was more common in lower social strata, when in fact the privacy afforded to more advantaged people allowed their abusive behaviors to go undetected. In addition, Sutherland and Cressey (1970) showed that the criminal justice system is biased against minorities. Minorities are more likely to be involved in visible crimes; they are arrested more frequently, convicted more frequently, and have poorer probation, when

actual transgressions are held constant. On the other hand, more affluent people have positions of trust and access to corporate resources,
and they commit "white-collar crimes" such as embezzlement.

Hollingshead and Redlich's (1958) study of social class and mental
illness found that, given the same configuration of symptoms, people
from lower social classes were more often diagnosed as schizophrenic
and those from more affluent social classes were diagnosed as manic-
depressive, a much more optimistic diagnosis. This example illustrates
the ideologically biased nature of the diagnostic process.

Taken to its extreme by Thomas Szasz (1961), the social constructivist perspective progressed to saying that mental illness was only the
label and that mental illness existed in the eye of the labeler. Szasz believed that the term "mental illness" was a misapplied and potentially
harmful metaphor, and he preferred the term "problems in living." His
work was not well-received by bioreductionist psychiatrists intent on
denying the importance of social and psychodynamic processes. Nevertheless, Szasz's work should raise concern about the validity of psychiatric diagnoses and the biological model of mental illness.

Within contemporary society, relegating authority to medicine followed from the recognition that punitive measures for many criminals
did not deter or correct criminal behavior. Partly, concern about the
secondary effects of criminal labels and institutionalization sparked
humanitarian efforts for change, particularly in situations involving
"victimless crimes," such as homosexuality (Schur, 1965). Often, less
stigma is attached to being sick, rather than criminal, because sickness
is presumed to be beyond the control of the individual. Social interventions based on biomedical models, in fact, made life substantially less
stressful for many people, most notably homosexuals (Bayer, 1987) and
substance abusers (Conrad & Schneider, 1985).

Although social constructivist studies circulated widely, generated
much discussion, and increased awareness of the contribution of social
factors to mental illness, this perspective faded, and psychiatry increased the number and types of diagnoses in its nosological system.
Witness the progression from DSM-I (1952) to DSM-II (1968) to DSM-
III (1980) to DSM-III-R (1983) and to DSM-IV (1994), plus ICD-9 and
ICD-10, all with increased numbers of categories. The medicalization
of social deviance is increasing, despite cogent and compelling arguments against it (Conrad, 1980).

As the number of forms of mental illness increases, more categories
fall into the domain of biological psychiatry. For example, many forms
of substance abuse are regarded as caused by a problem with neurotransmitters. Into this category falls such questionable substance abuse

as caffeine intoxication (Spitzer & Williams, 1987). Not only does this new diagnosis protect professional interests, it demonstrates the moral authority of psychiatry.

Deviance from norms implies biological abnormality in a medicalized social system. Because norms are established through political processes, deviance from norms is socially constructed. Psychiatry is in charge of this process in many areas, as is obvious in situations such as the diagnosing of political dissidents as mentally ill in the former Soviet Union, in order to confine them. Serious study of the medicalization of deviance has not persisted beyond the early 1980s, unfortunately.

When biological psychiatry is the authority, the mechanism of social control is medication and other somatic treatment, and physicians are the agents of social control. Medicalization of social deviance allows us a pretense of humanitarianism by removing connotations of immorality that characterized previous systems of social control. It shifts the locus of confinement from prison or purgatory to hospital, and shifts the emphasis from punishment to rehabilitation. Medicalization shifts the emphasis from "mending ways" to "healing," and from encouraging remorse to restoring chemical balances. In many cases, coarse physical constraints, like bars on windows and locked doors, direct personal restraint, and physical isolation continue to exist, but these are accompanied by more effective and more subtle constraints: behavior-altering drugs. These constraints are viewed as therapeutic rather than punitive measures.

SOCIAL DIVERSITY OR BIOLOGICAL ABNORMALITY?

When, where, and to whom we are born profoundly affects our lives. These conditions create the vantage points from which we view ourselves, others, and life in general. Reality differs depending on gender, race, social class, ethnicity, culture, and age. In this section, I discuss the second way in which biological psychiatry performs its mission: the manner in which biological psychiatry medicalizes behavior presumed to be abnormal based on stereotypical ideas about human behavior. There is a collateral process: biological psychiatry medicalizes behavior that deviates from expectations based on the dominant social class's ideology and viewpoint.

When psychiatry took on a "protector" role on behalf of society, it became responsible for making distinctions between acceptable and unacceptable behavior. What is acceptable and moral within a society depends on the characteristics of those who are powerful. When psychiatry recognizes diversity, then (where diversity means having characteristics that differ from dominant elites), this diversity is often labeled "deviant." To label someone is to attribute to that person a characteristic that an observer will insist is there, even if the person does not see it. When the labeled person can see the reason for the label, because of an internalization of social norms, it is much more difficult to discount the label's importance. Although all societies, as a part of social organization, have a dominant class that defines deviance, it is a peculiarity of this society that we rely so heavily on psychiatry for this task (Pam, personal communication, 1993).

Attributions about behavior associated with gender and race are most often made on the basis of physical characteristics. The behaviors are assumed to be biologically based. Often, these differences are presumed to be dichotomized: either you are a man or not, either you are white or not. Although there is gradual recognition of other interacting factors, such as level of education and the nature of socialization, dichotomized thinking persists about gender and race. This is as true for the social sciences as it is for psychiatry.

In this section, from a sociology of knowledge perspective, I examine information about gender and race that brings into question the assumptions of biomedical psychiatry. Then, I discuss subtle characteristics associated with social class, culture, and ethnicity, and the potential for biomedical psychiatry to misinterpret normal differences and label them pathological.

Gender as a Source of Diversity: Women's Bodies as Faulty

Throughout the history of psychiatry, the majority of "victims'" bodies have been female: women have been the primary clientele within psychiatry. The patterns associated with emotional distress mirror those associated with physical distress: women report more symptoms, seek treatment more frequently, receive more diagnoses, take more medications, and have more frequent hospitalizations (Chesler, 1972; Nathanson, 1975; Showalter, 1987; Tavris, 1992).

Women's bodies have been blamed for producing distinctly different and "weaker" psyches. It is true, as well, that stages in women's life cycles, particularly those associated with reproductive stages and cycles, have been treated as biomedically abnormal, rather than as life events or as the normal physical processes they are. Women's bodies, and indirectly their minds, have been the focus of medical intervention for childbirth, menstruation, sexuality (too much or too little), and menopause.

These internal biological faults in women's bodies require biomedical attention and treatment, as do associated psychiatric conditions, such as hysteria, postpartum depression, involutional melancholia, and late luteal phase mood disorder (Spitzer & Williams, 1987).

However, physical assaults against women, such as battery, rape, and incest, have been trivialized and often denied or treated inappropriately by general medicine and psychiatry. Women have been abused "for their own good" by the ideology and somatic treatments of biological psychiatry. Stories abound about psychosurgery and electroshock therapy prescribed for women who were unhappy with traditional roles, in order to render them more tractable (Chesler, 1972).

At the other end of the spectrum, intellectual and physical activity by women has been viewed as the cause of reproductive "failure." Some researchers still search for evidence to support arguments that when women step beyond the bounds of traditional roles, they will suffer for it either physically or mentally, or will fail their children (Ussher, 1989). In contrast to these arguments, research findings have consistently found, over time, that women are most satisfied with their lives when traditional roles are not the primary focus, and that women in more traditional roles tend to have more depression (Mirowsky & Ross, 1989). Most recently, Crosby (1991) discovered that, contrary to common assumptions, women who "juggle" many responsibilities, though more tired, are more satisfied with their lives and the more mentally stable compared to those with less diverse lifestyles.

For many women, biology has been destiny in psychiatry. Although there has been progress in medical understanding, this problem persists. How and why does this occur? There are biological gender differences; the question is whether these biological differences are symptoms that require treatment by psychiatric medicine. It is often not biology, but the presumed biological differences, the social constructions, that differentiate and separate the sexes.

Psychiatric theory developed predominantly from case studies of women, but with definitions of symptoms and normality, interpretations of symptoms, definitions of cure, and methods of treatment created almost exclusively by men. Historically, socially powerful males defined the boundaries of normality and abnormality. But women, effectively prevented for most of history from participation in the political economy, except in small numbers and in marginal positions, have as their predominant reality the world of the everyday, the mundane—a world not familiar to, valued, or even validated by the "fathers" of psychiatry. Psychiatry, by constructing its knowledge based on experiences of the socially dominant, by defining and enforcing appropriate behavior without adequate knowledge of women's realities, perpetuated male standards for femininity and female roles, often to its own benefit.

Worse, the denial of women's experiences and needs at times exacerbated mental illness. Chesler (1972) presented biographical material about Zelda Fitzgerald and case information from other women who, having ambitions other than being a wife and mother, were chastised and otherwise treated to redirect their attention properly. Each became emotionally disturbed, was institutionalized, and continued to deteriorate with more treatment. The life and emotional history of Charlotte Perkins Gilman (Ehrenreich & English, 1981) reflected clear associations between her mental state and her traditional roles. Seeking help for emotional distress, she told her physician that when she was away from her child, home, and husband, and when she was writing, she felt fine. The prescribed treatment was to rest, pay attention to her family, and avoid intellectual work. She became seriously mentally ill. In contemporary society, she might receive medication to help her to redirect her attention.

As a result of the emergence of a general concern for human rights, feminist movements of the past few decades, more educational opportunities for women, and a lot more noise, knowledge about women has begun to accumulate in psychiatry. For the first time, women have had sufficient power to set some research agendas, to get funding, and to base theory on women's realities. The results have discredited cherished beliefs about women that were based on underlying assumptions within psychiatry. Still, biological psychiatry flourishes and many women receive too much chemical treatment. The stated rationale is not overtly gender-biased, which would cause protest, but is instead based on posited somatic deficiencies that seem unrelated to the oppression or exploitation of women. In this respect, biological psychiatry perpetuates and reinforces social values that keep women in traditional roles.

Literature from the feminist movement that began during the 1960s, too varied and prolific to describe here, created awareness of the oppression and the general exclusion of women from public processes (Farganis, 1986; Mitchell, 1966). This awareness, plus politicization of the personal, a focus considerably different from the previous women's movement, created a favorable environment for a theory and practice of women's psychology. Recognizing that the construction of reality is the result of political processes allows the possibility of change.

Developments in the field of women's psychology arise from a post-positivist model of science. Researchers are redefining what were previously regarded as symptoms, indicative of deviance and defective bodies, as responses, sometimes exaggerated, to realistically distressing situations. For example, women's tendency to seek affiliation may now be seen as a healthy and natural behavior, rather than as an obstacle to healthy separation and as dependency (Surrey, 1991).

Nancy Chodorow's feminist psychoanalytic theory (1974) reinterpreted Freudian concepts by considering the impact of women's almost exclusive responsibility for child rearing on so-called "feminine" and "masculine" identities, and the manner in which gender-biased realities perpetuate inequality (1978, 1989). For example, Chodorow argued that children's initial intense relationships with mother promote feminine identities for girls and impede development of masculine identities for boys. At the same time, males are more likely to individuate, encouraged to do so by their mothers; the need to separate from mother is not such an issue for girls. This leads to development of more complex and extensive patterns of affiliation for girls than for boys. There is little room in this viewpoint for biological determinism, except for the fact that the reproductive capabilities of women unavoidably shape their roles.

Jean Baker Miller's *Toward a New Psychology of Women* (1976) addressed the impact of sexism and its concomitant powerlessness on the identities and psychological health of women. As a psychiatrist who became aware of the poverty of information about women in psychiatry, Miller, along with Irene Stiver, Judith Jordan, Alexandra Kaplan, and Janet Surrey, founded The Stone Center at Wellesley College. This research, education, and clinical center focuses on women's developmental psychology. From the resulting body of work has come the argument that, given patriarchal systems that systematically shape and define women's realities, there has been much pathologizing of women's normal experiences. These theorists argue, for example, that the male model for mature health—separation and individuation—differs from women's experience, which is to seek affiliation. Women's self develops in relation, not in separation. Because women's behavior did not conform to the male model for health, it was labeled immature and unhealthy. This body of theory, like Chodorow's, is called cultural feminism, and its thrust is that structural, not biological characteristics shape psychodynamics. A research agenda at the Stone Center is to uncover and to destigmatize some of these normal experiences of women.

Belenky, Clinchy, Goldberger, and Tarule (1986) added to the literature about women's reality by examining specifically how women's experiences affect ability to acquire and feel confident about knowledge of the external environment and the self. They described the multiple, nonlinear ways that women learn and the processes through which women construct knowledge. They showed how education designed by and for upper-class white men devalues "women's ways of knowing" and handicaps women further by depriving them of opportunities to learn and grow. They explained the interactions between social situations and identity, growth, and the construction of knowledge. Again, models based on elite men's characteristics are presented as normative, and many women are set up to "fail."

Women who become demoralized because of academic difficulties might be treated somatically by biological psychiatry, when what they need is validation of their worth, encouragement, and a different style of teaching. Commonalities among these researchers are findings that women have distinctly different self-conceptions than men, and that relationships are central in women's lives. For women, these relationships must have a sense of mutuality and equality. Equally important, gender-biased social structures have silenced women (Olsen, 1982) and rendered many invisible, and they have perpetuated stereotyped beliefs about women's mental health. Biological psychiatry perpetuates sexist beliefs and stereotypes by using medication to mask symptoms originating from psychodynamic and structural processes. It thereby further silences and invalidates women's realities. These stereotypes can create mental illness.

Emanating from the contemporary women's movement have been a growth in alternative therapeutic models and an increased acceptance of already established alternative modalities, for example, meditation, co-counseling, and various types of body work. Many contemporary approaches to women's therapy include increasing political awareness and activism. For example, aware that breast cancer was more widespread and fatal than previously believed, and aware of discriminatory practices in awarding research funding for women's conditions, women pressured the federal government for research funding. The personal becomes political. This is quite different from submerging the political in a bioreductionist psychiatric ideology that individualizes social problems and blames women's bodies for socially caused symptoms. An example of this misuse of psychiatry to defuse political situations occurred when welfare demonstrators were institutionalized in a psychiatric hospital in New York, and large numbers of women, unhappy with traditional roles, were given prescriptions for valium (Ehrlich & Abraham-Magdamo, 1978).

Currently, in feminist literature, there are conflicts surrounding these newly discovered, socially created gender differences and their significance. Cultural feminists, who applaud the differences, work toward accumulating knowledge specifically about women, arguing that too little has been known about women for too long, or that mistreatment of women's emotional problems resulted from failure to hear or validate women's truths, for example, concerning incest and sexual assault. Many women who exhibit intense emotions (especially anger), mistrust authority, and have difficulty with relationships, receive the diagnosis *borderline personality disorder,* and a great deal of medication that doesn't help, when their symptoms are caused by childhood trauma. These women became more powerless and silent as a reaction to invalidation, blaming, and the victimization they encounter within biological psychiatry. Borderline personality disorder *is* due to a problem with women's bodies, but the problem is more childhood sexual abuse than inherent biochemical abnormalities (Herman, 1982). These feminist theorists and clinicians have pressed traditional psychiatry to reexamine psychiatric diagnoses and treatments (Cauwels, 1992). Borderline personality disorder illustrates the political nature of psychiatric diagnosis and treatment.

A different feminist position is voiced by other women, who point out the dangers of dichotomizing gender differences, reifying them, and recreating stereotypes (Epstein, 1988). Also, they emphasize the diversity of characteristics within each gender, many of which overlap the two dichotomized categories. This group of feminists views gender as more fluid, but constrained by socially constructed roles. Research from this perspective focuses on diversity among women. Variations among women become more obvious, too, as women gain voice and political power.

This "women are different" versus "women are not different" conflict mirrors the dilemma faced by any marginalized group in society: Whether to retain distinctive characteristics of one's own group, or to work toward acculturation and assimilation into the mainstream, is the problem. The difference is that this particular marginalized group constitutes over half of the population!

Both approaches have in common a concern about the systematic, structural oppression of women and its impact on women's minds. From this research and discussion, we gain new approaches to defining and managing emotional problems, whether we take a reformist approach or a radical one. For example, what had been defined as codependency in women is viewed now as women's frantic attempts to form mutual relationships with people who cannot form mutual relationships. This puts the psychiatric shoe on the other foot!

Meanwhile, now, as has generally been the case historically, gender differences in psychiatry persist. Women express more distress, even under extreme and unusual situations (Ritchey, McGory, & Mullis,

1991); women use more services; and women take more prescribed drugs (Travis, 1988). Men are more prone to violence; men use more alcohol and street drugs; and men more often commit suicide in this country. Bioreductionist psychiatry supports and perpetuates these roles by failing to address social factors in mental illness.

The message for biological psychiatry is clear: not all psychiatric symptoms can be treated with medication. Masking social sources of mental illness by relieving symptoms with medication can do harm.

Racial Difference as a Source of Diversity

Fernando (1991) defined race as a physical characteristic with a social function. As with gender differences, racial differences in behavior are presumed by bioreductionists to have a genetic base. Racial stereotypes often influence—color, one might say—interactions with the medical system and psychiatric diagnoses. However, there is no medical reason to assume that racially specific behaviors are genetically determined. There is no evidence that melatonin levels determine behavior through biological mechanisms.

Racism and discrimination are pervasive in our culture; they produce misunderstanding at best, and gross mistreatment at worst, in society at large and in biological psychiatry. For example, following the civil disorder of the 1960s, physicians from a prestigious Massachusetts hospital advanced the theory that racial violence was the result of a neurological defect, to be brought under control by lobotomy (Mark & Ervin, 1970).

A more recent example is a speech, given in February 1992, by Dr. Frederick Goodwin, current director of the National Institute of Mental Health (NIMH). Goodwin compared violent behavior in over-populated inner cities to the behavior of monkeys in jungles (Hiltz, 1992; Leary, 1992; *New York Times*, 1992). His speech provoked protest about the racial analogy, and Goodwin got into further trouble by attempting to set up a conference on "The Biological Roots of Aggression" at NIMH. He was blocked by the Black Caucus in Congress because this was viewed as a way to blame and control African Americans, not social conditions, for the violence in their communities. Goodwin argued that his remarks were distorted.

When attitudes are based on stereotype, the important sources, the genuine sources of diversity, simply are not considered. Historically, psychiatry associated psychopathology with being "uncivilized," and Black people were believed to be uncivilized (Fernando, 1991). Stress, anger, and social problems that are the result of racism and discrimination become medicalized through diagnoses such as paranoia and schizophrenia, which are overdiagnosed in Blacks and Hispanics; depression, usually mistaken for lack of ambition and of a sense of responsibility, is not diagnosed or treated (Baker, 1988; Fernando, 1991).

For Black people, hospitalizations are more frequent and longer, with more seclusion and fewer privileges; there is less therapy, more drug and electroshock therapy, and a higher rate of premature discharge from therapy (Fernando, 1991). There is also a stereotypical view of Black families as having single mothers and absent fathers and as living in poverty, with little recognition of the diversity of family forms and social class differences (Hines & Boyd-Franklin, 1982).

There are problems in treatment, too. In a recent study of staff interactions with patients on an inpatient unit, Kavanaugh (1991) found that staff did not directly acknowledge racist or sexist attitudes, nor did they recognize discriminatory behaviors. Their actions told a different story. There was less frequent interaction between staff and patients of opposite gender or different race. Staff often referred to these same patients as having a lack of self-control, and then distanced themselves from them further. In addition, doctors did not acknowledge nurses' contributions, particularly their influence on decision making. Nurses were disgruntled, but they did not confront the issue directly. What they did was exert more control over patients. The result was that socially marginalized people, already relatively powerless, and rendered less powerful in an institutional setting, were further marginalized and disempowered by staff behavior (Kavanaugh, 1991). Unfortunately, this process is not unusual, nor is it confined to institutional settings. Within biological psychiatry, racial stereotypes further disempower patients through the message, "You have no control. It's in the genes."

A treatment bias in psychiatry is the tendency to assume a biological basis for symptoms that are caused by social–racial factors, and therefore to deal with these symptoms somatically. In addition, it has been said that less educated people are not suitable for psychotherapy. Frank (1974) has shown that this is not the case. Still, it has been more likely for minorities to come into contact with the police, not the medical system, and for their deviance to be labeled "criminal." With the democratization of psychiatry, and with increased access to the health care system for upwardly mobile minorities, there most likely will be larger numbers of minority people receiving psychiatric diagnoses. In a review of admissions to state hospitals between 1970 and 1986, Thompson, Belcher, DeForge, Myers, and Rosenstein (1993) found that admission patterns have shifted toward Black, indigent males, so several racially based trends may be occurring at once.

Social Class as a Source of Diversity

. . . the privileges of the professional extend beyond the workplace to a whole way of life. I call this way of life "respectability." To treat people with respect is to be prepared to listen to what they have to say or to do what they request because they have some authority, expertise, or influence.

—Iris Marion Young, 1990:57

Each of us stands in a unique position created by the intersection of many social categories. One of the most salient categories is social class. Social class affects opportunities, expectations, coping mechanisms, and exposure to trauma. Other class distinctions relevant for psychiatry, but not considered seriously or systematically by biological psychiatry, are variations in attributions of meaning, beliefs about health care, language, patterns of expressing distress, degree of alienation or social integration, and perceived power.

Resources, including capital, not only affect the ease with which it is possible to negotiate complex systems, but also represent ways to make clear distinctions between "us" and "them." Social reference groups affect self-esteem and self-evaluation (Webster & Sobieszek, 1974). They also orient the individual to class-appropriate reality.

Just as there is not an equitable distribution of resources within society, there is not an equitable distribution of mental illness across social classes. Generally, the relation is inverse—that is, the lower the social class, the higher the rates of mental illness. This relationship has been steady over time, despite somewhat different measurement tools and different definitions of mental illness (Dohrenwend et al., 1992; Hollingshead & Redlich, 1958).

Although the link between social class and psychiatric condition is established, the process that forges that link continues to provoke debate. The two main arguments in the debate are that factors associated with social class cause psychiatric conditions (social causation hypothesis), or that psychiatric conditions constitute barriers to life opportunities for upward social mobility, or could cause downward mobility between parents' social class and the social class of the psychiatrically impaired offspring (social selection hypothesis).

A huge body of literature in social psychiatry attests to the number of mechanisms posited to explain social causation. For example, recognition, interpretation, and presentation of symptoms differ across class: the higher the social class, the more likely that people will present to psychiatrists with psychologically defined symptoms. Less advantaged people tend to express emotional concerns somatically and to seek and get treatment from a general practitioner.

Patterns of help-seeking and routes into treatment differ across social class: there is less tolerance for bizarre behavior prior to medical encounters in higher social classes, which means a somewhat shorter delay in help-seeking, but high tolerance for the same behavior after diagnosis. A medical label confers legitimacy: "She is sick; she is not herself." In contrast, working-class and poor people generally have a higher tolerance for bizarre behavior prior to medical encounter, but low tolerance for the same behavior once there is a psychiatric diagnosis. Here, the label carries stigma. Historically, people from lower social classes have been more likely to enter the medical system from places such as police stations. For out-of-control behavior, and when tolerance wears thin, lower-class families are more likely to call the police for control. For them, it is one small step from a cell to a hospital room.

Medical encounters are class-biased, in terms of degree of social distance between patient and practitioner, language similarity, and expectations on both sides of the relationship about the role of the other. The lower the patient's social class, the less similarity there is between patient and physician, and the more the power differential between the two expands and becomes skewed in favor of the physician. In biological psychiatry, this means prescription, not discussion and choice, and it means a high likelihood of compliance, at least initially.

Patterns of emotional expression and intimacy differ by social class. Emotional expressiveness is associated with higher education. Family dynamics, communication, child rearing, and coping patterns within families differ substantially by social class (Rubin, 1976). Based on these different patterns of expression, assumptions are formed about "appropriateness" for psychotherapy. It is more likely that, given similar symptoms, people from upper-class backgrounds get psychotherapy and those from lower classes get custodial care or medication (Mechanic, 1978). Historically, psychoanalysis has been the treatment of the social elite.

People in lower social classes are doubly disadvantaged. They have fewer overall resources, and often the lack of resources is itself a stressor. In addition, they are exposed to higher levels, greater constancy, and more types of stress. Regardless of attitude or resiliency, living with chronic stress takes its toll on the human psyche (Lin, Dean, & Ensel, 1986). Because mastery and personal power contribute to well-being, the poor need opportunities to exercise power and to develop mastery, not simply diagnoses that medicalizes social problems, or psychotropic drugs.

The link between social class and mental illness is part of our history. Just prior to the Civil War, medical attention shifted away from "chronic fever" as a condition of the wealthy that required a calm environment

(Jiminez, 1987), to the poor as most at risk for mental illness. The link between poverty and illness began with the assumption that an innate quality was responsible for crime and illness among the poor; recognition of the impact of poverty on behavior came much later. Historically, we went through a period of recognizing the impact of poverty on mental health, but with the shift to biological psychiatry, poverty has become irrelevant again and innate characteristics, framed in politically correct ways, have taken center stage once more.

Psychiatry redefines a great deal of normal human behavior as medically deviant by pathologizing people who are socially marginal in any way. For example, we try to "cure" or isolate those who are disruptive, embarrassing, or different; for a long time, handicapped people were isolated, ostensibly for treatment purposes. A significant minority of old people are institutionalized for medical reasons, although the precipitant for institutionalization often is an adult daughter's exhaustion. For a time, homosexuals were labeled medically deviant. In some countries and during certain historical periods, political dissidents were institutionalized as medically deviant. Slaves in this country were labeled medically deviant when they did not behave in subservient ways. Whereas discrimination and censorship are illegal methods of containing and controlling diversity, in this country "inappropriate behaviors," including speech, can be attributed to biological misfortune and treated with drugs. This allows us to maintain the facade of having a society that tolerates diversity, respects human rights, and provides equal opportunities. It directs attention away from social inequalities and barriers to achievement, so that when someone does not "make it," we can blame biochemical processes or genes, and need not feel guilt or redistribute resources.

Diverse Cultural Realities: History, Geography, and Heredity

Healing has become increasingly marginal to the West's dominant healing system.
Arthur Kleinman, M.D., 1988:139

Culture is an ethos, a way to look at life and make sense of it; it is a shared, distinct way of being, knowing, and doing (Erickson, 1976). Culture shapes and constrains the way we construct knowledge. For example, the constructed self in modern cultures, argued Kleinman (1988), is secular and self-reflexive. In our society, we are aware of psychiatric symptoms (although this varies by social class), but have all but lost our ability to understand the spiritual and poetic. Our reductionist ideology disallows full participation in life (Hochschild, 1983). In contrast to ours, many non-Western cultures place a higher value on community, philosophy, and religion than on individuals. In some of these societies, not only is there a fuller participation in life, but religious trances are common and considered normal (Kleinman, 1988). An emphasis on community versus individual, on spiritual versus secular, and on morality versus efficiency will affect who will most likely enter the psychiatric system, and for what reason. In general, greater cohesiveness and sense of community mean less difficulty with emotional distress. On the other hand, for people who have migrated here and have brought different cultural experiences, there is likely to be conflict. Historically, biological psychiatry has not had to deal with cultural differences, except at upper social class levels. For people in other strata, as has been the case for racial minorities, contact with authority systems has been predominately with the police. Biological psychiatry has not been very concerned with cultural differences, and has defined behavioral norms based on White male American and urban models. Those who deviate are at risk of being defined as "sick" and treated with somatic remedies. This has been the case for all immigrant groups.

We define health and illness differently across cultures. Early studies by Zborowski (1952) and Zola (1966) on cultural differences in the presentation and interpretation of physical symptoms began a tradition of studying the cross-cultural salience of particular types of expression. Studies of expressed emotion across a wide range of cultures, although originally designed to gain an understanding of families' responses to schizophrenia, also provided important information about the cultures' emotions, beliefs, and attitudes (Jenkins & Karno, 1992).

In non-Western cultures, there is likely to be more expression of distress through somatic symptoms, religion, and spells and witchcraft (Kleinman, 1988). Contrast this with our tendency, in the psychodynamically oriented West, to reinterpret bodily distress as psychological. Within our culture, tendency varies by categories such as gender and social class.

It is important not to be ethnocentric, and to understand cultural forms of expression and attributions of meaning. Without due care, people will get diagnoses they do not need. Developing countries have higher rates of brief reactive psychosis diagnosed as "schizophrenia" by American or U.S.-trained physicians (Guiness, 1992). In addition, many indigenous conditions have no counterparts in Western culture. Indigenous treatment systems exist to manage emotional problems, often with success. In fact, there is substantially greater chronicity in schizophrenia in Western cultures. Kleinman (1988) argued that psychiatric chronicity is related to the type of political system in which the patient lives.

Diagnostic categories and tests, developed by Western psychiatrists, are now used as screening instruments for research about incidence and prevalence of mental illness in many societies and cultures. Bioreductionist research, not surprisingly, shows that schizophrenia is schizophrenia is schizophrenia, regardless of culture, and that culture has only a minor effect at the level of symptom content. The counterargument is not that mental illness is a Western myth, but that misdiagnosis occurs when cultural differences are not taken into account.

Cultural differences between physician and patient in this country are another issue. Even when patient and physician are born and raised in the United States, there may be cultural differences between them. The first, more obvious difference between them emanates from physicians' education and training: there is the distinctive language of medicine. Within psychiatry, training does not eliminate the use of this distinctive language in interactions with patients. Psychiatrists translate patients' language, verbal and nonverbal, into something more meaningful for their work, such as a diagnostic category. While listening and observing, the psychiatrist mentally selects certain information and reframes it. What is said and done may be less relevant than the interpretation. This can occur because of the physicians' cultural authority (Starr, 1982). For the biological psychiatrist, information selection and reframing occurs within a bioreductionist model. Information not relevant for the model tends to be discarded. For instance, information provided about powerlessness or feeling victimized might be interpreted as "paranoid ideation," and the fact that the patient is an unemployed immigrant might not be relevant to the decision to medicate.

Ethnic differences affect treatment both culturally and psychologically through a variety of mechanisms. People have different levels of awareness of these effects on themselves and on others; each of us believes that our view of reality and our unique perspective is normal, and, generally, we are right, within our sociocultural context. A psychiatrist interacting with a patient raised in the same culture may assume shared meanings, but cannot do so when there are ethnic differences. Norms, values, beliefs, traditions, and family patterns can differ by ethnicity (McGoldrick, Pearce, & Giordano, 1982). The extent of the difference will depend on the degree of acculturation to the dominant culture. Ethnic differences, even when they are recognized, create distance between psychiatrist and patient. Rosenberg (1992) argued that the interpretation of behavior and the ability to empathize differ when sociocultural beliefs differ. Abel, Metraux, and Roll (1987) presented examples of difficulties with transference, countertransference, and dream interpretation when such differences were not considered.

These should be relevant issues for biological psychiatry. However, they are usually not considered important by biological psychiatrists, who will make diagnoses based on their professional definition of reality, after observing behavior such as "poverty of speech," which they treat with medication. In this way, the body is "cured" of an "ailment" that is really an ethnic difference.

In the presence of sociocultural differences, or with changing sociocultural conditions, the distinction between normal and abnormal becomes less clear (Offer & Sabshin, 1984), and behavior may be distorted or misinterpreted. In addition, acculturation can produce stress, both within families and intraphysically. Acculturation involves entering a new reality and transforming the self. What sounds or looks like a thought disorder to a biological psychiatrist may be part of a confusing transition.

CONSTRUCTING SIMILARITY: RALLYING AROUND THE BIOLOGICAL FLAG

Following the current medical ideals, much effort was wasted in attempting to square these phenomena (psychiatric conditions) with the terms of neurophysiology the irrelevance of which was first clearly indicated by Breuer and Freud . . . .
—*Harry Stack Sullivan, 1964:8*

It is inexcusable for a profession that markets self-examination not to scrutinize itself. Psychiatry developed and uses concepts like the unconscious and defense mechanisms, but fails to recognize its professional defenses and its barriers to change. Such is the nature of ideologies. The belief that biological explanations for mental illness exist is ingrained; it is part of the everyday, taken-for-granted reality of biological psychiatrists. How is it that a large group of intelligent people persist in defending and embracing a bioreductionist model of psychiatry in the face of evidence to the contrary? How does the ideology persist in the presence of critics?

As we have seen, one line of criticism examines, in a variety of intelligent and provocative ways, the relation of psychiatry to oppression.

Chesler (1972), Showalter (1987), and Tavris (1992), among others, have analyzed psychiatry's contribution to sexism. These critics of psychiatry conclude that, through a variety of processes, psychiatrists psychologically oppress and physically mistreat women and thereby maintain a male-ordered world, in which they benefit from women's subordination. Although this is seen as a radical position by some, it at least regards psychiatrists as human beings embedded in social matrices, rather than viewing them as detached, objective, scientific researchers.

Fernando's (1991) comprehensive review provided similar insights about the oppression and mistreatment of racial minorities—again, to maintain the current social order. Psychiatry's emphasis on genes and neurotransmitters hides this social control function, by using terms like "predisposition" or "high risk for violence."

Kleinman (1988) is another critic of psychiatry's lack of insight and its movement toward a biomedical model that dismisses the importance of sociocultural context and psychodynamics. He has provided a thorough analysis of the field, a review of the literature, and cross-cultural comparisons of psychiatric treatment, as well as a wide range of insights about unjustified practices within biological psychiatry. His focus is the cultural authority of psychiatrists to define what is regarded as illness and how it is treated.

Ingleby's (1980) analysis of the role of positivist ideology in biological psychiatry explained its legitimacy and cultural authority. Science is regarded in our culture as objective and value-free. A pretense of science justifies the clinical approach of biological psychiatry, its lack of contextual focus, and its lack of attention to issues of power—I say *pretense* because, in terms of its scientific status, biological psychiatry has fundamental flaws. In Kleinman's (1988) and Meyer and Rowan's (1977) view, positivist ideology provides the rituals, myths, and symbols that sustain biological psychiatry. As with all rituals, myths, and symbols, those of biological psychiatry take on a life of their own, and psychiatrists often forget to look beneath and beyond them.

All these perspectives add to our understanding of biological psychiatry by providing a piece of a multidimensional mosaic. But none quite explains how and why a relatively small and not very successful group of researchers transformed themselves into a large, international, influential field of medicine—nor how and why critics within the field, such as Laing, Szasz, and Kleinman, are largely ignored, while the search for genes and enzymes progresses with increasing vigor.

Is psychiatry like a religion? I do not think so. I do not see a passionate attitude about the ideology, except from its critics. There is no social movement on behalf of biomedical psychiatry. Psychiatrists go about their daily work with patients, in privacy for the most part, and most seem to believe that they are contributing to the well-being of individuals who seek their services. They treat the body's biochemistry. This view does not imply that there is no biological component to human misery; bioreductionism is simply an insufficient explanation. Psychotropic medication can relieve symptoms, just as antihistamines can relieve symptoms of hay fever, or analgesics can relieve pain. But psychotropic medications are too often used indiscriminately in place of supportive therapy, education, environmental change, and political activism. This is not a conspiracy of silence; it is much more subtle and routine. To illuminate the process underlying the successful spread of biological psychiatry, it is necessary to turn to organizational theory and to examine what Chandler (1977) called "The Visible Hand." What larger social forces were associated with the spread and acceptance of psychiatry? What organizational factors led to the adoption and persistence of the dominant biomedical model?

Starr (1982) detailed events, such as the invention of the stethoscope and statistics, as preconditions for medicine's legitimization, and said that a critical mass of population was necessary for medicine to become a viable organized occupation. In addition, he saw the birth of modern psychiatry occurring around World War II, as do other researchers, when substantial numbers of European refugee psychiatrists brought the practice of psychoanalysis with them to North America. During the war, psychiatrists in the military had great success in quickly getting servicemen back on their feet and fighting; Starr attributed subsequent success in psychiatry to success during the war.

Professions are social organizations that construct, as they form themselves, the means to perpetuate themselves by controlling access and knowledge, and by neutralizing social mechanisms that might control them. This requires political activity, both in relation to potential or actual competitors and within the larger society, in order to maintain professional status. If successful during their formational periods, professions develop legitimacy.

Starr pointed out that, in 1844, psychiatrists formed a professional association. When the American Medical Association (AMA) formed a few years later, psychiatrists did not wish to affiliate. At that time, medicine was not lucrative or prestigious, and psychiatrists, securely employed within organizations, had little in common with physicians who were in private practice within communities. There were no education requirements for physicians at that time. There was no basis for a common definition of reality between physicians and psychiatrists.

World War I was accompanied by higher rates of mental illness for military men and substantially lower rates than normal for women.

Showalter (1987) has explained that women were gainfully employed at this time and were less affected by feminine role explanations. Current research about women and depression corresponds well with this argument. But there is a factor not considered: many psychiatrists were in the military. We know that the supply of medical services generates demand, as in all sectors of the economy.

Until the end of World War I, there were no major changes in the organization and delivery of psychiatric care. Psychiatrists continued to provide administrative, custodial care within public and private institutions. Between the two World Wars, there were large numbers of psychiatrists in civilian life, some formerly employed by the military, plus refugee psychiatrists who set up private practices within the community.

During World War II, the number of psychiatrists employed in the military increased from 40 to 2,400 (Starr, 1982). Perhaps for the first time, a large amount of clinical attention within psychiatry focused on men. Unlike the situation with women, the military psychiatric focus was on psychological trauma, rather than on "constitutional" factors. In conjunction with social scientists, research by psychiatrists during the war led to new information, theories, and treatments of reactions to stress. This school of psychiatry gained visibility in the larger male-dominated society. This was undoubtedly important for gaining legitimacy: psychiatrists demonstrated treatment successes during the war and during rehabilitation afterward. Psychiatry began to show some utility. Further, military service was an important opportunity to form social contacts that would serve as referral networks when the military men went back to their communities.

Legitimacy and contacts, plus the large supply of psychiatrists, contributed to funding mechanisms that fostered further growth. Another contributing factor was the wage and price controls that led to demands for employee medical coverage. In 1946, The National Mental Health Act established the National Institute of Mental Health (NIMH), which began operations in 1949. This federal agency funded research and training for physicians and social scientists. The scope of psychiatry widened, and more categories of mental illness were "discovered." DSM-I, published in 1952, focused on reactivity to social and psychological issues.

According to Starr, expansion of the Veterans Administration hospital system and the Hill–Burton Act of 1946 led to construction of new hospital facilities and formation of organizational relations between hospitals and medical schools. Although these were general hospitals, the expansion of the hospital system was significant for the later development of psychiatry. During this period, too, medicine as a profession was supported by Congress and became more powerful politically

(Starr, 1982). Hospitals expanded in response to funding opportunities. Financing mechanisms, private and public, provided incentives for psychiatrists to hospitalize patients, which benefited individual practitioners and the hospitals. Hospital administrators at that time were physicians.

Legislation during the 1960s promoted the move toward community mental health care, which, analyzed retrospectively, worked better in theory than in reality. In 1956, amendments to the Social Security Act had prompted the shift of old people with dementia to nursing homes (Starr, 1982). In addition, the Mental Retardation Facilities and Community Mental Health Centers Construction Act of 1963 provided federal funds, used in combination with other sources of funding, to develop community facilities (Koran, Brown, & Ochberg, 1977). The results of these laws were: the expansion of nursing homes, the development of psychiatric facilities within general hospitals, and some development of outpatient psychiatric facilities. There was little true development of community facilities. However, further amendments in 1968, 1970, 1972, and 1975 mandated expansion of community programs to include children's services, substance abuse treatment, and coverage for the elderly (Koran et al., 1977). All of this activity dovetailed nicely with the NIMH's epidemiological studies of mental illness in the community. With federal government support, psychiatry expanded its boundaries and legitimacy, and its financial status improved. In addition, this legislation promoted brief outpatient services, and treatment for mental illness more closely resembled that for physical illness (Ehrenreich & Ehrenreich, 1971).

Success begets success, says the old saw, and that was true for psychiatry. Psychiatric boundaries expanded rapidly. DSM-II was published in 1968, DSM-III in 1980, and DSM-III-R in 1987, and each successive publication considerably increased the number of diagnostic categories, as well as the political processes involved in creating them.

Professions are defined partly by their ability to capture markets (Collins, 1990). They are able to do this by coopting adversaries or potential adversaries, by limiting participation of those with different approaches, and by socializing these "outsiders" to the dominant model. Professions also exert control over their members, by training them in the skills and attitudes of the profession and by admitting them to a guild that supports its interests vis-à-vis competitors. In the case of psychiatry, the biological model helps beat back the competition of clinical psychologists, social workers, and clinical nurse specialists.

Academia, other than in the natural sciences, has entered a postpositivist period, in which processes other than linear causality are the source of inquiry. Funding sources, editors, and other gatekeepers influence what gets studied and published, and departmental policies dictate what constitutes desirable areas of inquiry. Major changes in social tenor have occurred: there are increased opportunities for women and minorities; there is increased fragmentation of social movements, reflecting diversity within these movements; there is a general shift toward conservatism and away from encouraging and supporting social criticism, including that from research funding sources. Critics of biomedical psychiatry largely are coopted or have created their professional niches outside of the mainstream. Leaders of the feminist movement have also turned attention inward. For example, Gloria Steinem (1992) and Germaine Greer (1992) have recently focused on their menopausal experiences and psyches.

Changes in the financing of psychiatric services have altered treatment patterns, as has the shift toward a biomedical approach to treatment. Expanded financing for psychiatric services once meant increased access for a range of services, including alcohol and drug treatment programs. With a contracting economy and emphasis on cost containment, plus the decreased power of unions, payment for psychiatric services has decreased substantially. Brief intervention and crisis management are more likely to get financed today. Not only has biological psychiatry expanded its market, it has found its niche in a climate of cost containment: it is less expensive to provide drugs than to provide therapy. A powerful pharmaceutical industry encourages this trend.

Bioreductionist psychiatry cannot possibly account adequately for mental illness. It is clinically and intellectually limiting, based on pseudoscience, and politically motivated. Although biological psychiatry in its current form appears to be a good marketing strategy for the profession, the rapid pace of social change in our world will soon make this model self-defeating for psychiatry. A number of large literatures provide compelling critiques of the negative effects of bioreductionism on patient care. It is hoped that a more adequate model, paying more than lip service to psychological, social, and cultural factors, will soon come to the fore.

REFERENCES

Abel, T. M., Metraux, T., & Roll, S. (1987). *Psychotherapy and culture*. Albuquerque: University of New Mexico.

Baker, F. M. (1988). Afro-Americans. In L. Comes-Diaz & E. E. H. Griffith (Eds.), *Chemical guidelines in cross-cultural mental health* (pp. 151–181). New York: Wiley.

Bayer, R. (1987). *Homosexuality and American psychiatry: The politics of diagnosis.* Princeton, NJ: Princeton University Press.

Belenky, M. F. B., Clinchy, B. M., Goldberger, N. R., & Tarule, J. M. (1986). *Women's ways of knowing. The development of self, voice, and mind.* New York: Basic Books.

Berger, P. L., & Luckmann, T. (1967). *The social construction of reality.* New York: Anchor Books.

Cauwels, J. M. (1992). *Imbroglio: Rising to the challenges of borderline personality disorder.* New York: Norton.

Chandler, A. (1977). *The visible hand.* Cambridge, MA: Belknap.

Chesler, P. (1972). *Women and madness.* New York: Avon.

Chodorow, N. J. (1974). Family structure and feminine personality. In M. Z. Rosaldo & L. Lamphere (Eds.), *Woman, culture, and society* (pp. 43–66). Palo Alto, CA: Stanford University Press.

Chodorow, N. J. (1978). *The reproduction of mothering.* Berkeley: University of California Press.

Chodorow, N. J. (1989). *Feminism and psychoanalytic theory.* New Haven, CT: Yale University Press.

Collins, R. (1990). Market closure and the conflict theory of the professions. In M. Burrage & R. Torstendahl (Eds.), *Professions in theory and history* (pp. 29–43). London: Sage.

Conrad, P. (1980). On the medicalization of deviance and social control. In D. Ingleby (Ed.), *Critical psychiatry* (pp. 102–223). New York: Free Press.

Conrad, P., & Schneider, J. W. (1985). *Deviance and medicalization.* Columbus, OH: Merrill.

Crosby, F. J. (1991). *Juggling: The unexpected advantages of balancing career and home for women and their families.* New York: Free Press.

Dohrenwend, B., Levak, I., Shrout, P., Schwartz, S., Navek, G., Link, B., Skodol, A., & Stueve, A. (1992). Socioeconomic status and psychiatric disorders: The causation–selection issue. *Science, 255,* 946–952.

Ehrenreich, B., & Ehrenreich, J. (1971). *The American health empire.* New York: Vintage Books.

Ehrenreich, B., & English, D. (1981). The sexual politics of sickness. In P. Conrad & R. Kern (Eds.), *The sociology of health and illness* (pp. 327–350). New York: St. Martin's Press.

Ehrlich, A., & Abraham-Magdamo, F. (1978). Caution: Mental health may be hazardous. In H. D. Schwartz & C. S. Kart (Eds.), *Dominant issues in medical sociology* (pp. 64–71). Reading, MA: Addison-Wesley.

Epstein, C. F. (1988). *Deceptive distinctions: Sex, gender and the social order.* New Haven, CT: Yale University Press.

Erickson, K. (1976). *Everything in its path.* New York: Simon & Schuster.

Farganis, S. (1986). *The social construction of the feminine character.* Totowa, NJ: Rowman and Littlefield.

Fernando, S. (1991). *Mental health, race, and culture.* New York: St. Martin's Press.

Frank, J. (1974). *Persuasion and healing.* New York: Schocken.

Goffman, E. (1961). *Asylums.* New York: Anchor Books.

Goffman, E. (1963). *Stigma: Notes on the management of spoiled identity.* Englewood Cliffs, NJ: Prentice-Hall.

Greer, G. (1992). *The change: Women, aging and the menopause.* New York: Knopf.

Guiness, E. A. (1992). Patterns of mental illness in the early stages of urbanization. *British Journal of Psychiatry, 160* (Suppl. 11), 4–72.

Herman, J. L. (1992). *Trauma and recovery.* New York: Basic Books.

Hiltz, P. J. (1992, February 22). Federal official apologizes for remarks on inner cities. *New York Times,* 1, 6:5.

Hines, P. M., & Boyd-Franklin, N. (1982). Black families. In M. McGoldrick, J. K. Pearce, & J. Giordano (Eds.), *Ethnicity and family therapy* (pp. 84–107). New York: Guilford Press.

Hochschild, A. R. (1983). *The managed heart.* Berkeley: University of California Press.

Hollingshead, A. B., & Redlich, F. C. (1958). *Social class and mental illness.* New York: Wiley.

Ingleby, D. (1980). Understanding "mental illness." In D. Ingleby (Ed.), *Critical psychiatry* (pp. 23–71). New York: Pantheon Books.

Janowitz, M. (1960). *The American soldier.* New York: Free Press.

Jenkins, J. H., & Karno, M. (1992). The meaning of expressed emotion: Theoretical issues raised by cross-cultural research. *American Journal of Psychiatry, 149,* 9–21.

Jiminez, M. A. (1987). *Changing faces of madness.* Hanover, NH: University Press of New England.

Kavanaugh, K. H. (1991). Invisibility and selective avoidance: Gender and ethnicity in psychiatry and psychiatric nursing staff intervention. *Culture, Medicine, and Psychiatry, 15,* 245–274.

Kleinman, A. (1988). *Rethinking psychiatry.* New York: Free Press.

Koran, L. M., Brown, B. S., & Ochberg, F. M. (1977). Community mental health centers: Impact and analyses. In L. Corey, M. F. Epstein, & S. E. Saltman (Eds.), *Medicine in a changing society* (2nd ed., pp. 141–150). St. Louis: Mosby.

Laing, R. D. (1960). *The divided self.* London: Tavistock.

Laing, R. D., & Esterson, A. (1964). *Sanity, madness and the family.* London: Tavistock.

Leary, W. E. (1992, March 8). Struggle continues over remarks by mental health official. *New York Times,* 1, 34:1.

Lemert, E. M. (1951). *Social pathology.* New York: McGraw-Hill.

Lin, N., Dean, A., & Ensel, W. M. (1986). *Social support, life events, and depression.* Orlando, FL: Academic Press.

Mannheim, K. (1936). *Ideology and utopia.* New York: Harvest.

Mark, V., & Ervin, F. (1970). *Violence and the brain.* New York: Harper & Row.

McGoldrick, M., Pearce, J. K., & Giordano, J. (1982). *Ethnicity and family therapy.* New York: Guilford Press.

Mechanic, D. (1978). *Medical sociology* (2nd ed.). New York: Free Press.

Meyer, J. W., & Rowan, B. (1977). Institutionalized organizations: Formal structure as myth and ceremony. *American Journal of Sociology, 83,* 340–363.

Miller, J. B. (1976). *Toward a new psychology of women.* Boston: Beacon Press.

Mirowsky, J., & Ross, C. E. (1989). *Social causes of psychological distress.* New York: de Gruyter.

Mitchell, J. (1966). *Women: The Longest Revolution.* Somerville, MA: New England Free Press (reprint).

Nathanson, C. A. (1975). Illness and the feminine role: A theoretical review. *Social Science and Medicine, 9,* 57–62.

New York Times (1992, February 28). Health official quits after harsh criticism, A12:6.

Offer, D., & Sabshin, M. (1984). *Normality and the life cycle: A critical integration.* New York: Basic Books.

Olsen, T. (1982). Silences. New York: Delacorte Press.

Ritchey, F. J., LaGory, M., & Mullis, J. (1991). Gender differences in health risks and physical symptoms among the homeless. *Journal of Health and Social Behavior, 32,* 33–48.

Rosenberg, M. (1992). *The unread mind: Unraveling the mystery of madness.* New York: Lexington Books.

Rubin, L. (1976). *Worlds of pain.* New York: Basic Books.

Scheff, T. J. (1966). *Being mentally ill.* Chicago: Aldine.

Schur, E. (1965). *Crimes without victims.* Englewood Cliffs, NJ: Prentice-Hall.

Showalter, E. (1987). *The female malady: Women, madness, and English culture 1830–1980.* New York: Penguin Books.

Spitzer, R. L., & Williams, J. B. W. (1987). *Diagnostic and statistical manual of mental disorders* (3rd ed., rev.). Washington, DC: American Psychiatric Association.

Starr, P. (1982). *The social transformation of American medicine.* New York: Basic Books.

Steinem, G. (1992). *Revolution from within: A book of self-esteem.* Boston: Little, Brown.

Sullivan, H. S. (1964). *The fusion of psychiatry and social science.* New York: Norton.

Surrey, J. L. (1991). The self-in-relation: A theory of women's development. In J. V. Jordan, A. G. Kaplan, J. B. Miller, I. P. Stiver, & J. L. Surrey (Eds.), *Women's growth in connection* (pp. 51–66). New York: Guilford Press.

Sutherland, E. H., & Cressey, D. R. (1970). *Criminology* (8th ed.). Philadelphia: Lippincott.

Szasz, T. (1961). *The myth of mental illness.* New York: Harper & Row.

Tavris, C. (1992). *The mismeasure of woman.* New York: Touchstone.

Thompson, J. W., Belcher, J. R., DeForge, B. R., Myers, C. P., & Rosenstein, M. J. (1993). Changing characteristics of schizophrenic patients admitted to state hospitals. *Hospital and Community Psychiatry, 44,* 231–235.

Travis, C. B. (1988). *Women and health psychology. Biomedical issues.* Hillsdale, NJ: Hove and London.

Ussher, J. M. (1989). *The psychology of the female body.* London: Routledge.

Webster, M., & Sobieszek, B. (1974). *Sources of self-evaluation: A formal theory of significant others and social evaluation.* New York: Wiley.

Young, I. M. (1990). *Justice and the politics of difference.* Princeton, NJ: Princeton University Press.

Zborowski, M. (1952). Cultural components in responses to pain. *Journal of Social Issues, 8,* 16–30.

Zola, I. K. (1966). Culture and symptoms: An analysis of patients' presenting complaints. *American Sociological Review, 31,* 615–630.

6

PSYCHIATRIC EDUCATION: LEARNING BY ASSUMPTION

Susan S. Kemker
Ali Khadivi

Biology clearly offers the only comprehensive scientific basis for psychiatry, just as it does for the rest of medicine. (p. 318) . . . I believe that continuing debate about the biological basis of psychiatry is derived much more from philosophical, ideological, and political concerns than from scientific ones. (p. 322)
— Guze (1989), *"Biological psychiatry: Is there any other kind?"*

INTRODUCTION

Susan S. Kemker

Guze (1989) stated what most of us have been taught to believe: biology is the science of psychiatry. The fact that I believed this dogma made Pam's (1990) critique of biological psychiatry especially unsettling. When I read his work, I felt that my entire education as a psychiatrist was subject to question. Some of the studies being scrutinized were known to me as major contributions to the field. I was shocked to find not a single "landmark" study emerging as methodologically sound. Definitions of terms alone rendered many of their conclusions invalid. The twin studies began with very questionable definitions of "reared apart," "same environments," and even "schizophrenia." There were biases in patient selection and interviews. Results were almost invariably overstated, with much confusion between correlation and cause.

With virtually no regard for the flaws described, these studies were cited to my class of residents as "proof" of the genetics of such disorders as schizophrenia and alcoholism, as well as for such theories as the dopamine hypothesis. They laid the foundation for a "medical model" of mental illness, which espoused the comforting faith that medical solutions would be found. These studies were regarded as part of an effort to develop psychiatry as a science. They were presented to me in textbooks and lectures with much authority, and I took them in—not the studies per se but their "bottom lines": that mental illness was determined by genes and neurotransmitters, to be eventually conquered by precise pharmacology.

How could I have accepted so much pseudoscience uncritically? How could I have learned so much by rote, as if what I was learning was the truth rather than assertions to be questioned? As I examine these questions, I have had to review the education I and, perhaps, all residents have received. I believe that we have learned important *skills* for patient care, but our *understanding* of our own field remains naive, based on what we have been told by supervisors and a few "experts." The purpose of this chapter is to provide an account of the impact of biomedical reductionism on the training of psychiatrists, and to describe biological psychiatry in operation in the clinic.

RESIDENCY AND PSYCHIATRY: ASSUMPTIONS WE LEARN

Susan S. Kemker

Psychiatrists must learn . . . the conceptual issues associated with interpreting raw data as well as the methodological problems and limitations of current work. (Guze, 1989, p. 320)

Throughout most of my residency, I took for granted the medical model of psychopathology. I did not always grasp the fine points of biological research, but I certainly respected it. As far as I knew, biology was the "science" of psychiatry. There was no other science to consider.

If studies of genetics and neurotransmitters were reaching publication, then their methodology *had* to be sound—especially if the journal or the investigators were considered eminent. The underlying assumptions and the conclusions that followed *had* to be equally sound. Otherwise, we would not be taught them in our residency training.

In essence, my learning was based on the following assumptions:

1. If it is being taught, it is true and important;
2. If it reaches print in a major journal, it is scientific;
3. If it is scientific, it is both worthwhile and objective, free of cultural or political bias;
4. The conclusions are more important than the methodology.

These assumptions, which were also adhered to by my instructors, allowed me to avoid thinking about the material I was being taught: residency training tends to discourage critical appraisal of biomedical reductionism.

In psychiatry, residents learn primarily through clinical experience, observing and emulating the practice of others in a kind of apprenticeship. They are thrown into clinical settings, assigned to a group of patients, and instructed to ask for help when they think they need it. Contact with patients shapes their learning—applied, practical knowledge is more immediately useful than theory or research. In this setting, supervisors tend to focus on helping the resident take care of a particular patient. The goal is the development of clinical skills. Rarely are current research findings the focus of supervision. When articles are handed out, they are generally pragmatic in nature.

For many residents, there is tension between academic and clinical responsibilities. The patients are ill, at times in crisis, regardless of the timing of classes or conferences. From the outset, residents must choose between going to a particular lecture and taking care of a particular patient. When faced with a crisis, they generally will skip the lecture. When classes do not pertain to the residents' immediate needs, they tend to be skipped too. One chief resident remarked that his interns almost never attended Grand Rounds—they chose instead to finish their clinical work.

When I was a resident, I viewed clinical experience as my primary source of learning. I sought out supervisors who could help me integrate my experience in the here-and-now. My goal was to develop into a strong clinician, with skills in all the different areas of treatment: individual, group, and family therapy; medical procedures; psychopharmacology; case management; and functioning as part of a multidisciplinary team. I found working with patients compelling and consuming. I learned what I was expected to know of neurotransmitters, genes, and cell receptors, but I did not feel curious or excited about these things. Theoretical constructs and research findings, impressive as they were, could not help me when confronted with acutely suicidal or psychotic individuals. As Lipowski (1989) pointed out, "Neuroscience offers precious little that we could apply in our daily work with patients" (p. 253). How much more true for the pressured resident!

On the other hand, the PRITE and Psychiatry Boards loomed as necessary rites of passage for all residents. Respecting these imperatives, I absorbed the required number of "facts" about research findings in the field. I attended review courses and consulted the usual synopses of modern psychiatry. Neither examining nor questioning the material set before me, I "crammed." I suspect that most residents used fairly similar coping measures. Turning to the literature was not my usual practice. In one survey, 58% of residents reported spending less than one hour per week reading the current literature (Schweizer & Shtasel, 1990)! Psychiatry residents do not tend to read—they learn by absorbing information from authorities.

Most residents develop into psychiatrists by learning in clinical settings. We are not taught the skills necessary to read the research literature critically. Our medical training taught us how to absorb large amounts of information, rather than to think analytically about what was being presented. Now, unable to fully apply the scientific method, we find ourselves in a poor position to evaluate the implications of what we are hearing, much less the methodology of the research. Even when we have the tools, most of us are unable to invest the time and energy necessary to truly evaluate the literature—especially given the current state of information overload described by Lipowski (1989). When we are under pressure to "keep up," we find out what we're supposed to know in various review courses and outlines.

Thus, we depend on various "experts," many of them primarily researchers, to do what we cannot do—evaluate, integrate, and present the latest developments in our field. As a result, we adopt a language and set of assumptions, largely weighted toward biological psychiatry, with a minimum of debate and self-examination. We passively and unwittingly become part of the culture of biological psychiatry.

The next section examines how the values and ideology of biological psychiatry are transmitted in our clinical language and educational institutions. Largely unquestioned, these ideas form the basis on which our field trains future psychiatrists.

LANGUAGE AND PSYCHIATRY: ASSUMPTIONS WE SPEAK

The words "science" and "scientific," which we all revere and freely use to endorse our pet beliefs, are ambiguous and have at times been used to sanction man's inhumanity to man (Lipowski, 1989, p. 250)

Perhaps the greatest obligation of science is objectivity. "Pure" or "basic" science is expected to transcend bias and cultural values. Its language is supposed to be neutral. In the field of psychiatry, however, terms that appear scientific are fraught with "metameaning" and buried assumptions, promoting biology as the primary determinant of human behavior. The terms we have chosen to describe here are *genetic loading*, *chemical imbalance*, and *noncompliance*.

Genetic Loading

Every psychiatrist "knows" that a family history is crucial in case evaluations and presentations. Those who omit this information will either fail their boards or risk shame in front of their peers. These incentives alone give significance to the family history for residents in training. But what is the *clinical* importance of this information?

Family history provides clues about how a patient grew up, receptiveness of the family group to professional help, response to illness, and, *maybe*, genetics. In its narrowest sense, family history is a statement of correlation—the presence of *some* shared genes and the presence of shared mental illness. Correlation, as we know, does not imply causality. Shared genes are not necessarily a cause of mental illness; they simply cannot be *ruled out* as one cause in this particular case or family.

In the past few years, the term *genetic loading* has become widely used in clinical psychiatry. When asked about "genetic loading," residents are expected to discuss the patient's family history of a particular mental illness. More and more, it has become acceptable (and even enlightened) to make the statement, "He has a genetic loading for schizophrenia."

On casual examination, genetic loading appears to be a benign term with a technical ring. However, it is precisely the "scientific" quality of the term that makes it less than benign. When residents describe genetic loading in their patients, they have made a jump from correlation to cause, although they do not question the legitimacy of the term they are using. Most are unaware that any jump in logic has occurred.

A consequence of the term genetic loading is the weight that it implicitly gives to genetic factors in the family psychiatric history. Psychotic individuals are more likely to receive the diagnosis of schizophrenia if they have a positive family history of schizophrenia, regardless of their symptoms. In contemporary psychiatry, the "environmental loading" of schizophrenia is relatively neglected, and, in fact, that term is never used. For example, "genetic loading for schizophrenia" tells us nothing about the environmental pressures on a girl whose mother believed she was the devil. "Genetic loading for alcoholism" tells us nothing about the effect of an eight-year-old's being recruited as a parent's "drinking buddy," which could fully account for the alcoholism diagnosed when this child became an adult.

The term genetic loading fosters racism, in which behaviors observed in certain ethnic groups are interpreted as being constitutional, with little corresponding analysis of sociological or cultural factors. In one recent case conference, an eminent consultant remarked on genetic loading for alcoholism in the case, based partly on the patient's being American Indian. This remark met with no protest or challenge from the audience.

Genetic loading is now being claimed for homosexuality, and there has been much publicity about this in the lay press. Recently, residents in a large New York program received an article on the genetics of homosexuality with no accompanying class discussion or opposing articles. In this program, the heritability of homosexuality is regarded as a given for residents to learn, rather than a possibility being investigated. This language and this method of teaching result in residents' using the term "genetic loading for homosexuality" without questioning its validity.

Chemical Imbalance and Noncompliance

As a psychiatric resident, I (SSK) found these terms helpful when talking with patients and their families. Taking the lead of various mentors, I would explain that mental illness is caused by a chemical imbalance in the brain. Mental illness resembles diabetes, which involves a chemical imbalance in the body, I would explain. The patient's psychiatric disorder is chronic, I would say, and requires medication every day for the rest of the person's life. I would then assure the patient that if he took the medication, he would probably live a more normal life.

I sincerely believed what I was saying. The notion of a chemical imbalance seemed understandable enough—my patients just did not seem to accept it. If they would, they would not be suffering so much.

Relief was as close and easy as a pill. In a similar manner, I viewed *noncompliance* as the primary precipitant of acute illness.

Later in my training, I was surprised to be challenged on my case presentation of a patient's acute psychosis. My supervisor refused to accept noncompliance as the cause of a decompensation. Insisting that "something happened," he made me examine recent life events experienced by that patient, and later I did so in other cases as well. Since then, I have encountered a great variety of noncompliant patients, including a young woman whose estranged husband called her "crazy" and threatened to take custody of their child; a man too sedated to get to work in the morning; a woman recently being refused reentry into her teaching job; and a young man whose mother died. Noncompliance is a behavior that occurs within a social context. Within the chemical imbalance model, it is usual to view noncompliance as occurring *without* a social context.

Residents, given the stresses and demands of training, are understandably inclined to view suffering as a purely chemical construct. Chemicals are then defined as the source of healing, and noncompliance as the cause of relapse. This model can alleviate much anxiety in trainees by simplifying the task of treatment. However, the model radically narrows the range of clinical inquiry.

In his article on psychiatric education, Reiser (1988) expressed concerns about how patients were being understood by psychiatrists, with the growing emphasis on chemical intervention. He found a number of his residents remarkably "unpsychological" in their approach and mindset. "Once they had done the DSM-III 'inventory' and had identified target symptoms for pharmacotherapy, the diagnostic workup and meaningful communication stopped. Worse than that, to my mind, so did the residents' curiosity about the patient as a person. Most of these residents could and would have learned more about a stranger who was sitting next to them for an hour on an airplane trip" (p. 151). Residents are increasingly led to think of treatment as pharmacotherapy; they miss the richest aspects of the patient–therapist interaction.

Regarding chemicals as the cause of mental illness is a growing trend, despite flaws in the logic of this model. Lipowski (1989) described difficulties in the model, pointing out that a term like chemical imbalance "confuses the distinction between etiology and correlation, and cause and mechanism, a common confusion in our field. It gives the patient the misleading impression that his or her imbalance is *the* cause of his or her illness, that it needs to be fixed by purely chemical means, that psychotherapy is useless, and that personal efforts and responsibility have no part to play in getting better" (p. 252).

Terms such as genetic loading, chemical imbalance, and noncompliance are far from being neutral, or free of value and bias. They communicate a narrow model of mental illness, one that is determined by chemicals and genes alone. The power of these terms lies in their ordinary, "everyday" quality. They are uttered daily by residents and other clinicians, without context and without ever being challenged.

CLINICAL PSYCHIATRY: ASSUMPTIONS IN PRACTICE

Ali Khadivi

Traditionally, the ultimate focus of the physician's concern has been (and should continue to be) the patient as a person, not diseases, instruments, rating scales, or laboratory data. (Reiser, 1988, p. 148)

Just as the assumptions of biological psychiatry have permeated our language, they have shaped our practice and our attitudes toward patients. Residents have been especially sensitive to this shift to a biomedical model of psychiatric illness, because they have limited experience with competing models. This section deals with behavior observed in residents who adhere primarily to a biological model of illness. Their underlying assumption is that psychiatric illness is analogous to medical illness. Diagnostics and treatment in psychiatry are thought of as being similar to practice in internal medicine. Although this assumption is superficially benign and often made by well-meaning residents, it is simplistic and reductionistic. It ignores other dimensions of illness, including psychological factors that contribute to illness, the patient's reaction to his illness, and the meaning of being ill. Furthermore, the bioreductionist model underestimates the stigma of mental illness, the power of denial, and resistance on the part of patients.

I recently observed an interview in which a psychiatric resident asked a patient to describe his "psychopathology." To the resident's surprise, the patient replied, "I do not have any psychopathology." A more sensitive interviewer would have received a different response, but many residents speak to patients as if they are taking a medical history. They expect patients to accept that they are mentally ill, and to provide historic details as if discussing an episode of appendicitis. The residents do not appreciate that, from the vantage point of the patient, mental illness does not have the same status as a medical condition; instead, it has a very unique, often shameful connotation. Residents frequently find themselves surprised and frustrated by patients' intense negative affects and their refusal to cooperate during diagnostic interviews.

I have observed trainees having similar difficulties when proposing treatment to patients. They underestimate the symbolic meaning of medications and the emotional reactions that medications elicit. The offering of psychotropic medication is far more analogous to giving a psychotherapeutic interpretation or suggestion than it is to any medical procedure, in my view. In prescribing medication, we are asking the patient to abandon a prior view of himself or herself, and to entertain a new perspective.

Medicine has become increasingly interested in the psychological dimension of illness, and has taken steps to train physicians in becoming more sensitive to a patient's reaction to his or her illness, and in improving physician–patient relations (Reiser, 1988). However, psychiatry, because it is dominated by biomedical reductionism, is moving in the opposite direction. Currently, residency programs are placing less and less emphasis on the teaching of psychotherapy and psychosocial theory. Reiser (1988) warned us that the focus of psychiatry residency programs has been increasingly shifted away from the patient as a person and toward disease. Gabbard (1990) has also observed that many contemporary residents lack skills in approaching patients therapeutically. The clinical struggles of our residents are showing us that a bioreductionist model of mental illness is not a sufficient framework for working clinically with psychiatric patients. Without appropriate training in psychotherapy, residents are apt to be left frustrated and mystified by their patients, who in turn feel misunderstood and alienated from those charged with their care.

ACADEMIC PSYCHIATRY: ASSUMPTIONS WE BUILD

> It would be a great irony if, as medicine works frantically to set its house in order and restore the doctor–patient relationship, psychiatry, in its romance with science and remedicalization, lost its heart and gave up its interest in the patient's live experience. (Cooper, 1989, p. 20)

In the previous section, we described how biological psychiatry has shaped the clinical behavior of residents. In a similar manner, it has dramatically altered our institutions. Academic psychiatry is increasingly espousing the principle of "medicalization," placing a premium on biological research and funded researchers. Clinicians and teachers are being demoted or replaced, in order to fuel the scientific "mission" of the institution. The role of the clinical psychiatrist is being reshaped and is increasingly narrowed to that of psychopharmacologist and administrator. Residents still receive some psychodynamic training, but psychotherapy has been generally devalued and is considered an adjunct to "medical" treatment. Although at times charged with supervising other disciplines, psychiatrists are increasingly divorced from the role of therapist, which is considered for them largely "obsolete." Teaching and clinical supervision are also being deemphasized; they compete for time with activities more directly related to the survival of the faculty (Cooper, 1989). This section describes the psychiatric hospital as it undergoes the process of medicalization, and the effects of pseudoscientific medicalization on the psychiatrists within its walls.

Recently, a psychiatrist was given notice from her job at an academic hospital we will call "the Hall." This happened despite strenuous efforts to prove herself valuable to the institution: she worked over 50 hours a week taking care of patients; she developed a clinical research project; she taught residents and medical students in extra hours; and she did not complain. Her supervisors considered her competent and hardworking. However, she was "shocked but not surprised" when she and 10 other junior faculty, who had invested similar hours, were informed that they were no longer part of the Hall's mission. They were to leave in 8 months. Other, more senior faculty were either demoted or pressured to leave, or both. One unit chief was advised to enroll in a 2-year research fellowship if he wished to stay at the Hall. Former training directors and senior supervisors were reassigned to inpatient wards to replace the ousted junior faculty.

These measures could be viewed as a desperate attempt to maintain financial solvency under growing economic pressures, but the shuffling of staff did not necessarily follow lines of economics or seniority. Individuals with biological research interests were kept, regardless of their seniority, and junior faculty are significantly less expensive than the senior staff who were demoted to replace them. Further, the changes were announced as a step toward progress, not as unavoidable sacrifices for survival. With a new focus and channeling of resources, the Hall was now to flourish as a center for biological psychiatric research.

Despite the cuts, the Hall describes patient care as moving in the direction of greater efficiency and more specialized programs. In other words, fewer psychiatrists can and *should* be caring for more patients, with increasing turnover, and in less time. As this occurs, more resources are to be devoted to the "academic mission" of the hospital, defined as biomedical research.

The Hall maintains that the teaching of residents will be preserved, or even improved. However, a substantial number of teaching faculty were demoted or transferred to other positions. No longer functioning primarily as senior supervisors, they are directing wards or managing caseloads of patients. There are going to be changes in who does the teaching and in what is being taught. Teaching will shift even further toward the bioreductionist medical model.

This story is not unique. The entire field of psychiatry is shifting its emphasis toward biological research. Cooper (1989) remarked on the "transformation of the university medical school into a vast research corporation and the parallel rise of biomedical science" (p. 17). He was most concerned with how this development affected the survival of teachers and residency education in psychiatry. He wrote:

> Full-time psychiatry faculties are under enormous, unrelenting pressure to sustain themselves through external funding. In effect, the departments, unsupported by general funds for education, have increasingly subordinated psychiatric education to research funding and profitable patient care activities. (p. 17)

Cooper described power in medical schools as tilting "heavily towards the researcher and administrator, less towards the clinical caretaker who is increasingly seen as part of a profit center rather than a source of teaching, and least towards the teacher" (p. 17). He maintained that there is a parallel shift in numbers of faculty—an increase in those with fundable biological interests, and a corresponding decrease in those with psychotherapeutic and psychodynamic interests. Teachers, especially teachers of psychotherapy, are an "endangered species" in the academic institution.

After teachers, clinicians identified with psychotherapy are the next most endangered species. Almost all of the personnel cut at the Hall were clinical. In another program, a resident quoted his chairman as stating that "psychiatry will not be the same" in the foreseeable future; psychiatrists would be expected to deal with many more patients in a much shorter time. Their role would be to act as supervisors and administrators—not as psychotherapists.

Training directors seem to be in agreement that psychotherapy is being deemphasized as a skill to be learned by residents. Verhulst (1991) stated:

> Psychiatry's return to medicine has been a return to science, with a denouncement of psychodynamic psychotherapy. Academic psychiatry intends to develop a data-based construction of the reality of the brain, rather than an empathic understanding of the reality of experience. (p. 122)

As psychotherapy diminishes in perceived value, clinical psychiatrists are narrowing their roles. Viewed essentially as "medical consultants," they are expected to make diagnoses and initiate treatment quickly and efficiently. The "therapeutic alliance" is no longer considered a legitimate concept—at least not when it comes to time demands. Clinicians are serving patients in greater numbers, but from a greater distance. They are being laid off or given notice with the expectation that their "survivors" are capable of increased productivity.

The work of academic psychiatry has evolved into a struggle involving the ever-increasing tensions of research, clinical, and teaching responsibilities. In this setting, only the "fittest"—those who can generate funded biological research—are able to survive. The ruling assumption is that this evolution is progress. The question is—progress for whom?

CONCLUSION

Most psychiatric residents have developed first and foremost as clinicians. They entered the field to become clinical psychiatrists, not researchers. They recognize and often endorse research efforts, but are neither inclined nor trained to analyze technical papers. In the meantime, economic forces and the ballooning of biological research have contributed to the medicalization of psychiatry, with a corresponding devaluation of psychotherapy. As a result, many clinicians and teachers have been rendered "obsolete," sometimes by developments funded by their own labor. Resources are being siphoned away from direct patient care and teaching into basic research, whose worth is being taken for granted.

If, as clinical psychiatrists, we continue uncritically to accept these developments as "scientific," we will find ourselves becoming mere technicians, practicing the principles of dopaminology and serotonology. We will be treating our patients as sets of errant genes and neurotransmitters, to be "corrected" by genetic counseling and neurochemicals. We will be speaking the language of medicalization, instead of analyzing its biases. We will be learning by assumption, basing our learning on assumptions that are unproven and, worse yet, unchallenged.

REFERENCES

Cooper, A. M. (1989). The teacher: An endangered species? *Academic Psychiatry*, *13*(1), 13–23.

Gabbard, G. O. (1990). *Psychodynamic psychiatry in clinical practice.* Washington, DC: American Psychiatric Press.

Guze, S. B. (1989). Biological psychiatry: Is there any other kind? *Psychological Medicine*, *19*, 315–323.

Lipowski, Z. J. (1989). Psychiatry: Mindless or brainless, both or neither? *Canadian Journal of Psychiatry*, *34*, 249–254.

Pam, A. (1990). A critique of the scientific status of biological psychiatry. *Acta Psychiatrica Scandinavica*, *82* (Suppl. 362), 1–35.

Reiser, M. (1988). Are psychiatric educators "losing the mind"? *American Journal of Psychiatry*, *145*, 148–153.

Schweizer, E., & Shtasel, D. (1990). The role of current literature in psychiatric residency education. *Academic Psychiatry*, *14*(2), 92–98.

Verhulst, J. (1991). The psychotherapy curriculum in the age of biological psychiatry: Mixing oil with water? *Academic Psychiatry*, *15*(3), 120–131.

7

TRAUMA-RELATED SYNDROMES

David K. Sakheim
Susan E. Devine

There is a need in psychiatry for a more broad-based understanding of trauma-induced syndromes. Unfortunately, psychiatry to date has medicalized the victims of social problems, portraying traumatized patients as helpless, defective, and in need of "expert" intervention. There is a clear need to critically evaluate currently accepted assessment and treatment methods within psychiatry, in order to explore their impact on traumatized individuals who seek assistance. This chapter presents a critique of current approaches and a new diagnostic category for the assessment and treatment of Trauma-Related Syndromes.

In recent years, it has become apparent that psychiatry focuses our attention on people injured by abuse, but because this etiology is minimized or ignored, the primary effect is to pathologize and stigmatize these survivors instead of understanding them as individuals who have been coping with external stressors. A bioreductionist focus on the individual deflects attention away from social problems such as rape, war, child abuse, wife battering, and violent crime. This leads to a channeling of resources toward understanding the "pathology" of the victim rather than focusing attention on those who perpetrate abuse or on exploring the "pathology" present in the social systems that allow such abuses to occur.

If the field does not attend to trauma as the cause of many psychiatric symptoms, it risks doing great harm to the individuals involved. For example, if a consultant had been asked in 1944 to make recommendations about how society should deal with the Nazi death camps in Germany, it would have been bizarre if his attention was devoted to researching and treating the interpersonal and intrapersonal problems of the camp inmates, with no attempt to connect these to the atrocities with which the inmates were forced to live on to address the pathology of the guards; no focus on the camps themselves; and no mention of the pathology of the social and political systems that allowed the camps to be created in the first place.

A focus on the psychopathology of the inmates would not have been misguided; they would clearly have needed help to deal with the horrors of their experiences. However, if that were the only focus, or even the primary focus, it would clearly have political and social implications. Where one directs one's attention will often determine where subsequent resources and efforts are expended, as well as how the problem becomes defined. Ignoring social pathologies that create and enable such victimization could actually end up contributing to them. The situation would be made still worse if this theoretical concentration camp consultant not only ignored the social factors, but, in his focus on the inmates, used psychiatric labels that medicalized their reactions instead of describing the problems as resulting from abuse and trauma (if, for example, the inmates were diagnosed as having personality disorders because they had difficulties with trust, self-soothing, and closeness). When the focus is on the psychopathology of individuals, one is least moved to advocate social change.

With respect to the Holocaust, we would be outraged by a bioreductionist approach, yet this is what biological psychiatry does today to survivors of child abuse and other forms of trauma. We focus primarily on individuals, give them psychiatric diagnoses that do not mention trauma or abuse, and devote virtually all of our resources to the identification and treatment of survivors. We have few specific diagnoses for perpetrators of abuse, and we fail to address the social factors that create and enable such problems.

We do not label violence, war, sexism, and persecution as "crazy," only those who get injured by them (Ahrendt, 1964; Borovasky & Brand, 1980). Instead of acknowledging how common abuse appears to be (which would likely lead to decreased secrecy and shame for the victims, and corresponding attempts at social change), we tend to do the opposite and support secrecy, shame, and hiddenness by acting as though such abuse is unusual. When the prominent psychiatric treatment of trauma is individual psychotherapy or psychopharmacology, we give the implicit message that survivors should deal with their experiences individually, rather than encouraging social action to change external problems.

It is important to recognize the impact that trauma can have on an individual, and to study how many of our social institutions routinely expose people to such experiences. In today's world, it is not really "outside the range of usual human experience" to experience trauma. For example, in addition to traumas caused by war, crime, accidents, poverty, and illnesses, between 1947 and 1973 there were 836 major disasters in the world, each of which involved over 100 injuries or deaths (Glesser, Green, & Winget, 1981). Thus, it is very important for mental health professionals to recognize how often trauma is a part of a person's significant history, and to take this into account when trying to understand the symptoms displayed.

Not all adult psychiatric problems are caused by trauma. However, when symptoms do result from such events, it is a disservice to the patient to minimize this fact. Despite statistics about the frequency of child abuse, rape, battering, violent crime, murder, and sexual harassment, bioreductionist psychiatry does not seriously consider the psychological impact of such trauma. Nowhere in DSM-IV is there a discussion of syndromes resulting from sexual or physical abuse in childhood, nor of the impact of living in a society in which 5% to 10% of women are raped, and 20% to 30% of married women are battered (Coons, Cole, Pellow, & Milstein, 1990). In her large random-sample retrospective study of adult women in the general population, Russell (1986) found that 38% of women had experienced sexual abuse before they were 18 years old, and 16% were victims of incestuous abuse.

Although statistics on abuse vary, it has been estimated that well over a million children are victims of abuse in the United States each year; that 2,000 to 5,000 children die each year as a result of this abuse; that 1 in every 7 married women report having been raped by their spouse; and that at least 2,000 women are killed each year by husbands or boyfriends. This does not even mention other types of potentially traumatic political and social experiences, such as living in poverty (a state of affairs for 1 in 4 children in the United States) or facing various types of discrimination (Breggin, 1991; Finkelhor, 1979; Gelles & Cornell, 1985; Horton & Williamson, 1988; National Center on Child Abuse and Neglect, 1982; Russell, 1982).

These issues and their consequences tend to remain hidden, veiled in secrecy and shame. Within bioreductionist psychiatry, as occurs in the larger society, the problem primarily is viewed as internal to the victim, especially if he or she breaks the code of silence. This occurs despite the fact that there is overwhelming evidence that such external factors can play a major role in the development of psychiatric symptoms. For example, in 1978, the President's Commission on Mental Health provided official recognition of the "normalcy" of the oppression of women in our society. One of their conclusions was as follows:

> Circumstances and conditions that society has come to accept as "normal" and "ordinary" lead to profound unhappiness, anguish, and mental illness in women. Marriage, family relationships, reproduction, childbearing, divorce, work, and aging all have a powerful impact on women. Since there is no scientific evidence to suggest that women are innately more vulnerable to mental illness, we conclude that our usual social institutions have a differential and more stressful impact on women. Compounding these ordinary events are the extraordinary events to which women are routinely subjected such as rape, marital violence, incest, and other traumas. (Davis, R. & Freidman, L., 1985)

It is time that psychiatry acknowledged social factors in the construction of its diagnostic categories. Although we have emphasized the trauma experienced by women in this discussion, men clearly experience a major amount of trauma in our society through urban violence, child neglect, war, workplace injuries, physical abuse, and sexual abuse.

How one views the problem that a patient presents determines the interventions that will be considered. Central to every school of psychiatric diagnosis and treatment are beliefs about what people are like and what they might become, as well as a conceptual framework that helps to order and understand human experience. Such models enable a clinician to make sense of a person's life story. The point of view taken by the clinician will affect what is defined as the problem, what can be considered in the way of appropriate interventions, and what constitutes success when evaluating treatment outcome.

THEORY

In psychiatry, there are presently a wide variety of "points of view," but biological psychiatry is the dominant paradigm. Bioreductionist psychiatry fails to take into account very important aspects of the experience of traumatized patients. For example, if one is attempting to make a DSM-IV diagnosis (American Psychiatric Association, 1994), one is usually not going to attend to etiology, because the categories in DSM-IV are deliberately designed to be phenomenological, or symptom-oriented. Clinicians need to be consciously aware of the assumptions underlying their point of view, and the conceptual framework they have chosen, because the choice will appreciably affect their work.

For example, when assessing a patient with borderline personality disorder, a clinician using a family systems model might focus on the family dynamics that maintain the symptoms; a biological psychiatrist might look for genetic factors that would predispose the person to exhibit such behaviors; a behaviorist would look for reinforcements of maladaptive responding; an analyst might focus on early developmental arrests; and a feminist therapist might look for a history of childhood physical and/or sexual abuse to explain the current experience of the patient. The "findings" or clinical data will be different for each of these clinicians because the models that guide their search are different, and no one model alone is adequate. Each clinician will come to a different conclusion, in part as a result of the different data collected, but also in part as a result of the differential importance placed on the same data. The model used will influence any subsequent intervention.

These differences can be seen in the daily practices of mental health professionals. For example, a colleague described attending a seminar in which a well-known psychodynamic clinician was asked what he made of the fact that so many patients with borderline personality disorder report childhood sexual and physical abuse. The expert replied that the abuse histories are "irrelevant" but earlier developmental experiences are significant. In a similar fashion, a biological psychiatrist might regard child abuse merely as proof of the fact that the patient's parents were also psychiatrically disturbed. Thus, rather than understanding the trauma as causative of later symptoms, a bioreductionist model would regard the disturbance as inherited (Stone, Kahn, & Flye, 1981). Unlike other approaches, a trauma model would regard the trauma itself as a cause of the patient's current symptoms (Browne & Finkelhor, 1986; Bryer, Nelson, & Miller, 1987; Gelinas, 1983; Herman, 1992). The inter- and intrapersonal problems of the patient would be viewed as a response to the violations of trust and boundaries that the abuse involved.

The history of psychiatry reveals a stark contrast in the interventions chosen, depending on the paradigm adhered to by the clinician. When Freud changed his theory regarding the causes of hysteria from the seduction theory to the fantasy theory, approaches to conceptualization and treatment, as well as clinical perspectives about childhood trauma in general, all changed dramatically (Masson, 1984). As a trauma model of the dissociative disorders has re-emerged in the late 20th century (Kluft, 1985; Putnam, 1989), therapy has reverted back to an approach in which the patient's experiences of trauma is the most important factor to be understood. However, the pendulum may swing back in the other direction once again. Greaves (1992) pointed out that the recent controversy about the veracity of reports of severe abuse (such as ritualized maltreatment) threaten to move the field back toward an internal view, in which trauma memories are viewed primarily as internal creations serving various conscious and unconscious motivations.

Trauma memory is not a simple issue. The recent controversies concerning the veracity of recovered trauma memories demonstrate how complex this area can be (Greaves, 1992; Loftus, 1993; Richardson, Best, & Bromley, 1991; Sakheim, 1993; Tavris, 1993). Just as the field is being forced to accept that trauma can create psychiatric symptoms, it is also being faced with examples in which other kinds of psychiatric problems can create distortions in reports of trauma memories. Sakheim (1993) pointed out the complexity of this area of psychiatry; not only must we appreciate that patients presenting as trauma survivors can be a very heterogeneous group psychiatrically, but we must understand that, for any given patient, different trauma memories may have distinct psychological significance and defensive values. For example, besides providing information about actual traumatic experiences, a recovered memory of trauma could also involve malingering for secondary gain, delusional material, metaphoric communication, incorporated material, exaggeration, symbolic meanings, confusion, misperception, and distortion. It is important not to swing from extreme denial about the role of trauma to an extreme and simplistic view of trauma as the root of all problems. The purpose of the Trauma-Related Syndromes diagnostic category is not to suggest that all psychiatric problems are rooted in trauma.

Instead, it is to point out that because many symptoms can have such an etiology, it is important for clinicians to have this understanding. For example, just as a clinician needs to know that, among other things, a tumor or a blow to the head can cause later memory problems, that clinician should also be aware that a severe psychological trauma can result in the defense of dissociation, which can produce later memory problems. The goal is not for clinicians to always come to a singular conclusion, but rather to broaden awareness and consideration of one set of potentially important etiological factors.

LANGUAGE

In addition to the impact of a theory, model, or paradigm, it is important to examine the meaning of individual words that are used when professionals talk about patients. This is far more than an exercise in semantics. How one talks about others influences how one thinks about them. To view individuals as "depressed" or "borderline" is to think of them within a particular paradigm. For example, one reacts very differently to someone described as having "AXIS I: 296.2 Major Depressive Disorder V61.1 Partner Relational Problem," than to someone described as being "battered by an abusive partner." However, these could be descriptions of the same person and the same symptoms, using two different ways of speaking. The terms represent more than merely a minor semantic difference. The influence of the two ways of speaking—on the patient, the clinician, and anyone else involved in treatment—would likely be significant. Clinicians' reactions to someone being "depressed" are often different from their reactions to someone being "oppressed." Breggin (1991) gave many examples of battered women who have been "treated" with shock, drugs, and lobotomy because their symptoms were understood within a bioreductionist paradigm, while their abuse histories were unexplored.

Psychiatric diagnoses and other psychological terms often function as a way of maintaining distance from the patient. Although it is important to be objective, such terminology also can serve to preclude clinical understanding. Clinical language often does not capture the reality of trauma. For example, "dissociative disorder" does not by itself evoke the abuse and suffering that are almost universally at the root of these disorders. It is important for the field to question why such terms are so often selected. Language can foster or foreclose empathy in the clinician. Diagnoses can also unduly limit one's understanding of a person by focusing attention only on certain facets of the whole self. For example, the diagnosis "multiple personality disorder" (MPD) captures only one aspect of a person's psychological defense against horrendous abuse and torture. It does not focus on the specific traumas. The diagnostic term also fails to say anything about the rest of the person's self, including his or her creativity, intellect, courage, humor, compassion, ability to function, and other defenses. Mental health professionals often fail to appreciate the serious, socially stigmatizing effects of psychiatric diagnoses. It is not unusual for such a diagnostic label to interfere with relationships, jobs, housing, and other important life issues.

Words can also be used by professionals to hide problematic aspects of a situation or procedure. It is interesting to note how many hospitals give benign names to coercive procedures like "specialing," "quiet room," and "special attention." These interventions are often experienced by patients as if they were Orwellian phrases from *1984* (such as "The Ministry of Peace")—bizarre reversals of what they really involve (Orwell, 1949). Deegan (1990) discusses the impact of military language used by human service professionals, such as sending staff out "into the field" to provide "front-line" services to "target populations" (p. 302).

THE SYMPTOM–TRAUMA CONNECTION

All clinicians are familiar with patients who have developed lifelong careers as treatment failures despite various experts' interventions, and who have accumulated a plethora of diagnoses and been multiply hospitalized and therapized. Often, this has been caused by a failure to attend to the traumatic etiology of the person's symptoms. Beck and van der Kolk (1987) demonstrated that a very large percentage of chronically hospitalized psychotic patients have incest histories; unfortunately, these histories are rarely addressed. There is a need for a diagnostic approach that provides descriptive information about symptoms and ties them to abuse experiences, but does not medicalize the patient. We do not need just one more new diagnosis.

PERPETRATORS

If approximately $1/4$ to $1/10$ of people in North America are abused in childhood, then there must be many as-yet-unidentified abusers in our society. Psychiatric approaches that are endogenous-reductionistic do not compel us to realize that there are many perpetrators living and working among us. Why is there not a major psychiatric movement to identify and treat the perpetrators, rather than their victims? This is a social issue.

As professionals and as a society, we make it very hard for abusers to be identified and stopped. Such crimes are usually denied or minimized unless the evidence becomes impossible to ignore. If someone is actually convicted of rape or child abuse, he is viewed as an aberrant and a terrible monster, even by other convicts in prison. Society distances itself from such an individual, considering him to be "deviant" and unlike its other members. The truth appears to be very different from this view. It would appear from the statistics on abuse that rapists and child molesters comprise a significant part of our population. Until we recognize this, it will be difficult to change the social conditions that allow such abuse to occur, or to treat the large number of perpetrators among us. If we view people who commit sexual harassment, rape, and child abuse as monsters, we won't notice when these actions are being perpetrated by a friend, neighbor, stepfather, father, mother, brother, teacher, doctor, or therapist.

The types of treatment offered sexual offenders are often punitive. The perpetrator's abuse history is rarely acknowledged and even less commonly seen as important to address in a safe and supportive, but limit-setting treatment program. Treating childhood sexual abuse as an aberrant and monstrous act only serves to maintain denial about its true prevalence. The usual reaction of friends and neighbors to the arrest of an abuser is, "He seemed like such a normal guy." In fact, if one attends to the statistics about child abuse, rape, marital violence, and sexual harassment in our society, it would appear that this assessment is not far wrong.

If one accepts the prevalence data about child abuse, then it can no longer be viewed as an individual disorder for either the child victim or the adult perpetrator. Like slavery, it must be viewed as a social and historical phenomenon that has roots in many of the existing social, religious, and political institutions. This is very important. As frightening as it may seem, child abuse appears to be fairly normative behavior in our society. Using the parallel of slavery, society could not have eliminated the practice by offering individual diagnosis and therapy to slaves and slave owners. Imagine if the slaves were diagnosed as "passive" or as having "a wish to be exploited." Imagine if the slave owners were diagnosed as "exploiters" or "domineering." This would make no more sense than it would to make similar diagnoses for factory workers and business executives in the present day. Slavery was abolished by political and social action. Treating slavery as a problem of individual brutality or oppression would miss the fact that it was accepted and widely practiced.

In looking back from our perspective and with our values today, wanting to own a slave seems deviant, yet it was accepted and normative behavior in that historical context. Rather than defining a phenomenon as being one of individual psychopathology, it is important to attend to prevalence data, which show that the problem is widespread and is social and institutional in nature. The social pathology is what needs to be changed. This is not to rule out a place for individual therapy in helping people deal with the impact of their life experiences. However, individual psychotherapy alone for slaves and slave owners would never have ended the practice of slavery, any more than it could eradicate child abuse and urban violence.

HISTORICAL PRECEDENTS

The oppression of women and children has a long history and has been practiced and accepted in most countries. For example, in India, women have been burned alive at their husbands' funeral pyres; in China, the practice of footbinding for women is an exotic ritual with terribly disfiguring and crippling effects; in Africa, genital mutilation is a procedure done to young women's genitals to make them more appealing to their sexual partners; and both Europe and America have at one time sanctioned witch burning in which thousands of women were murdered (Daley, 1978). Children have received few protections and many abuses in most countries. The cruelty of these and other practices was certainly not widely understood in these societies.

It is important to understand that psychiatry is prone to the same social and historical forces as is the larger society. For example, women who refused or were unable to adjust to childhood and/or adult traumas have not fared well historically. In Victorian times, women who showed symptoms of posttraumatic stress disorder were understood under the rubric of "hysteria" and were put to bed for extended periods of time as a "rest cure." During the Renaissance, it was believed that women who showed certain special abilities (such as midwives or others who could "heal the sick") were possessed or were "witches" and could be cured only by torture or deserved death. In the not too distant past, willful, obstinate women have been "treated" with unnecessary hysterectomy, clitorectomy, or oopherectomy (Masson, 1986). In many psychiatric settings, often against their will, women have been treated with tranquilizing medications, beatings, bleeding, electroconvulsive therapy, lobotomy, and sterilization (Breggin, 1991).

Too often, the current use of forced biomedical treatment is too similar to these past atrocities. Involuntary commitments, restraint, forced drugs, or shock treatments can be violations of basic civil liberties. Many survivors of childhood abuse encounter brutality in the mental health system that only adds one more trauma to their experience. Breggin (1991) pointed out that "those whose lives are least treasured in the society are the most likely to be afflicted with psychiatry's most destructive treatments" (p. 193). It is essential that we examine the values embedded in our diagnostic and treatment models so that we do not continue to ignore the psychological and biological impact of trauma.

Psychiatry tends to define "normal" according to what is presently "usual" or socially valued. This causes the mental health profession to maintain the social status quo. For example, masturbation used to be viewed by the field as pathological (even as a cause of mental illness) because it was viewed in society as an unacceptable behavior, and some very extreme attempts were made to control it (Zambaco, 1882). However, in recent times, masturbation has not only been considered "healthy," but failure to masturbate has now become a sign of mental illness (sexual dysfunction), and masturbation has been prescribed as treatment (Lobitz & LoPicolo, 1972). Thus, the values that drive psychiatric theory and practice are not purely scientific, they are also social and political in nature. It is therefore critical to examine and consciously determine which values we wish them to be.

POLITICAL ISSUES

Future generations may well look back on our current practices and point out how bioreductionist psychiatry focused on diagnosing individual victims of abuse rather than on identifying and changing the social conditions that create or allow abuse to occur. Thus, we may well be seen primarily as agents of social control who helped to maintain the status quo by focusing on the "pathology" of victims and thereby supporting the secrecy and shame that enable such abuses to continue. If current clinicians were to carefully consider this issue, it is likely that most would prefer to see their role as being more than social control and the maintenance of a problematic status quo.

Unfortunately, contemporary psychiatry does not have the social and political will to address such issues. The recent debate about whether homosexuality is a disorder pointed this out very clearly. Deciding such an issue involved a debate, intensive lobbying, and, ultimately, a deciding vote. It did not and could not involve scientific or medical research as the primary determiner of outcome. Similar confrontations are still occurring about the recently proposed diagnostic categories of rapism disorder, self-defeating personality disorder, and late luteal phase disorder. How we decide what is abnormal or pathological is not a purely scientific question. It appears to be very hard for us to learn from our history that certain aspects of psychiatry are political and social in nature.

TRAUMA-RELATED SYNDROMES

There is a need for a diagnostic framework that helps provide an understanding that child abuse, as well as other types of victimization, can produce psychiatric symptoms. Although it has been well argued that trauma does not produce a specific psychiatric disorder (Breslau & Davis, 1989), many types of previously confusing psychopathology become clear (the symptoms no longer appear psychotic nor confusing) when one is aware of their traumatic origins (Braun, 1983; Bryer et al., 1987, Kluft, 1985; McCann, Sakheim, & Abrahamson, 1988; Putnam, 1989). However, this insight causes major problems for a diagnostic system, such as the current DSM-IV (American Psychiatric Association, 1994), that is strictly based on observable symptoms rather than etiology. As the field of psychiatry comes to know more about the etiology of such disorders as borderline personality disorder, posttraumatic stress disorder, the dissociative disorders, brief psychotic reactions, adjustment disorders, and even some anxiety disorders, psychotic disorders, affective disorders, eating disorders, substance abuse disorders, and paraphilias, it is becoming increasingly clear that there needs to be more recognition of the potential impact of trauma in the formation of these later symptoms (Beck & van der Kolk, 1987; Bryer et al., 1987; Herman, 1992; Jacobson & Richardson, 1987). There is clearly a need for an overarching diagnostic category such as "Disorders of Extreme Stress" (Pelcovitz, 1990), "Syndromes of Traumatic Etiology" (Sakheim, 1990; Sakheim & Devine, 1992a), or "Complex Post-Traumatic Stress Disorder" (Herman, 1992) that would specifically reflect the traumatic etiology, as well as the areas of functioning that have been affected by the trauma.

Currently, DSM-IV, in an attempt to increase diagnostic reliability and validity, has tried to utilize observable symptoms rather than unobservable motives, defenses, assumed etiologies, or dynamics. In addition to enhancing the reliability of diagnostic categories, the advantage of starting out with a purely observational system is to be able to see patterns from research and clinical experience that can then help to organize thinking about etiology, course, and prognosis. However, the field of psychiatry is now at the point where enough is known about trauma that it should be reflected in the diagnostic categories that are utilized. If one is going to utilize diagnosis at all, it certainly makes sense to have a category that reflects the knowledge that trauma is responsible for certain types of posttraumatic responses. At present, no current diagnostic grouping sufficiently acknowledges traumatic etiology or the wide variety of diagnostic categories in which trauma can have an impact. This is despite the fact that research and clinical practice have shown that many areas of life can be affected by trauma (Browne & Finkelhor, 1986; Bryer, et al., 1987; McCann & Pearlman, 1990; McCann, Pearlman, Sakheim, & Abrahamson, 1988; van der Kolk & Greenberg, 1987). There is a need for a category that would allow for notation of just how injurious events have disrupted various aspects of the person's functioning.

Thus, the development of a new diagnostic category, "Trauma-Related Syndromes," is proposed here. Briere (1993) suggested that a diagnostic label should reflect that these are really syndromes resulting from confronting overwhelming pain. In her recent book, Herman (1992) frequently used the phrase "the traumatic syndromes," which ultimately may be the simplest and clearest name for such a new diagnostic category; however, Trauma-Related Syndromes has been retained for the present chapter because it stresses the connection between the history of trauma and the present symptoms. Regardless of the name chosen, there is a very important assumption inherent in such a diagnostic category: those choosing to use it will simultaneously be studying the larger social systems and attempting to understand the experiences of trauma survivors; the category will not be used as another way to medicalize them.

The category of Trauma-Related Syndromes would not be a single disorder, but would encompass the diagnoses most commonly affected by trauma. Because each person is different, effects of the trauma might be found in many aspects of a person's life, but the initial search for how the trauma influenced later functioning would be guided by the diagnostic category and current research and clinical data. The coded diagnosis would allow for communication of the presence of a trauma history, as well as information about the specific areas most impacted by the trauma.

Instead of being just another diagnostic category, Trauma-Related Syndromes would provide both informative description and an understanding that the observed symptoms are psychologically connected to earlier experiences. This is not a minor difference from current categories; it has many implications. For example, it is currently not unusual for therapists to react very negatively to patients diagnosed as having borderline personality disorder. This is especially true when the clinician is aware of only the problematic interpersonal patterns of the patient, without understanding their causes. If, on the other hand, the therapist is aware that many of the inter- and intrapersonal symptoms represent the impact of childhood trauma, the countertransference reaction is quite different. Seeing that someone flees from closeness because he was hurt by a parent who was supposed to protect him produces a different response than does noting that the patient "pathologically flees from closeness." Similarly, appreciating that "manipulative" behavior by a patient may have been the only way to survive in the family of origin produces less likelihood of a retaliatory response from a clinician than does the view that such behavior is the result of "primitive character pathology" (Sakheim & Devine, 1992b).

In our psychiatric institutions, present approaches often foster an attitude of hostility toward traumatized patients: one might contrast how many times professionals discuss among themselves the courage of a borderline patient in her struggle to overcome her background, with how many times the patient is discussed in condescending or belittling ways. Despite the fact that an appreciation of someone's courage often enables a real connection with that person, this is not a part of many professional discussions in psychiatry, in large part because information about the traumas that are being overcome have been removed from traditional diagnosis and treatment.

The proposed new diagnostic category would also help to clarify some of the confusion that currently arises about diagnosis. For example, clinicians frequently struggle with such questions as "Is this patient borderline or dissociative?" The new classification would help clinicians to see that someone who has been traumatized can experience later interpersonal and intrapersonal problems (such as one sees in borderline personality disorder) as well as defenses such as dissociation (Schultz, Kluft, & Braun, 1986). Studies have shown a considerable overlap between diagnoses such as histrionic personality, antisocial personality, borderline personality, dissociative identity disorder, and somatization disorder, because all of these contain aspects of the trauma response (Herman, 1992). Differential diagnosis does not have to be an "either/or" question; more usefully, it should involve a broad-based understanding of how this particular individual was affected by the traumatic events in his or her history. The proposed change in diagnostic approach would also reinforce awareness that successful treatment is going to have to focus on the traumas that caused a variety of disturbances in functioning.

In general, a category like Trauma-Related Syndromes would allow a more wholistic view of an individual. An example might help to clarify this point. When someone is currently diagnosed with multiple personality disorder, the diagnosis often has the unfortunate effect of stigmatizing him or her. Many of us who work in the field had hoped that the diagnosis of multiple personality disorder for traumatized patients would lead to more humanistic approaches, a decrease in stigma, and an increased awareness of the role of trauma in the patient's disorder. However, even though the diagnosis of MPD has done this to some degree, the diagnosis tends to place the patient outside of the mainstream of human problems and conditions. It often conveys a certain circus sideshow quality rather than leading to increased understanding. Whether the DSM-IV term *dissociative identity disorder* will change this situation is unknown at present.

Continuing with MPD as an example, it is important to understand that everyone has different ego states. These can be more or less walled off from each other, depending on many factors (Beahrs, 1982; Watkins & Watkins, 1982). In extreme cases, there is a defensive need for strong, nonpermeable walls to keep separate from everyday functioning knowledge of terrible abuse and overwhelming feelings. In less extreme situations, there may merely be a sense of a "child within" who is connected to memories of abuse but does not feel completely separate from the rest of the person. In fact, varying degrees of such experiences are not abnormal. DSM-IV suggests that 70% of young people experience some type of depersonalization at least once, and the New Harvard Guide to Psychiatry (1988) states that "depersonalization is not only common, but should not be viewed as evidence of emotional illness."

Other recent studies are beginning to document the high prevalence of other dissociative defenses within the "normal" population (Devine, 1991). Such data help prevent the trauma survivor from believing that his or her internal experiences are completely out of the realm of usual human experience. Instead of attempting to diagnose "multiple personalities," which seems, at best, unusual, one wants to know how the trauma affected the degree of fluidity of the person's ego states. In fact, it is probably important to study those individuals at the other extreme of this continuum who do not have the flexibility to have different ego states in different situations, and who always present rigidly the same way (one patient cleverly referred to this condition as "Singular Personality Disorder (SPD)"). In a more wholistic approach, one would note where the person is on this continuum of dissociation, but it would also become clear that this is only one facet of a complex person who has many other qualities, problems, and strengths.

In summary, there is a need for a more comprehensive diagnostic approach in which clinicians do not overlook the traumatic etiology of many mental disorders. Therapists need to understand that what patients have to say about the details of their lives, their personal histories, and their failures has significance and validity, both for diagnosis and treatment. One must remember that, no matter how complex and encompassing a diagnostic system becomes, it can never take the place of listening to the patient's experience. Any diagnostic system can only be a guide to the clinician, and can never replace the patient's own understanding of his or her life.

REFERENCES

Ahrendt, H. (1964). *Eichmann in Jerusalem: A report on the banality of evil* (2nd ed.). New York: Penguin Books.

American Psychiatric Association. (1994). *Diagnostic and Statistical Manual of Mental Disorders* (4th ed.). Washington, DC: The Association.

Beahrs, J. O. (1982). *Unity and multiplicity: Multilevel consciousness of self in hypnosis, psychiatric disorder and mental health.* New York: Brunner/Mazel.

Beck, J. C., & van der Kolk, B. A. (1987). Reports of childhood incest and current behavior of chronically hospitalized psychotic women. *American Journal of Psychiatry, 144,* 1474–1476.

Borovasky, G., & Brand, D. (1980). Personality organization and psychological functioning of the Nuremberg war criminals. In J. Dimsdale (Ed.), *Survivors, victims and perpetrators* (pp. 359–403). New York: Hemisphere.

Braun, B. (1983). Psychophysiological phenomena in multiple personality and hypnosis. *American Journal of Clinical Hypnosis, 26,* 124–137.

Breggin, P. R. (1991). *Toxic psychiatry.* New York: St. Martin's Press.

Breslau, N., & Davis, G. (1989). Chronic posttraumatic stress disorder in Vietnam veterans. *The Harvard Medical School Mental Health Letter, 5,* 3–5.

Briere, J. (June 1993). *Tension reduction behaviors.* Paper presented to the Fifth Regional Conference on Abuse and Multiple Personality. Washington, DC.

Browne, A., & Finkelhor, D. (1986). Impact of child sexual abuse: A review of the literature. *Psychiatric Bulletin, 99,* 66–77.

Bryer, J., Nelson, B., & Miller, J. (1987). Childhood sexual and physical abuse as factors in adult psychiatric illness. *American Journal of Psychiatry, 144,* 1426–1430.

Coons, P. M., Cole, C., Pellow, T. A., & Milstein, V. (1990). Symptoms of posttraumatic stress and dissociation in women victims of abuse. In R. P. Kluft (Ed.), *Incest-related syndromes of adult psychopathology* (pp. 205–221). Washington, DC: American Psychiatric Press.

Daley, M. (1978). *Gynecology: The metaethics of radical feminism.* Boston: Beacon Press.

Davis, R., & Freidman, L. (1985). Emotional aftermath of crime and violence. In Figley (Ed.), *Trauma & Its Wake: The Study and Treatment of Post Traumatic Stress Disorder* (p. 90). New York: Bruner/Mazel.

Deegan, P. E. (1990). Spirit breaking. *The Humanistic Psychologist, 18,* 301–313.

Devine, S. (1991). A validation study of dissociative experiences scale, Master's Thesis, Yale University School of Nursing, New Haven, CT.

Finkelhor, D. (1979). *Sexually victimized children.* New York: Free Press.

Gelinas, D. L. (1983). The persisting negative effects of incest. *Psychiatry, 46,* 312–322.

Gelles, R. J., & Cornell, C. P. (1985). *Intimate violence in families.* Beverly Hills, CA: Sage.

Glesser, G., Green, B., & Winget, C. (1981). *Prolonged psychosocial effects of disaster: A study of Buffalo Creek.* New York: Academic Press.

Greaves, G. (1992). Alternative hypotheses regarding claims of satanic cult activity: A critical analysis. In D. K. Sakheim & S. E. Devine (Eds.), *Out of darkness: Understanding satanism and ritual abuse.* Lexington, MA: Lexington Books.

Herman, J. (1992). *Trauma and recovery: The aftermath of violence—From domestic abuse to political terror.* New York: Basic Books.

Horton, A., & Williamson, J. (1988). *Abuse and religion: When praying isn't enough.* Lexington, MA: Lexington Books.

Jacobson, A., & Richardson, B. (1987). Assault experiences of 100 psychiatric inpatients: Evidence of the need for routine inquiry. *American Journal of Psychiatry, 144,* 908–913.

Kluft, R. (Ed.). (1985). *Childhood antecedents of multiple personality.* Washington, DC: American Psychiatric Press.

Lobitz, W. C., & LoPicolo, J. (1972). The role of masturbation in the treatment of orgasmic dysfunction. *Archives of Sexual Behavior, 2,* 163–171.

Loftus, E. F. (1993). The reality of repressed memories. *American Psychologist, 48,* 518–537.

Masson, J. M. (1984). *The assault on truth: Freud's suppression of the seduction theory.* New York: Farrar, Straus & Giroux.

Masson, J. M. (1986). *A dark science.* New York: Farrar, Straus & Giroux.

McCann, I. L., & Pearlman, L. A. (1990). *Psychological trauma and the adult survivor: Theory, therapy and transformation.* New York: Brunner/Mazel.

McCann, I. L., Pearlman, L., Sakheim, D. K., & Abrahamson, D. (1988). Assessment and treatment of the adult survivor of childhood sexual abuse within a schema framework. In S. M. Sgroi (Ed.), *Vulnerable populations: Vol. I.* Lexington, MA: Lexington Books.

McCann, I. L., Sakheim, D. K., & Abrahamson, D. (1988). Trauma and victimization: A model of psychological adaptation. *The Counseling Psychologist, 16,* 531-594.

National Center on Child Abuse and Neglect, U.S. Department of Health and Human Services. (1982). *Executive summary: National study of the incidence and severity of child abuse and neglect.* Washington, DC: Government Printing Office.

Nemiah, J. C. (1988). *Harvard Guide to Psychiatry.* Cambridge, MA: Belknap, Armand Nicholi, p. 254–255.

Orwell, G. (1949). *1984.* San Diego: Harcourt, Brace, Jovanovich.

Pelcovitz, D. (1990). *The effects of abuse and implications for treatment.* Paper presented to Hartford Hospital Conference on disorders of extreme stress. Diagnostic, treatment, legal, and ethical issues. Hartford, CT, December.

Putnam, F. (1989). *Diagnosis and treatment of multiple personality disorder.* New York: Guilford Press.

Richardson, J., Best, J., & Bromley, D. (1991). *The satanism scare.* New York: Aldine de Gruyter.

Russell, D. (1982). *Rape in marriage.* New York: Macmillan.

Russell, D. (1986). *The secret trauma.* New York: Basic Books.

Sakheim, D. (1993). Clinical aspects of sadistic ritual abuse. In W. J. Ray & L. K. Michelson (Eds.), *Handbook of dissociation.* New York: Plenum Press.

Sakheim, D., & Devine, S. (1992a). Conclusion. In D. K. Sakheim & S. E. Devine (Eds.), *Out of darkness: Understanding satanism and ritual abuse* (pp. 295–299). Lexington, MA: Lexington Books.

Sakheim, D., & Devine, S. (1992b). Bound by the boundaries. In D. K. Sakheim & S. E. Devine (Eds.), *Out of darkness: Understanding satanism and ritual abuse* (pp. 279–293). Lexington, MA: Lexington Books.

Sakheim, D. (1990). *Multiple personality disorder and other syndromes of traumatic etiology.* Paper presented to Hartford Hospital Conference on disorders of extreme stress. Diagnostic, treatment, legal, and ethical issues. Hartford, CT, December.

Schultz, R., Kluft, R., & Braun, B. (1986). The interface between multiple personality disorder and borderline personality disorder. In B. Braun (Ed.), *Dissociative disorders.* Chicago: Rush University Press.

Stone, M., Kahn, E., & Flye, B. (1981). Psychiatrically ill relatives of borderline patients: A family study. *Psychiatry, 53,* 71–84.

Tavris, C. (1993, January 3). Beware the incest-survivor machine. *New York Times Book Review.*

van der Kolk, B., & Greenberg, M. (1987). The psychobiology of the trauma response: Hyperarousal, constriction, and addiction to traumatic reexposure. In B. A. van der Kolk (Ed.), *Psychological trauma.* Washington, DC: American Psychiatric Press.

Watkins, J. G. & Watkins, H. H. (1982). Ego-state therapy. In L. E. Abt & I. R. Stuart (Eds.), *The newer therapies: A source book.* New York: Van Nostrand Reinhold.

Zambaco, D. A. (1882). Masturbation and psychological problems in two little girls. In J. Masson (Ed.), *A dark science.* New York: Farrar, Straus & Giroux.

8

CONCLUSION:
A TRAUMA MODEL

Colin A. Ross

It is evident from the preceding chapters that biological psychiatry is dominated by pseudoscience and reductionist ideological bias. The purpose of this concluding chapter is to outline a trauma model of psychopathology that is truly biopsychosocial in nature and, if accepted, would result in a paradigm shift in psychiatry. The model offers a corrective to the expenditure of tens of millions of dollars on bioreductionist research projects that cannot yield meaningful results because of the blinders biological psychiatry in its current form has imposed on psychiatric thinking. The purpose of the chapter is *not* to marshal evidence in favor of the proposed model, but only to present it as an alternative way of thinking about psychopathology.

The trauma model is medical, biological, psychiatric, and scientific, and it generates testable hypotheses.

The core assumption of the trauma model is that chronic, severe childhood trauma is a major driver of serious psychopathology. In North America, the most common forms of such trauma are physical and sexual abuse, severe emotional abuse, and neglect. In other parts of the world, war, famine, and natural disaster might be the major forms of severe childhood trauma, with resulting variations in symptomatology caused by the different types of trauma and by cultural factors.

Within any given DSM-IV diagnostic category, the severely traumatized subgroup has a distinct onset, course, phenomenology, psychobiology, response to psychotherapy and psychopharmacology, and pattern of family transmission. Patients with dissociative identity disorder illustrate the normal human response to chronic childhood trauma to the most extreme degree, because they are the most traumatized diagnostic category in DSM-IV. In the absence of rigorously demonstrated genetic factors, the trauma response of dissociative identity disorder patients is assumed to be psychobiologically normal, and based on a normal genetic endowment.

It will not be possible to identify a gene for depression, if any such gene exists, until trauma-driven cases, who may be genetically normal, are removed from analysis in family studies. The total dose of depression in the general population driven primarily by genetic factors is swamped out by the contribution of psychosocial trauma, including early childhood loss of a parent. If this is correct, bioreductionist psychiatry dooms itself to a futile search for genes for mental illnesses by retaining too much noise in its pedigrees, in the form of trauma-driven psychopathology.

Empirically testable predictions can be derived from the trauma model. Examples of these are:

1. Certain disorders that are highly trauma-related, such as dissociative identity disorder, borderline personality disorder, and posttraumatic stress disorder, would yield findings of extremely high statistical and clinical significance in family and twin studies. Cross-fostering studies with abusive and nonabusive biological and adoptive parents would yield high levels of significance, as would twin studies. There would be no cases of twins concordant for dissociative identity disorder who were discordant for severe childhood trauma, and no difference in the concordance rates of monozygotic and dizygotic twins for the disorder when trauma dose was controlled for. Concordance for the absence of dissociative identity disorder in the absence of trauma would be perfect.

In family studies, the risk for complex dissociative identity disorder in daughters of affected mothers adopted at birth into nonabusive families would be zero. Daughters of unaffected mothers adopted at birth into abusive families would have risks for the disorder dozens of times higher (actually, infinitely higher) than their cross-fostered opposites. In the absence of severe trauma, cases would not occur no matter what the fostering pattern.

2. Many of the biological markers currently under study in psychiatry are in fact markers of the psychobiology of trauma. Within any diagnostic category, the marker will appear more frequently in the traumatized subgroup.

3. Severely traumatized individuals introduce considerable noise into all drug studies in psychiatry by virtue of their more variable, inconsistent, fleeting, and paradoxical responses. These affect both the placebo and medication response rates. Exclusion of severe trauma survivors from standard drug studies would markedly reduce pharmaceutical development costs and provide much cleaner data, while identifying a large subpopulation for specific drug studies.

4. A trauma pathway to positive symptoms of schizophrenia confounds all studies of medication response, biological markers, and family transmission of schizophrenia spectrum disorders, including schizophrenia itself. Schizotypal personality disorder criteria are highly contaminated by trauma-driven paranormal experiences and dissociative symptoms. The rates of severe childhood trauma are higher in schizotypal than schizoid personality disorder.

5. Unrecognized trauma-driven dissociative symptoms result in false-positive diagnoses of major mental illness. For instance, about 10% of subjects in published clinical and research studies of schizophrenia would prove to have false-positive diagnoses of schizophrenia and false-negative diagnoses of dissociative identity disorder, if carefully screened with structured interviews for dissociative disorders.

6. Taken as a prototype of the new model, dissociative identity disorder has the highest interrater reliability and treatment validity of any major mental illness, because it has a specific etiology.

7. Normal adults exposed to acute catastrophic trauma will exhibit the symptom profile of dissociative identity disorder to a milder degree in a dose-dependent fashion.

8. The biopsychosocial symptom and marker profile of dissociative identity disorder is trauma dose-dependent with respect to childhood trauma.

9. The frequency of different DSM-IV comorbid diagnoses in dissociative identity disorder occurs in a hierarchy, with the most common forms of comorbidity at the top, and those at the bottom having frequencies no different from the general population. The order of diagnoses in this hierarchy is the same as the risk ratio for the disorders in the general population, when the rate of the disorder in adults subjected

to severe childhood trauma is compared to the rate in nontraumatized individuals. This is because dissociative identity disorder patients best illustrate the relationship between childhood trauma and the different DSM-IV Axis I and II disorders.

10. Severe trauma survivors are overrepresented in treatment failures of standard treatments throughout DSM-IV.

11. Combining trauma-specific psychotherapy with standard treatments for true comorbidity is synergistic, and results in better outcomes than either modality alone. This is true for antidepressant treatment of depression, group therapy of substance abuse, and individual cognitive-behavioral therapy of bulimia, to mention a few examples.

12. Severe childhood trauma is the most powerful identifiable risk factor for depression.

A number of observations and predictions about somatic aspects of the trauma response can be made:

13. Somatization disorder diagnostic criteria must be redefined. The conceptualization of the disorder in terms of sick role and medical help-seeking is based on secondary sociological artifacts. The disorder is primarily one of autonomic/physiological trauma memory.

14. Biological markers of trauma can be used rationally in clinical triaging decisions based on empirical treatment outcome studies. Triaging may be to pharmacotherapy, psychotherapy, or a combination of the two.

15. Biological markers of trauma are diagnostically specific in proportion to the average lifetime trauma dose for different disorders.

16. Biological markers of severe trauma will be manifest by early to mid-adolescence, before a substantial lifetime dose of Axis I or II morbidity has been accumulated, demonstrating that the relationship is with the trauma, not with disorders such as depression.

17. The psychobiology of trauma in psychiatric disorders is directly related to a large body of literature on mammalian physiology. The hypothalamic-adrenal-pituitary axis is a key candidate for such relationships.

18. There is an identifiable sleep architecture of trauma.

Finally, three implications of the trauma model for the health care system can be defined:

19. Primary prevention of major mental illness through prevention of severe child abuse is possible. This can be shown by intervention studies.

20. Long-term sequelae of severe child abuse are generating over $100 billion in psychiatric and medical health care costs per year in North America. The vast majority of these costs are unrecognized and misattributed.

21. Trauma-specific psychotherapy is the most financially cost-effective intervention in psychiatry.

The purpose of listing these 21 predictions of the trauma model, in this context, is to demonstrate that a radically different biological psychiatry—one that is medical and scientific—is possible. The ideology of contemporary reductionist psychiatry is not essential to biology, science, or medicine, and places highly restrictive blinders on the field. It drives a considerable portion of organized psychiatry's resistance to serious consideration of the role of childhood trauma in psychopathology.

Allowing psychiatry to be dominated by pseudoscience and ideological bias cannot be good medicine, cannot be good for psychiatric patients, and, in the long term, cannot be anything but bad public relations for psychiatry. Part of the purpose of this book is to document the current state of the field, but it is also to demonstrate that a different, nonreductionist biological psychiatry is possible and that it could find its place within a truly biopsychosocial paradigm.

AUTHOR INDEX

SUBJECT INDEX

Abuse, *see specific types of abuse*
Acetazolamide, panic disorder and, 151
Acute stress disorder, diagnostic criteria, 124
Adrenergic receptor genes, 150
Affective disorder:
  Alzheimer's Disease and, 170
  schizophrenia and, 179
  ventricular abnormalities in, 145
Affective spectrum disorders, 186–191
Agglutinin autoantibodies study, 158–159
Agoraphobia, panic disorder and, 168
Akinetic mutism, 141
Alcoholics:
  adult children of, 181
  brain transmission in, 166
  GABA levels study, 146
  REM latency study, 153–154
Alcoholics Anonymous (AA), 96
Alcoholism:
  biological markers for, 48
  biopsychosocial model, 54
  as a disease, 48, 96–99
  family studies, 50, 178
  genetic linkage, 199
  imipramine treatment, 167
  longitudinal studies, 54
  major depression study, 172
  marital dysfunction and, 51
  neuropsychological-neurophysiological findings, 47–54

pedigree studies, 49–50
twin studies, 22, 52
Alprazolam, 93
Alzheimer's Disease:
  affective disorder and, 170
  amino acids and, 149–150
  familial vs. nonfamilial, 162
  impairment and progression of, 144
  magnetic resonance imaging study, 149
  neuropathological findings, 183
The American Journal of Psychiatry:
  affective spectrum disorders, 186–191
  bias in, 130–140
  doubtful clinical significance, 151–169
  family studies, 169–183
  genetic studies, 169–183
  severe childhood trauma, 183–186
  symptoms correlates, 140–151
  twin studies, 169–183
American Medical Association, formation of, 233
Amino acids:
  Alzheimer's Disease and, 149–150
  psychiatric disorders and, 191
Amotivation syndrome, 141
Anorexia nervosa:
  cholecystokinin study, 150–151
  temporal lobe epilepsy and, 184–186
ANOVA, 168
Anticonvulsant medication, 119

287

GETTYSBURG COLLEGE

3326800 0278638 6

DATE DUE

DEC 1 0 1999			
MAY 3 0 2000			

Demco, Inc. 38-293